The Impact of Neurologic Disease on the Urinary Tract

Editors

JOHN T. STOFFEL
YAHIR SANTIAGO-LASTRA

UROLOGIC CLINICS
OF NORTH AMERICA

www.urologic.theclinics.com

Consulting Editor
SAMIR S. TANEJA

August 2017 • Volume 44 • Number 3

ELSEVIER

1600 John F. Kennedy Boulevard • Suite 1800 • Philadelphia, Pennsylvania, 19103-2899

http://www.theclinics.com

UROLOGIC CLINICS OF NORTH AMERICA Volume 44, Number 3
August 2017 ISSN 0094-0143, ISBN-13: 978-0-323-53261-7

Editor: Kerry Holland
Developmental Editor: Alison Swety

Urologic Clinics of North America (ISSN 0094-0143) is published quarterly by Elsevier Inc., 360 Park Avenue South, New York, NY 10010-1710. Months of issue are February, May, August, and November. Business and Editorial Offices: 1600 John F. Kennedy Blvd., Suite 1800, Philadelphia, PA 19103-2899. Periodicals postage paid at New York, NY and additional mailing offices. Subscription prices are $360.00 per year (US individuals), $680.00 per year (US institutions), $100.00 per year (US students and residents), $415.00 per year (Canadian individuals), $850.00 per year (Canadian institutions), $515.00 per year (foreign individuals), $850.00 per year (foreign institutions), and $240.00 per year (Canadian and foreign students/residents). Foreign air speed delivery is included in all *Clinics* subscription prices. All prices are subject to change without notice. **POSTMASTER:** Send address changes to *Urologic Clinics of North America*, Elsevier Health Sciences Division, Subscription Customer Service, 3251 Riverport Lane, Maryland Heights, MO 63043. **Customer Service: 1-800-654-2452 (US). From outside the United States, call 1-314-447-8871. Fax: 1-314-447-8029. E-mail: JournalsCustomerServiceusa@elsevier.com (for print support)** and **JournalsOnlineSupport-usa@elsevier.com (for online support)**.

Reprints. For copies of 100 or more, of articles in this publication, please contact the Commercial Reprints Department, Elsevier Inc., 360 Park Avenue South, New York, New York 10010-1710. Tel.: 212-633-3874; Fax: 212-633-3820; E-mail: reprints@elsevier.com.

Urologic Clinics of North America is covered in MEDLINE/PubMed (*Index Medicus*), *Excerpta Medica, Current Contents/ Clinical Medicine, Science Citation Index,* and *ISI/BIOMED.*

PROGRAM OBJECTIVE

The goal of Urologic Clinics of North America is to keep practicing urologists and urology residents up to date with current clinical practice in urology by providing timely articles reviewing the state of the art in patient care.

TARGET AUDIENCE

Practicing urologists, urology residents and other health care professionals practicing in the discipline of urology.

LEARNING OBJECTIVES

Upon completion of this activity, participants will be able to:
1. Review injections, surgery, and other management methods of neurologic diseases of the urinary tract.
2. Discuss the economic impact of neurologic disease on the urinary tract.
3. Recognize the effects of acute and degenerative neurologic disorders on the lower urinary tract.

ACCREDITATION

The Elsevier Office of Continuing Medical Education (EOCME) is accredited by the Accreditation Council for Continuing Medical Education (ACCME) to provide continuing medical education for physicians.

The EOCME designates this enduring material for a maximum of 15 *AMA PRA Category 1 Credit*(s)™. Physicians should claim only the credit commensurate with the extent of their participation in the activity.

All other health care professionals requesting continuing education credit for this enduring material will be issued a certificate of participation.

DISCLOSURE OF CONFLICTS OF INTEREST

The EOCME assesses conflict of interest with its instructors, faculty, planners, and other individuals who are in a position to control the content of CME activities. All relevant conflicts of interest that are identified are thoroughly vetted by EOCME for fair balance, scientific objectivity, and patient care recommendations. EOCME is committed to providing its learners with CME activities that promote improvements or quality in healthcare and not a specific proprietary business or a commercial interest.

The planning committee, staff, authors and editors listed below have identified no financial relationships or relationships to products or devices they or their spouse/life partner have with commercial interest related to the content of this CME activity:

Shree Agrawal, BS; Ravi R. Agrawal, BA; Humphrey O. Atiemo, MD; Lori A. Birder, PhD; Anne P. Cameron, MD, FRCSC, FPMRS; Diana Cardona-Grau, MD; George Chiang, MD; William C. de Groat, PhD; Elizabeth V. Dray, MD; Sean P. Elliot, MD, MS; Anjali Fortna; Ronak A. Gor, DO; Thomas L. Griebling, MD, MPH; Priyanka Gupta, MD; Kerry Holland; Amitabh Jha, MD, MPH; Katsumi Kadekawa, MD, PhD; Sidhartha Kalra, MD; Anthony J. Kanai, PhD; Aaron Kaviani, MD; Rose Khavari, MD; Takoya Kitta, MD, PhD; Adam P. Klausner, MD; Sara M. Lenherr, MD, MS; Meredith Metcalf, MD; Minoru Miyazato, MD, PhD; Jeremy B. Myers, MD; Unwanaobong Nseyo, MD; Isaac D. Palma-Zamora, MD; Zachary Panfili, MD; Darshan P. Patel, MD; Paholo G. Barboglio Romo, MBBS, MPH; Seiichi Saito, MD, PhD; Yahir Santiago-Lastra, MD; Nobutaka Shimizu, MD, PhD; John T. Stoffel, MD; Randy A. Vince Jr, MD; Vignesh Viswanathan; Naoki Wada, MD, PhD; Blayne Welk, MD, MSc; Katie Widmeier; Hadley M. Wood, MD; Naoki Yoshimura, MD, PhD.

The planning committee, staff, authors and editors listed below have identified financial relationships or relationships to products or devices they or their spouse/life partner have with commercial interest related to the content of this CME activity:

Benjamin M. Brucker, MD is a consultant/advisor for Allergan, a consultant/advisor for Cook MyoSite and Medtronic, and an investigator for Covance Inc.

John T. Stoffel, MD has research support from Cogentix Medical; Patient-Centered Outcomes Research Institute, and the U.S. Department of Defense.

UNAPPROVED/OFF-LABEL USE DISCLOSURE

The EOCME requires CME faculty to disclose to the participants:
1. When products or procedures being discussed are off-label, unlabelled, experimental, and/or investigational (not US Food and Drug Administration [FDA] approved); and
2. Any limitations on the information presented, such as data that are preliminary or that represent ongoing research, interim analyses, and/or unsupported opinions. Faculty may discuss information about pharmaceutical agents that is outside of FDA-approved labelling. This information is intended solely for CME and is not intended to promote off-label use of these medications. If you have any questions, contact the medical affairs department of the manufacturer for the most recent prescribing information.

TO ENROLL

To enroll in the *Urologic Clinics of North America* Continuing Medical Education program, call customer service at 1-800-654-2452 or sign up online at http://www.theclinics.com/home/cme. The CME program is available to subscribers for an additional annual fee of USD $270.

METHOD OF PARTICIPATION

In order to claim credit, participants must complete the following:

1. Complete enrolment as indicated above.
2. Read the activity.
3. Complete the CME Test and Evaluation. Participants must achieve a score of 70% on the test. All CME Tests and Evaluations must be completed online.

CME INQUIRIES/SPECIAL NEEDS

For all CME inquiries or special needs, please contact elsevierCME@elsevier.com.

Contributors

CONSULTING EDITOR

SAMIR S. TANEJA, MD
Division of Urologic Oncology, Smilow
Comprehensive Prostate Cancer Center,
Department of Urology, New York University
Langone Medical Center, New York, New York

EDITORS

JOHN T. STOFFEL, MD
Professor, Department of Urology, University
of Michigan, Ann Arbor, Michigan

YAHIR SANTIAGO-LASTRA, MD
Clinical Assistant Professor, Department of
Urology, University of California, San Diego,
La Jolla, California

AUTHORS

RAVI R. AGRAWAL, BA
Boston University, Boston, Massachusetts

SHREE AGRAWAL, BS
Case Western Reserve University School of
Medicine, Cleveland, Ohio

HUMPHREY O. ATIEMO, MD
Clinical Associate Professor of Urology,
Vattikuti Urology Institute, Henry Ford Hospital,
Detroit, Michigan

LORI A. BIRDER, PhD
Professor, Department of Medicine, University
of Pittsburgh School of Medicine, Pittsburgh,
Pennsylvania

BENJAMIN M. BRUCKER, MD
Assistant Professor, Female Pelvic Medicine
and Reconstructive Surgery, Associate
Residencey Directomy, Director of
Neurourology at MS Comprehensive Care
Center, Departments of Urology, and Obstetrics
and Gynecology, New York University Langone
Medical Center, New York, New York

ANNE P. CAMERON, MD, FRCSC, FPMRS
Associate Professor, Division of Neurourology
and Pelvic Reconstruction, Department of
Urology, University of Michigan, Ann Arbor,
Michigan

DIANA CARDONA-GRAU, MD
Fellow, Pediatric Urology, University of
California, San Diego, Rady Children's
Hospital, San Diego, California

GEORGE CHIANG, MD
Chief and Associate Professor of Surgery,
Department of Pediatric Urology, University
of California, San Diego, Rady Children's
Hospital, San Diego, California

WILLIAM C. DE GROAT, PhD
Professor, Department of Pharmacology and
Chemical Biology, University of Pittsburgh
School of Medicine, Pittsburgh, Pennsylvania

ELIZABETH V. DRAY, MD
Fellow, Female Pelvic Medicine and
Reconstructive Surgery, Division of
Neurourology and Pelvic Reconstruction,
Department of Urology, University of Michigan,
Ann Arbor, Michigan

SEAN P. ELLIOTT, MD, MS
Cloverfields Professor, Vice Chair of Urology,
Director of Reconstructive Urology,
Department of Urology, University of
Minnesota, Minneapolis, Minnesota

RONAK A. GOR, DO
Fellow and Instructor, Department of Urology, University of Minnesota, Minneapolis, Minnesota

TOMAS L. GRIEBLING, MD, MPH
Department of Urology, The Landon Center on Aging, The University of Kansas School of Medicine, Senior Associate Dean for Medical Education, John P. Wolf 33° Masonic Distinguished Professor of Urology, Faculty Associate, The Landon Center on Aging, The University of Kansas, Kansas City, Kansas

PRIYANKA GUPTA, MD
Assistant Professor, Neurology and Pelvic Reconstruction Division, Department of Urology, University of Michigan, Ann Arbor, Michigan

AMITABH JHA, MD, MPH
Department of Physical Medicine and Rehabilitation, Salt Lake City Veterans Medical Center, University of Utah, Salt Lake City, Utah

KATSUMI KADEKAWA, MD, PhD
Research Fellow, Department of Urology, University of Pittsburgh School of Medicine, Pittsburgh, Pennsylvania

SIDHARTHA KALRA, MD
Clinical Instructor, Female Pelvic Medicine and Reconstructive Surgery, Department of Urology, New York University Langone Medical Center, New York, New York

ANTHONY J. KANAI, PhD
Professor, Department of Medicine, University of Pittsburgh School of Medicine, Pittsburgh, Pennsylvania

AARON KAVIANI, MD
Research Associate, Department of Urology, Houston Methodist Hospital, Houston, Texas

ROSE KHAVARI, MD
Assistant Professor, Department of Urology, Houston Methodist Hospital, Houston, Texas

TAKEYA KITTA, MD, PhD
Research Fellow, Department of Urology, University of Pittsburgh School of Medicine, Pittsburgh, Pennsylvania

ADAM P. KLAUSNER, MD
Associate Professor and Warren W. Koontz Jr Professor of Urologic Research, Division of Urology, Department of Surgery, Virginia Commonwealth University School of Medicine, Richmond, Virginia

SARA M. LENHERR, MD, MS
Assistant Professor, Genitourinary Injury and Reconstructive Urology, Division of Urology, Department of Surgery, University of Utah, Salt Lake City, Utah

MEREDITH METCALF, MD
Urology Resident, Department of Urology, The Landon Center on Aging, The University of Kansas School of Medicine, Kansas City, Kansas

MINORU MIYAZATO, MD, PhD
Associate Professor, Department of Urology, Graduate School of Medicine, University of the Ryukyus, Okinawa, Japan; University of Pittsburgh School of Medicine, Pittsburgh, Pennsylvania

JEREMY B. MYERS, MD
Genitourinary Injury and Reconstructive Urology, Division of Urology, Department of Surgery, University of Utah, Salt Lake City, Utah

UNWANAOBONG NSEYO, MD
Resident, Department of Urology, UC San Diego Health, University of California, San Diego, San Diego, California

ISAAC D. PALMA-ZAMORA, MD
Pre-Clinical Urology Fellow, Vattikuti Urology Institute, Henry Ford Hospital, Detroit, Michigan

ZACHARY PANFILI, MD
Urology Chief Resident, Department of Urology, The Landon Center on Aging, The University of Kansas School of Medicine, Kansas City, Kansas

DARSHAN P. PATEL, MD
Genitourinary Injury and Reconstructive Urology, Division of Urology, Department of Surgery, University of Utah, Salt Lake City, Utah

PAHOLO G. BARBOGLIO ROMO, MBBS, MPH
Fellow, Female Pelvic Medicine and Reconstructive Surgery, Neurology and Pelvic Reconstruction Division, Department of Urology, University of Michigan, Ann Arbor, Michigan

SEIICHI SAITO, MD, PhD
Professor and Chair, Department of Urology, Graduate School of Medicine, University of the Ryukyus, Okinawa, Japan

YAHIR SANTIAGO-LASTRA, MD
Clinical Assistant Professor, Department of Urology, University of California, San Diego, La Jolla, California

NOBUTAKA SHIMIZU, MD, PhD
Research Fellow, Department of Urology, University of Pittsburgh School of Medicine, Pittsburgh, Pennsylvania

JOHN T. STOFFEL, MD
Professor, Department of Urology, University of Michigan, Ann Arbor, Michigan

RANDY A. VINCE Jr, MD
Division of Urology, Department of Surgery, Virginia Commonwealth University School of Medicine, Richmond, Virginia

NAOKI WADA, MD, PhD
Research Fellow, Department of Urology, University of Pittsburgh School of Medicine, Pittsburgh, Pennsylvania

BLAYNE WELK, MD, MSc
Assistant Professor, Department of Surgery (Urology), Schulich School of Medicine, Western University, London, Ontario, Canada

HADLEY M. WOOD, MD
Glickman Urological and Kidney Institute, Cleveland Clinic, Cleveland, Ohio

NAOKI YOSHIMURA, MD, PhD
Professor, Departments of Urology, and Pharmacology and Chemical Biology, University of Pittsburgh School of Medicine, Pittsburgh, Pennsylvania

Contributors

RANDY A. VINCE Jr, MD
Division of Urology, Department of Surgery, Virginia Commonwealth University School of Medicine, Richmond, Virginia

NAOKI WADA, MD, PhD
Research Fellow, Department of Urology, University of Pittsburgh School of Medicine, Pittsburgh, Pennsylvania

BLAYNE WELK, MD, MSc
Assistant Professor, Department of Surgery (Urology), Schulich School of Medicine, Western University, London, Ontario, Canada

HADLEY M. WOOD, MD
Glickman Urological and Kidney Institute, Cleveland Clinic, Cleveland, Ohio

NAOKI YOSHIMURA, MD, PhD
Professor, Departments of Urology, and Pharmacology and Chemical Biology, University of Pittsburgh School of Medicine, Pittsburgh, Pennsylvania

PAHOLO G. BARBOGLIO ROMO, MBBS, MPH
Fellow, Female Pelvic Medicine and Reconstructive Surgery, Neurology and Pelvic Reconstruction Division, Department of Urology, University of Michigan, Ann Arbor, Michigan

SEICHI SAITO, MD, PhD
Professor and Chair, Department of Urology, Graduate School of Medicine, University of the Ryukyus, Okinawa, Japan

YAHIR SANTIAGO-LASTRA, MD
Clinical Assistant Professor, Department of Urology, University of California, San Diego, La Jolla, California

NOBUTAKA SHIMIZU, MD, PhD
Research Fellow, Department of Urology, University of Pittsburgh School of Medicine, Pittsburgh, Pennsylvania

JOHN T. STOFFEL, MD
Professor, Department of Urology, University of Michigan, Ann Arbor, Michigan

Contents

Neurogenic bladder is a chronic and disabling condition associated with multiple co-morbidities and a widespread economic impact. Literature on cost of care and resource utilization is sparse and heterogeneous. Nonstandardized approaches, impact perspectives, and types of costs are used to describe the economic implications of neurogenic bladder. The financial toll is difficult to ascertain due to indirect and intangible costs exacerbated by the underlying disability. Health resource utilization based on clinical manifestations of neurogenic bladder may serve as an alternative measure. Understanding the multifold economic implications and health resource utilization patterns of neurogenic bladder may guide improvement of treatment strategies.

There is an evolving role for quality-of-life measures and patient-reported outcomes in the evaluation of neurogenic lower urinary tract dysfunction. We review available health-related quality-of-life instruments and patient-reported outcomes measures used in the assessment of patients with neurogenic bladder. We also discuss considerations for incorporation of these measures into clinical and patient-reported research. Emphasizing patient-reported outcomes in neurogenic bladder research will guide clinicians and other stakeholders to improve quality of life in this patient population.

It is widely accepted that neurogenic lower urinary tract dysfunction, when left untreated, has a natural history that has a potential for causing deterioration of renal function over time. However, certain patient profiles are at higher risk for this and other complications. This can be linked to their underlying neurologic disease process. Identifying risk profiles allows the provider to determine what surveillance strategies might be adopted. Risk factors for upper urinary tract deterioration include loss of bladder compliance, repeated bouts of pyelonephritis, and chronic indwelling catheterization. Other long-term complications include nephrolithiasis, refractory urinary incontinence, and malignancy.

Patients with neurogenic lower urinary tract dysfunction (NLUTD) experience significant morbidity and mortality due to urological complications including upper tract
damage and bladder malignancy. This has led to increased surveillance in patients
NLUTD. This article discusses the methods available for surveillance of patients with
NLUTD and pulls information from the largest and most established organizations
that have produced evidence-based surveillance guidelines for NLUTD. These organizations include the Paralyzed Veterans of America (PVA), US Department of Veterans Affairs, European Association of Urology (EAU), The NICE organization from the
UK, and cites additional literature not been included in these documents.

Neurologic diseases often affect the urinary tract and may be congential or acquired.
The progressive nature of many neurologic diseases necessitates routine surveillance and treatment with a multidisciplinary approach. Urologic treatments may
interact with pharmacologic or procedural interventions planned by other specialists, mandating close coordination of care and communication among providers.
Primary care and nursing often can serve as the quarterbacks of the multidisciplinary
team by identifying when a slowly progressive condition warrants further investigation and management by specialists.

In the United States, there are an estimated 25,000 children ages 0 to 19 years and
about 166,000 of all ages currently affected by spina bifida. Management is multimodal and can be complex. Management techniques vary throughout a child's lifetime, but the goals remain the same: prevention of urinary tract infections and
establishing acceptable continence. Continence is addressed as the child reaches
school age. Additional considerations such as development of urolithiasis and the
associated burden are highlighted in adolescence and into adulthood. These complex medical needs become more challenging as patients age and need to transition
to adult providers.

Stroke is an extremely common clinical entity, and poststroke incontinence is a major cause of morbidity for stroke survivors. Although patients can experience a wide
variety of lower urinary tract symptoms, detrusor overactivity is among the most
common clinical findings following stroke. All forms of lower urinary tract symptoms
can negatively impact physical and psychosocial function for affected patients and
their caregivers and loved ones. Careful evaluation is critical for successful management. Treatment is tailored to the goals and needs of each individual patient. Improvements in continence status can help to enhance overall and health-related
quality of life.

Parkinson's disease (PD) and atypical Parkinsonism are the second most common neurodegenerative movement disorders. Lower urinary tract dysfunction is among the most common types of associated autonomic dysfunctions. Differentiating the subtypes of PD is important for symptom management and understanding prognosis, because lower urinary tract symptoms (LUTS) can evolve differently depending on the primary disease. LUTS are caused by storage and/or voiding dysfunctions. Urodynamics is a key investigative tool. The complex pathophysiology of this bladder dysfunction is not responsive to levodopa, and add-on therapy is necessary. Newer interventions hold promise as therapy to improve bladder dysfunction.

Many multiple sclerosis (MS) patients are affected by urinary retention. Common causes include neurogenic underactive bladder and/or bladder outlet obstruction from detrusor sphincter dyssynergia. Systemic review of contemporary MS urodynamic studies demonstrates that 53% of MS patients have detrusor overactivity, 43% have detrusor sphincter dyssynergia, and 12% have atonic bladder (12 studies, 1524 patients). There is no standard definition of MS-related urinary retention, but greater than 300 mL is a proposed threshold value for the condition based on literature review. Treatment should be based on stratifying patients by risk from morbidity from retention and by symptoms caused by retention.

More than 12,000 spinal cord injuries occur annually in the United States; more than 80% of these individuals will experience urinary tract dysfunction. Despite the clinical demand, there is a paucity of guidelines for the care of these patients. Although most urologists are familiar with dangerous urodynamic parameters and the benefits of clean intermittent catheterization, these patients face a myriad of risks that may go unrecognized. In this article, the authors discuss the impact of specific neurologic diseases on the urinary tract, examine the risks inherent to each, and determine strategies for screening, prevention, and treatment of these complications.

Sacral and peripheral neuromodulation are minimally invasive surgical procedures that are third-line therapy options for the treatment of patients with idiopathic overactive bladder syndrome. There has been interest in their efficacy in the management of neurogenic lower urinary tract dysfunction (NLUTD). Contemporary data suggest promising outcomes for urinary and bowel symptoms in carefully selected patients with spinal cord injury and/or multiple sclerosis. This article reviews the current literature regarding urinary and bowel outcomes in patients with NLUTD and also discusses contemporary studies that suggest that treatment during particular stages of neurologic injury may prevent long-term urinary sequelae.

Intradetrusor injection of botulinum toxin A (BTX-A) is an effective option for managing patients with neurogenic detrusor overactivity (NDO) who do not respond to or tolerate oral pharmacologic agents. There is level I evidence that intradetrusor injection of onabotulinumtoxinA for refractory NDO in patients with multiple sclerosis and spinal cord injury is associated with a significantly greater achievement of goals and improved performance in urodynamic studies than placebo. Pilot studies or small case series support BTX-A for NDO in patients with Parkinson's disease and cerebrovascular accident. BTX-A seems to be effective in children with myelomeningocele. However, no adult data exists.

Surgery for patients with neurogenic urinary tract dysfunction (nLUTD) is indicated when medical therapy fails, to correct conditions affecting patient safety, or when surgery can enhance the quality of life better than nonoperative management. Examples include failure of maximal medical therapy, inability to perform or aversion to clean intermittent catheterization, refractory incontinence, and complications from chronic, indwelling catheters. Adults with nLUTD have competing risk factors, including previous operations, obesity, poor nutritional status, complex living arrangements, impaired dexterity/paralysis, and impaired executive and cognitive function. Complications are common in this subgroup of patients requiring enduring commitments from surgeons, patients, and their caretakers.

The lower urinary tract's main functions are storage and elimination. The micturition reflex pathway is modulated by the spinobulbospinal reflex pathway as well as higher brain centers involved in the voluntary micturition control. Micturition is sensitive to numerous injuries, resulting in various types of dysfunction. Animal studies indicate that lower urinary tract dysfunction partly depends on plasticity of the neural pathways. Reflex plasticity is associated with changes in ion channels, receptors, and numerous mediators. Animal models may aid in understanding the mechanisms leading to pathologic conditions and the plasticity in reflex pathways to the lower urinary tract after neurogenic lesions.

Patient-reported outcomes and quality of life assessments are essential to studying conditions such as neurogenic bladder in which multiple management strategies are approximately equally efficacious. Innovations for the treatment of neurogenic bladder need to be guided by both clinical and patient-reported outcomes that are rigorously tested via high-quality prospective cohort or randomized studies. Collaborative research groups in reconstructive urology are critical to the study of uncommon disease processes because they allow studies to be powered adequately, foster innovative treatment strategies through collaboration, and help moderate the risk of investigator and or institutional biases.

Foreword

The Impact of Neurologic Disease on the Urinary Tract

Samir S. Taneja, MD
Consulting Editor

Not only has the influence of neurologic injury and disease on the urinary tract been an intense subject of study throughout much of the history of modern urology but also much of our knowledge of the pathophysiology of normal voiding and voiding dysfunction emerged from observation of the neurologically impaired. Neurourology was my first exposure to urology as a medical student, while rotating on the neurology service. I was fascinated by the variations in voiding dysfunction observed upon injury to the nervous system at each level from the stroke patient to the spinal cord injured. It struck me that the urinary tract was a perfect organ system in which to study all forms of neurologic disease through their manifestations within a simple organ.

While my aspirations to be a neurosurgeon quickly melted away, it was that exposure that initially drove me to consider urology. While I ultimately settled on oncology, I recognize that in urology, I have perhaps the greatest change in the field of neurourology. A field once limited to aggressive operations to reduce bladder pressure and protect the upper tracts has evolved into a sophisticated practice of often individualized approaches to each patient, often based on a sustained evaluation of bladder behavior.

In this comprehensive issue of Urologic Clinics, our Guest Editors, Drs Yahir Santiago-Lastra and John T. Stoffel, have solicited a wide range of articles regarding bladder function specific to various neurologic disease from some of the field's most authoritative authors. In doing so, they have highlighted critical concepts pervasive to the evaluation and assessment of neurogenic bladder but also illustrated that the effects of each disease process of bladder function are unique, and as such, considerations in each patient are unique as well. As always, I am deeply indebted to each of the contributors for this fine issue and to Drs Santiago-Lastra and Stoffel for their hard work in making this issue of Urologic Clinics such fantastic resource for the practicing urologist.

Samir S. Taneja, MD
Division of Urologic Oncology
Department of Urology
NYU Langone Medical Center
150 East 32nd Street, Suite 200
New York, NY 10016, USA

E-mail address:
Samir.Taneja@nyumc.org

Urol Clin N Am 44 (2017) xv
http://dx.doi.org/10.1016/j.ucl.2017.06.001
0094-0143/17/© 2017 Published by Elsevier Inc.

Preface

Introducing "The Impact of Neurologic Disease on the Urinary Tract"

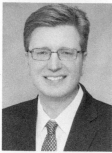

John T. Stoffel, MD   Yahir Santiago-Lastra, MD
Editors

We are very pleased to deliver a comprehensive issue of *Urologic Clinics*, focusing on "The Impact of Neurologic Disease on the Urinary Tract." We hope that this issue will serve as an excellent guide on the best and latest evidence on relevant topics within this theme, applicable to urologists and other health professionals spanning a wide range of expertise.

Neurogenic lower urinary tract dysfunction, more commonly referred to as neurogenic bladder, can affect all ages and can occur because of a congenital condition, acutely acquired event, or chronically degenerative condition. Almost all neurologic conditions can be associated with some degree of neurogenic lower urinary tract dysfunction. The basic principles of Neurourology are straightforward: protecting renal function, maintaining continence, ensuring a safe bladder that stores and empties well without stones or infections, and preserving quality of life in this vulnerable population. However, there are a limited number of providers who are well versed in the treatment of neurogenic bladder, and there is great need for more health care professionals that are able to see and treat these patients.

Our central theme for this issue was that neurogenic lower urinary tract dysfunction can be specific to the underlying neurologic condition. In short, not all patients with a diagnosis of neurogenic bladder are the same. Practitioners need an understanding of both how the underlying neurologic condition affects the lower urinary tract and how the neurologic condition could potentially change over time. Practitioners should then use this disease-specific knowledge to select treatments, surveillance strategies, and long-term supportive care for the patients with neurogenic lower urinary dysfunction. Our intent is for this issue to spark discussion around the concept that "neurogenic bladder" is too broad of a definition to adequately stratify risk morbidity and treatment outcomes for patients with neurogenic lower urinary tract dysfunction. Describing the heterogeneity of symptoms and treatment outcomes across neurogenic bladder conditions is a necessary step to drive this conversation forward.

We want to acknowledge and thank the many experts who contributed to this issue. They represent leaders in our specialty and the foremost medical institutions. The authors were eager to share their personal expertise with other providers caring for these patients, who wish to be up-to-date in this emerging field and who serve the patients seeking care for their neurogenic bladder. The authors excelled in presenting their information in a clear, easy-to-follow writing style while comprehensively covering the breadth of Neurourology and neurogenic bladder care. In addition, all of the articles include a *Key Points* section that highlights important conclusions made in the text.

urologic.theclinics.com

Urol Clin N Am 44 (2017) xvii–xviii
http://dx.doi.org/10.1016/j.ucl.2017.05.001
0094-0143/17/© 2017 Published by Elsevier Inc.

We hope you find this issue useful in your practice and research efforts.

John T. Stoffel, MD
Department of Urology
University of Michigan
3875 Taubman Center
East Medical Center Drive, SPC 5330
Ann Arbor, MI 48109, USA

Yahir Santiago-Lastra, MD
Department of Urology
University of California–San Diego
9444 Medical Center Drive, MC #7897
La Jolla, CA 92037-7897, USA

E-mail addresses:
jstoffel@med.umich.edu (J.T. Stoffel)
ysantiagolastra@ucsd.edu (Y. Santiago-Lastra)

Understanding the Economic Impact of Neurogenic Lower Urinary Tract Dysfunction

Isaac D. Palma-Zamora, MD, Humphrey O. Atiemo, MD*

KEYWORDS

- Neurogenic bladder (NGB) • Economic impact • Health care costs • Financial burden
- Resource utilization

KEY POINTS

- Neurogenic bladder (NGB) is a chronic and disabling condition that is associated with multiple co-morbidities and a widespread economic impact.
- There is a paucity of literature regarding the cost of care in patients with NGB due to methodological and practical challenges in estimating its economic footprint.
- NGB is an end-organ manifestation of an underlying disease process. Its associated health care costs may represent but a small portion of the total medical costs of the underlying disease process.

INTRODUCTION

Function of the lower urinary tract is governed by an intricate neurologic system that coordinates the storage and voiding of urine. Disturbances to the central nervous system, autonomic nervous system, or peripheral nervous system may result in neurogenic lower urinary tract dysfunction (NLUTD), a condition commonly known as NGB.

Multiple approaches have been used to define NGB based on functional, anatomic, and syndromic descriptions.[1,2] Functional assessments are based on urodynamic characterization. The presence, type, and severity of lower urinary tract dysfunction (LUTD) are influenced by the location of the underlying neurologic insult. Diseases involving the upper motor neurons or suprasacral cord most commonly lead to neurogenic detrusor instability, whereas injury to lower motor neurons typically manifest as urinary retention (UR). These symptoms can be identified in patients with multiple sclerosis (MS), spinal cord injury (SCI), traumatic brain injury, stroke, dementia, Parkinson disease, central nervous system tumors, diabetes mellitus, and pelvic surgery.[2,3] The onset and severity of the NGB symptoms remain variable and poorly understood.

One of the severe manifestations of NGB is poor bladder compliance. It involves the emergence of a high-pressure urine storage system and a propensity for developing urinary tract infections (UTIs) through various mechanisms, including ongoing catheterization, immunodeficiency, molecular structural changes in the bladder wall, UR, and dysfunction of the detrusor muscle and urethral sphincter complex.[4] Left untreated, deterioration of the urinary tract from recurrent renal injuries may progress to kidney failure.

Understanding the economic impact of NGB may guide the development of treatment strategies designed to improve the management of NGB. Available literature on the cost of care and

Disclosures: The authors have nothing to disclose.
Vattikuti Urology Institute, Henry Ford Hospital, 2799 West Grand Boulevard, Detroit, MI 48202, USA
* Corresponding author. Henry Ford Hospital, K-9 Urology, 2799 West Grand Boulevard, Detroit, MI 48202.
E-mail address: hatiemo1@hfhs.org

Urol Clin N Am 44 (2017) 333–343
http://dx.doi.org/10.1016/j.ucl.2017.04.001
0094-0143/17/© 2017 Elsevier Inc. All rights reserved.

resource utilization is sparse and heterogeneous. This article examines cost perspectives, resource utilization, health care costs, and implications of managing NGB patients by extrapolating from associated underlying neurologic conditions and similar forms of urinary dysfunction, such as overactive bladder (OAB) and urinary incontinence (UI), and where available, the assessment of pertinent literature.

UNDERSTANDING ESTIMATION STUDIES AND TYPES OF COST

A multitude of nonstandardized approaches have been used to estimate the economic impact of NGB, OAB, and UI. Cost-of-illness estimation methods have previously been described, including top-down or bottom-up approaches.[5] Longitudinal cohort studies often use a top-down approach that relies on health claims data or registries. A bottom-up approach may use cross-sectional surveys to estimate cost of care. Furthermore, studies may emphasize the cost perspective by the consumer, payer, society, or other.

Health care costs can be presented in various forms: direct, indirect, and intangible. The distinction between them is subjective and at times overlapping. For example, loss of employment due to health disability can be considered both an indirect and intangible cost. Cost estimates may reflect all medical expenses versus disease-specific costs. The latter may be difficult to ascertain in patients with chronic and disabling conditions, such as those with NGB, because the underlying neurologic disease may limit the ability to assess disease-specific costs due to confounding. An alternative is to extrapolate from similar conditions. For example, the costs associated with the management of UI may be similar between OAB and NGB.[5] Patients with NGB differ, however, from those with OAB and may view their NLUTD differently,[6] which limits the ability to generalize health resource utilization (HRU) patterns and treatment outcomes.

Patient encounters generate a trail of expenditures that can be used to estimate the direct and indirect costs associated with an illness. Direct costs are those associated with the delivery of medical services, such as medications, diagnostic work-up, and indicated procedures. Their cost is influenced by the acuity of the presenting condition and health care setting at which medical attention is sought. Indirect expenses, for example, include administrative costs for the payer and payments by the consumer in the form of premiums, deductibles, and copays.

INTANGIBLE COSTS

Similarly, the economic burden of an illness can be described by intangible costs. Patients with NGB may be physically incapacitated and unable to carry out activities of daily living due to their underlying disability. As a result, a series of arrangements may be necessary, such as transportation to and from health care settings or placement in long-term facilities, including assisted living and nursing homes. Furthermore, physical incapacitation limits a patient's ability to participate in forms of employment that lead to a loss of income and decreased earning potential stemming from permanent job loss, temporary unemployment, decreased productivity, or absenteeism. Unemployment rates at 1 year and 30 years postinjury in SCI patients are 86% and 58%, respectively.[7,8] NGB patients with Medicaid coverage and potential job opportunities often have a dilemma because increased income may compromise their eligibility for government assistance, including health coverage, with disability status providing higher levels of medical coverage than actual limited employment. Some investigators have estimated work productivity loss in patients with OAB and UI.[9-12] Their extrapolation to the NGB population, however, is inappropriate due to the different type and degree of underlying disability.

Bladder dysfunction is present in approximately 80% of patients with MS.[13] Hence, the economic repercussions in patients with MS and other NGB diagnosis may be similar. In MS, costs associated with the loss of employment exceed health care costs.[14] Estimation of decreased earning potential in MS patients relies on census data and labor statistics to estimate annual incomes based on age and national average of hourly wages.[15,16] Furthermore, the personal intangible costs are influenced by the natural history of the underlying neurologic condition. For example, the cumulative costs associated with NGB from Parkinson disease are different from those in patients with MS. A substantial portion of the negative economic impact in patients with MS falls under intangible costs because the condition presents during the most productive years of life and patients have a relative normal life expectancy.[14] In older populations, increasing costs may be driven by direct medical costs (ie, institutionalization) and less so by lost earning potential.[10] Unlike in the general population with OAB/UI, the disease-specific personal economic implications of NGB are unclear given their disability at baseline. Future approaches may consider, for example, comparing the incomes of patients with and without MS to derive the NGB-specific economic implications.

Repercussions extend to friends and family who may function as the primary caregivers for NGB patients. Doing so is time consuming, more so as the underlying condition progresses requiring lifestyle modifications by a caregiver to adjust to the patient's increasing needs. Such an undertaking by caregivers limits their participation in the workforce, which exacerbates the economic impact by NGB because caregivers may serve as the primary economic support for patients. There is also an emotional toll caused by pain, suffering, and diminished quality of life (QOL). Quantifying their impact is problematic given their subjective nature. Studies in the OAB/UI populations have used willingness to pay and quality-adjusted life years to estimate the emotional burden in patients with LUTD.[17] Using such measures to guide treatment may become problematic, raising the question, What is the goal of intervention: treating the disease or improving the human condition? Although available treatments and procedures may not cure the underlying disease, they may prove beneficial to patients and improve QOL. QOL improvement has been seen in patients with NLUTD treated with onabotulinumtoxinA (OBTA) or sacral nerve stimulation (SNM),[18,19] which may be clinically prohibitive due significant costs. Carlson and colleagues[20] argued that with a willingness to pay $50,000 per quality-adjusted life year, OBTA had a 97% probability of being cost-effective. Their assessment is problematic because it uses a flawed measure that derives costs from a payer's perspective and not the patient's.

CLINICAL IMPLICATIONS OF HEALTH CARE COSTS

Health care costs are influenced by geographic location and time. Cost of care varies across countries due to inherent differences in health care systems. As a result, direct comparison of cost-of-care studies between the United States and other countries is challenging. Furthermore, health care costs can vary across state lines due to marketplace competition, existing laws, and contractual agreements between providers, health systems, and suppliers of goods, such as pharmaceuticals and medical equipment. Additionally, health care costs change over time due to inflation and change in practices. This is particularly true with the NGB population. Over the past 2 decades the use of OBTA has become a third-line treatment of neurogenic detrusor overactivity. Its cost can become clinically prohibitive, especially in a population with limited financial means. Unit costs should be expected to remain high because the OBTA pharmaceutical maker is granted market

exclusivity under the Orphan Drug Act, thus monopolizing the drug's availability and price.[21,22] Such status can be extended if a new indication for a rare disease is found.[22] High costs may be offset by the development of standard and more efficacious dosing regimens. Using current procedural terminology (CPT) codes, the procedural cost at the authors' institution for OBTA injection is $760 (52287) at $16 (J0585) per unit.

Managing NGB patients is challenging. Providers have to navigate a world in which they meet patients' needs and caregivers' demands while being fiscally and clinically responsible regardless of health coverage. This may be frustrating to patients and caregivers, especially as indirect and intangible costs take their toll. The payer has a natural inclination to restrain costs by limiting coverage in the form of stratification of health plans and refusal to cover health care deemed unnecessary. This is to be expected given that a majority of direct costs lie with the payer (ie, insurance companies and government) or with the hospital (uninsured and/or outstanding bills).[23] And although the extent and complexity of health care costs are unknown to most patients, the intangible and indirect cost may persistently be underestimated and potentially neglected by providers and third parties alike.

HEALTH RESOURCE UTILIZATION

Health care costs are influenced by innumerable factors. HRU patterns provide a more stable approach than health care costs when examining the economic impact of NGB. Key contributors to HRU include the immediate postindex period, associated complications, and access to health care, including basic care and disease-modifying treatments (DMTs).

NDO elicits OAB-like symptoms in some NGB patients and may be associated with UI. Patients with restricted mobility may develop decubitus ulcers, which could be aggravated by UI, leading to further integumentary complications and risk for potentially life-threating infections. The chronic management of UI is simple and involves intermittent catheterization or an indwelling catheter. Yet, it is bothersome to patients and burdensome to caregivers. Patients are still at an increased risk of developing complicated UTIs and may also develop urethral erosions and strictures that further complicate their care. Managing such complications may prove challenging in patients with restricted mobility and have a negative impact on a patient's QOL.[3,7] Inadequate management of UI may have a negative impact on overall health and increase HRU and higher health-related costs.[3,24–26] In a Korean cohort with OAB, UI severity was associated with increased costs from pad use, decreased work productivity, and a greater interference with regular activities but not with visits to hospitals, clinics, or an emergency department (ED).[27] These findings are controversial because the relationship between HRU and UI has been widely established,[25] case in point that not all forms of cost increments affect patients.

Clinical complications may dictate HRU patterns, which may become more frequent with the progression of NGB and associated comorbidities. In patients with a recent NGB diagnosis, more than 50% of admissions during the 1-year postindex period were related to NGB sequelae where the overall contribution by UTI/UR accounted for approximately 30% of admissions.[7] Similarly, UTI/UR were responsible for 94% of ED visits by NGB patients (Sood A, Phelps J, Tarun J, et al, unpublished data, 2017). The former study included patients with commercial insurance or Medicare, whereas a majority of patients in the latter study (Sood A, Phelps J, Tarun J, et al, unpublished data, 2017) were uninsured or covered through Medicaid and Medicare. Furthermore, these data point out the relevance of comorbidities because they are responsible for almost half of the admissions.[7] A multitude of presenting comorbidities is not surprising given the complexity of NGB patients but could also represent a formality of assigning diagnoses to a clinical encounter. Therefore, the presence of an NGB diagnosis code associated with ED visits and admissions may not reflect an active issue but merely an unweighted diagnosis. Such trends could obscure and inflate the NGB-specific HRU patterns.

A period of high HRU ensues during the first year after the diagnosis of NGB.[7] Hospitalizations and ED visits are common, seen in one-third and one-fourth of the NGB patients, respectively.[7] They are infrequent during the 1-year postindex period, however, and average 0.5 during the first year.[7] It seems that at this stage resource utilization is not driven by clinical complications but by initial assessment and ensuing diagnostic workup as patients adjust to a new baseline and establish care with appropriate providers. During the first year after NGB diagnosis, the numbers of specialist visits, distinct diagnosis, and distinct prescription classes are 16.1, 13.8, and 11.1, respectively.[7] This points to one of the drawbacks of subspecialized medicine—patient shuttling. Visits to urology, neurology, nephrology, and physical and rehabilitation medicine account for 84% of all specialist outpatient visits.[7] The role of the primary care physician (PCP) in the management of NGB is not well defined. A recent review emphasized the importance of the PCP by functioning as gatekeeper and referring patients to a neurourologist when NGB decompensation is suspected.[28] Patients with chronic conditions may benefit from a PCP who coordinates care among subspecialists, home-based, and social services. This multidisciplinary approach may help reduce health care costs.[29]

The HRU trends in patients with NGB are influenced by the underlying neurologic condition. In the Manack and colleagues[7] cohort, patients with SCI had a higher number of office visits, hospitalizations, ED visits, and distinct diagnosis compared with patients with MS. It is unclear, however, if such differences are statistically different. This is supported by a similar study that investigated HRU patterns in patients with SCI during the first 12 months after the emergence of neuropathic pain.[30] The presence of renal and bladder conditions was more pronounced in patients with neuropathic pain (23% vs 20%, $P<.001$).[30] Numbers of admissions per patient and ED visits over the first year were noticeably higher in patients with SCI complicated by neuropathic pain (unknown bladder function) compared with SCI patients with NGB, which persisted in the SCI cohort without neuropathic pain.[30] The presence of neuropathic pain is noteworthy and a key factor that may explain the purported differences. The onset of neuropathic pain is variable and not necessarily present immediately after SCI. Therefore, the patients in the Margolis cohort may include patients with a more advanced form of SCI. Similarly, the differences in HRU in patients with SCI and MS may stem from the timeline in which NGB symptoms begin to appear. In SCI, spinal shock may delay the onset of NGB by months, whereas the emergence of NGB in the MS population may be insidious and become apparent only after the underlying condition has significantly progressed.

Cost shift is an important aspect of HRU. It is influenced by an aging population, health coverage, and current practices. During the 1990s, increased costs associated with the management of NLUTD were attributed to the emergence of ambulatory surgery.[31] It is unclear if such a trend contributed to current ED utilization patterns by NGB patients. It could be argued that the status quo prevents patients from benefiting from potential DMTs, such as OBTA, which may not be readily available through inpatient or acute care settings. Furthermore, limited access to health care is commonplace in the NGB population. Many patients are unemployed, lack insurance, or have limited coverage through Medicaid or Medicare.[8] As a result, increasing numbers of NGB patients use EDs as an entry point to health care (Sood A, Phelps J, Tarun J, et al, unpublished data, 2017). The economic impact of a shifting point of care setting is 2-fold because it increases costs in the acute care setting while decreasing inpatient costs (Sood A, Phelps J, Tarun J, et al, unpublished data, 2017). This trend may place an undue burden on the public payer sector and on the PCP as medically complex patients with potentially limited health coverage continue to present to the ED with increasing frequency (Sood A, Phelps J, Tarun J, et al, unpublished data, 2017). A similar paradigm takes place in older patients and/or with the progression of disease as costs shift from patient and the private sector to caregivers and public payers.[10] For example, young patients early in the disease process may still be able to participate in the workforce and benefit from employment-based health coverage, which may be compromised as their underlying disability progresses. Furthermore, routine care in the form of over-the-counter supplies used to manage UR and incontinence account for substantial expenses due to the chronicity of NGB. Inability to front out-of-packet expenses may lead to suboptimal management, leading to higher HRU as seen in patients with worsening UI.[25]

DMTs are considered second-line or third-line treatment of NGB and have the potential to drastically alter the progression of disease. They are not limited to surgical interventions but have varying degrees of invasiveness. There is no 1-treatment-fits-all option. Indications for DMTs have been discussed previously.[2,32] Pertinent literature emphasizes on comparisons involving any of the following: conservative management, OBTA, SNM, and more invasive surgeries, such as augmentation cystoplasty and forms of urinary diversion. Treatment outcomes tend to be variable and, as previously discussed, may improve patients' QOL but not improve their overall LUTD. In theory, they have the potential to curtail cost. In a German cohort, an OBTA regimen improved parameters and reduced costs associated with UI, UTI, and pad use.[26] Similar studies have shown improvement in associated complications and cost-effectiveness of OBTA in patients with LUTD.[33,34] DMTs are associated with cumulative costs, including treatment maintenance, escalation of care, and management of associated complications. Watanabe and colleagues[35] compared the cumulative costs between SNM, OBTA, and augmentation cystoplasty at 1 year and 3 years and showed that DMT-associated costs persist at 3 years, with SNM the most expensive option in patients with OAB.

NEUROGENIC BLADDER AND ITS ASSOCIATED MEDICAL COSTS

The multifaceted heterogeneity in NGB patients and cost-of-care studies makes the estimation of associated health care costs challenging, in part due to the lack of standardized forms of management strategies resulting in fragmented care. Best available guidelines from the European Association of Urology focus on the initial assessment and the evidence behind treatment modalities and management of associated complications.[2] Recommendations involving the escalation of care and disease monitoring, however, are less clear. Simplifying the classification of NGB based on its clinical manifestations may facilitate the standardization of care and offer an opportunity to assess the estimation of costs in a way that is more clinically relevant. Patients with NGB typically present with OAB, UI, UR, or a combination of these. A few authors have simplified the underlying LUTD or desired outcome to guide the selection of surgical candidates.[2,32] This could be expanded to include the clinical manifestations and HRU patterns to derive the NGB-specific direct medical costs (**Fig. 1**).

Formulating a management algorithm for NGB is beyond the scope of this review. The intent is to show that escalation of care differs based on the underlying clinical manifestation. In doing so, a certain commonality is assumed that can be exploited to provide a framework for future guidelines and circumvent the challenges associated with determining NGB-specific costs. The issue, however, is the timeliness with which escalation of care takes place. It is influenced by myriad factors, including the subjective nature of symptoms, access to health care, variable symptom onset, and nonlinear disease progression. The latter is particularly important. Clinicians use urodynamic parameters as markers of NLUTD and upper tract deterioration to guide urgency and mode of escalation of care. This should be done on a frequent basis because the lower urinary tract function is subject to change.[32] It has been proposed that urodynamic testing occur every 12 months to 24 months, or sooner, in patients with MS or SCI or when risk factors for urinary tract decompensation emerge,[2,32] because symptoms and urodynamic parameters do not correlate well in the MS population where the risk of upper urinary tract deterioration going unnoticed is considerable.[2] Another reason may include the inherent immunosuppressive state seen in NGB that may predispose patients to recurrent UTIs, more so in the MS population given their ongoing exposure to pharmacologic immunosuppression as part of their disease treatment.[4]

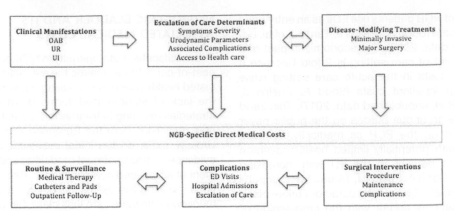

Fig. 1. The classification of NGB patients based on their clinical manifestations provides a framework for understanding the interrelationships between health care costs at different stages of disease. Exploiting this commonality simplifies management strategies and escalation of care pathways.

Conservative forms of management are the basis of NGB treatment. Escalation of care is indicated for those with refractory symptoms, associated complications, or lack of desired improvement after surgical intervention. Components of conservative management include behavioral modifications, forms of catheterization, absorbent incontinence aids, anticholinergics, and outpatient follow-up. Behavioral modifications include maneuvers (ie, Credé and Valsalva) to assist bladder emptying in addition to pelvic floor muscle exercises and biofeedback techniques that may require the involvement of a physical therapy specialist for an unknown length of time. A high-intensity physical therapy session costs $215 at authors' home institution based on CPT codes. In contrast, management involving forms of catheterization is limited to patients with neurogenic UR/UI. Clean intermittent catheterization (CIC) is recommended as opposed to an indwelling catheter. Costs associated with CIC depend on the frequency with which it is performed and preference for reusing catheters. At the authors' institution, the providing home care agency of CIC catheters offers a wide range of catheter options, with costs from $2 to $6, depending on brand, size, and model. If a patient performs CIC 3 times per day using a new 214 Self-Cath model (Coloplast, Minneapolis, MN, USA) catheter each time, it amounts to $6 per day. For Medicare patients, catheters are considered a form of durable medical equipment and as such 80% of the costs are covered under Part B. On the other hand, indwelling urethral catheters may not be ideal but are frequently used by patients with chronic incontinence because they are more convenient to caregivers and provide an increased sense of social acceptance to patients.

Variations of UI can be seen in neurogenic OAB/UR or it can be the primary clinical manifestation of NGB. The mainstay form of conservative management includes absorbent aids, such as pads and diapers. Unlike other forms of care, their related costs represent an ongoing out-of-pocket expense to patients because such products are available over the counter and often not covered by health plans. Overall costs depend on product preference and frequency of exchanging absorbent aids. In 2006, patient costs associated with the routine care of UI in the general population were estimated at approximately $412 per year,[36] whereas payer costs for total annual medical expenditures in patients with a primary diagnosis of UI were estimated at $12,357 in 1998.[24,31] Furthermore, UI results in higher costs to providers of long-term care where the presence of UI was responsible for $4834 to $6740 in added labor costs.[24]

Medical therapy is largely limited to the use of anticholinergics. Their use is common, variable, and associated with an unfavorable side-effect profile. More than 70% of NGB patients are started on anticholinergics during the 1-year postindex period with an average duration of 202 days.[7] Their use is continuous in less than one-third of patients,[37] and approximately 92% of patients with OAB fail therapy within 2 years.[38] There is no optimal anticholinergic regimen to guide treatment. Some investigators have argued that extended-release (ER)[39] formulations and combination[40] therapy may improve compliance. This comes at an increased cost, however, that some health plans do not cover. So it is not surprising that only 8% of NGB patients are on combination therapy.[7] Associated Medicare expenditures for the ER formulations of 2 commonly used anticholinergics were obtained from a publicly available dataset from the Centers for Medicare & Medicaid Services (CMS) Web site (**Table 1**).[41]

Table 1
Total Medicare expenditures of extended-release formulations of tolterodine and oxybutynin during 2015

	Claim Count	Total Spending	Beneficiary Count	Total Annual Spending Per User	Unit Count	Average Cost Per Unit (Weight)	Beneficiary Count No LIS	Average Beneficiary Cost Share No LIS	Beneficiary Count LIS	Average Beneficiary Cost Share
Tolterodine ER	880,243	$212,801,673	190,744	$1,115	37,871,801	$5.62	120,956	$163	69,788	$9.59
Oxybutynin ER	2,819,488	$268,430,003	593,530	$271	128,360,353	$1.25	360,272	$105	233,258	$7.02

Abbreviation: LIS, low income subsidies.
It is unclear if units represent number of tablets, grams, or refills. Beneficiary cost share represents the annual out-of-pocket contribution by a patient, which vary depending on the eligibility for low-income subsidies.

13. Chancellor MB, Anderson RU, Boone TB. Pharmacotherapy for neurogenic detrusor overactivity. Am J Phys Med Rehabil 2006;85(6):536–45.

14. Dunn J. Impact of mobility impairment on the burden of caregiving in individuals with multiple sclerosis. Expert Rev Pharmacoecon Outcomes Res 2010; 10(4):433–40.

15. Kobelt G, Berg J, Atherly D, et al. Costs and quality of life in multiple sclerosis: a cross-sectional study in the United States. Neurology 2006;66(11):1696–702.

16. Campbell JD, Ghushchyan V, Brett McQueen R, et al. Burden of multiple sclerosis on direct, indirect costs and quality of life: National US estimates. Mult Scler Relat Disord 2014;3(2):227–36.

17. Coyne KS, Wein A, Nicholson S, et al. Economic burden of urgency urinary incontinence in the united states: a systematic review. J Manag Care Pharm 2014;20(2):130–40.

18. Hamid R, Loveman C, Millen J, et al. Cost-effectiveness analysis of onabotulinumtoxinA (BOTOX((R))) for the management of urinary incontinence in adults with neurogenic detrusor overactivity: a UK perspective. Pharmacoeconomics 2015;33(4):381–93.

19. Siddiqui NY, Amundsen CL, Visco AG, et al. Cost-effectiveness of sacral neuromodulation versus intravesical botulinum A toxin for treatment of refractory urge incontinence. J Urol 2009;182(6):2799–804.

20. Carlson JJ, Hansen RN, Dmochowski RR, et al. Estimating the cost-effectiveness of onabotulinumtoxinA for neurogenic detrusor overactivity in the united states. Clin Ther 2013;35(4):414–24.

21. Health Resources and Services. Orphan Drugs. In: Orphan Drug List Governing January 1-March 31, 2017. Available at: https://www.hrsa.gov/opa/programrequirements/orphandrugexclusion/. Accessed March 15, 2017.

22. Kaiser Health News. Drugmakers manipulate orphan drug rules to create prized monopolies. In: The orphan drug machine. Available at: http://khn.org/news/drugmakers-manipulate-orphan-drug-rules-to-create-prized-monopolies/. Accessed March 15, 2017.

23. Flack C, Powell CR. The worldwide economic impact of neurogenic bladder. Curr Bladder Dysfunct Rep 2015;10(4):350–4.

24. Tapia CI, Khalaf K, Berenson K, et al. Health-related quality of life and economic impact of urinary incontinence due to detrusor overactivity associated with a neurologic condition: a systematic review. Health Qual Life Outcomes 2013;11:13.

25. Jimenez-Cidre M, Costa P, Ng-Mak D, et al. Assessment of treatment-seeking behavior and healthcare utilization in an international cohort of subjects with overactive bladder. Curr Med Res Opin 2014; 30(8):1557–64.

26. Wefer B, Ehlken B, Bremer J, et al. Treatment outcomes and resource use of patients with neurogenic detrusor overactivity receiving botulinum toxin A (BOTOX) therapy in germany. World J Urol 2010; 28(3):385–90.

27. Lee KS, Choo MS, Seo JT, et al. Impact of overactive bladder on quality of life and resource use: Results from korean burden of incontinence study (KOBIS). Health Qual Life Outcomes 2015;13:89.

28. Klausner AP, Steers WD. The neurogenic bladder: An update with management strategies for primary care physicians. Med Clin North Am 2011;95(1): 111–20.

29. Bardes CL. Defining "patient-centered medicine". N Engl J Med 2012;366(9):782–3.

30. Margolis JM, Juneau P, Sadosky A, et al. Health care resource utilization and medical costs of spinal cord injury with neuropathic pain in a commercially insured population in the united states. Arch Phys Med Rehabil 2014;95(12):2279–87.

31. Thom DH, Nygaard IE, Calhoun EA. Urologic diseases in america project: Urinary incontinence in women-national trends in hospitalizations, office visits, treatment and economic impact. J Urol 2005;173(4): 1295–301.

32. Taweel WA, Seyam R. Neurogenic bladder in spinal cord injury patients. Res Rep Urol 2015;7:85–99.

33. Game X, Castel-Lacanal E, Bentaleb Y, et al. Botulinum toxin A detrusor injections in patients with neurogenic detrusor overactivity significantly decrease the incidence of symptomatic urinary tract infections. Eur Urol 2008;53(3):613–8.

34. Wu JM, Siddiqui NY, Amundsen CL, et al. Cost-effectiveness of botulinum toxin a versus anticholinergic medications for idiopathic urge incontinence. J Urol 2009;181(5):2181–6.

35. Watanabe JH, Campbell JD, Ravelo A, et al. Cost analysis of interventions for antimuscarinic refractory patients with overactive bladder. Urology 2010; 76(4):835–40.

36. Subak L, Van Den Eeden S, Thom D, et al. Reproductive Risks for Incontinence Study at Kaiser Research Group. Urinary incontinence in women: direct costs of routine care. Am J Obstet Gynecol 2007;197(6):596.e1–9.

37. Lawrence M, Guay DR, Benson SR, et al. Immediate-release oxybutynin versus tolterodine in detrusor overactivity: a population analysis. Pharmacotherapy 2000;20(4):470–5.

38. Reynolds WS, Fowke J, Dmochowski R. The burden of overactive bladder on US public health. Curr Bladder Dysfunct Rep 2016;11(1):8–13.

39. Madhuvrata P, Cody JD, Ellis G, et al. Which anticholinergic drug for overactive bladder symptoms in adults. Cochrane Database Syst Rev 2012;(1): CD005429.

40. Cameron AP, Clemens JQ, Latini JM, et al. Combination drug therapy improves compliance of the neurogenic bladder. J Urol 2009;182(3):1062–7.

41. Centers for Medicare and Medicaid Services. CMS Drug Spending. In: 2015 Medicare Drug Spending Data. Available at: https://www.cms.gov/Research-Statistics-Data-and-Systems/Statistics-Trends-and-Reports/Information-on-Prescription-Drugs/2015 MedicareData.html. Accessed January 14, 2017.

42. Newman DK, Willson MM. Review of intermittent catheterization and current best practices. Urol Nurs 2011;31(1):12–28, 48; [quiz: 29].

43. Dieleman JL, Baral R, Birger M, et al. US spending on personal health care and public health, 1996-2013. JAMA 2016;316(24):2627–46.

How to Measure Quality-of-Life Concerns in Patients with Neurogenic Lower Urinary Tract Dysfunction

CrossMark

Darshan P. Patel, MD, Jeremy B. Myers, MD,
Sara M. Lenherr, MD, MS*

KEYWORDS

- Urinary bladder • Neurogenic • Patient-reported outcome measures • Health-related quality of life
- Urinary incontinence

KEY POINTS

- Patient-reported outcomes measurements are an important method of assessing bladder-specific quality of life in patients with neurogenic bladder.
- Recent instruments validated specifically in patients with neurogenic bladder allows more precise assessment of priorities pertinent to this population.
- Prospective utilization of patient-reported outcome measures will benefit further understanding of patient priorities as clinicians continue try to improve care of patients with chronic neurogenic bladder.

INTRODUCTION

Neurogenic lower urinary tract dysfunction, also classically described as neurogenic bladder (NGB), is a term used to describe lower urinary tract problems arising secondary to damage to the central nervous system, peripheral nervous system, and/or autonomic nervous system. Some causes include spinal cord injury (SCI), multiple sclerosis (MS), traumatic brain injury, cerebrovascular accident, spina bifida, cerebral palsy, and transverse myelitis.[1] There are many severe health long-term complications associated with NGB, including urinary tract infections, sepsis, and renal failure. Additionally, urinary symptoms have a significant impact on quality of life (QoL) in these patients.[2–4]

Globally, there is a growing interest in patient-reported outcomes and in patients' perspective on health and QoL. However, most assessments are validated for the general patient population and not for neurogenic patients specifically. For example, at the health care system level, the Centers for Medicare and Medicaid Services and the Agency for Healthcare Research and Quality developed the Hospital Consumer Assessment of Healthcare Providers and Systems (HCAHPS).[5] HCAHPS is a 27-question survey administered to patients at the time of discharge from the hospital to gather critical aspects of the patient's hospital

Disclosures: Authors report grant support from Patient-Centered Outcomes Research Institute during the preparation of this article (Patient-Centered Outcomes Research Institute CER14092138).
Division of Urology, Department of Surgery, University of Utah, 30 North, 1900 East, Room 3B420, Salt Lake City, UT 84132, USA
* Corresponding author. 30 North, 1900 East, Salt Lake City, UT 84132.
E-mail address: sara.lenherr@hsc.utah.edu

Urol Clin N Am 44 (2017) 345–353
http://dx.doi.org/10.1016/j.ucl.2017.04.002
0094-0143/17/© 2017 Elsevier Inc. All rights reserved.

urologic.theclinics.com

GENERAL BLADDER-SPECIFIC QUESTIONNAIRES AND NEUROGENIC BLADDER POPULATIONS

Perhaps the most commonly used PROM in urology to assess lower urinary tract symptoms is the American Urological Association symptom index (AUA-SI) and the closely related International Prostate Symptom Index (I-PSS).[14] The AUA-SI captures information about urinary storage, emptying, and irritative symptoms. The I-PSS asks an additional QoL question "If you were to spend the rest of your life with your urinary condition just the way it is now, how would you feel about that?" Interestingly, the AUA-SI does not ask about urinary incontinence. On many levels, the AUA-SI is not a practical survey to ask to those with NGB because most questions are based on voluntary voiding and sensations that those with NGB may not experience and there is no assessment of urinary incontinence, which is a common symptom in NGB.

Some commonly used urinary incontinence PROMs are the Incontinence Quality of Life (I-QOL)[15] and King's Health Questionnaire (KHQ).[16] These questionnaires have the advantage of asking very specific questions about the impact of urinary incontinence on activities, psychosocial situation, and feelings. The I-QOL and the KHQ each have more than 20 questions permitting increased sensitivity of detecting differences in impact on various aspects of function and QoL as compared with a general QoL measure. For example, a general QoL questionnaire might ask "How depressed are you?" and the answer for a given patient may be "some of the time." A bladder-specific questionnaire might ask "How much do your bladder problems contribute to your depression?" and the same patient with mild depression might state "all the time." The patient has mild depression in a general QoL question, but all of his or her depression is due to bladder problems. If bladder problems have a major impact on a group of patients' QoL, we would expect bladder-specific questions to be much more sensitive for the effects of the disease on a patient's perception.

The I-QOL is one of the most widely used incontinence PROMs and was also validated in a single, small, mixed population of patients with SCI or MS.[17] The I-QOL was used in 2 large randomized studies of the use of onabotulinum toxin A administration in SCI and MS, which were collectively called the DIGNITY trial.[17–19] In these studies, QoL was demonstrated to be improved in patients treated with onabotulinum toxin A compared with placebo. The DIGNITY trial is really the largest clinical study to use bladder-specific PROMs in NGB combined with objective clinical parameters measuring success. The investigators of the trial appropriately recognized that without combining patient perceptions about the impact of incontinence of their QoL with objective clinical evidence of improvement in bladder function, the results of the study would be much less impactful.

The KHQ has not been validated in NGB, but has been used in one study to identify lower QoL and worsened psychosocial impact in patients with SCI performing intermittent catheterization with assistance compared with independent intermittent catheterization.[20]

NEUROGENIC BLADDER–SPECIFIC QUESTIONNAIRES

As opposed to retroactively applying an instrument to the NGB population, several PROMs have been developed and validated for certain NGB populations (see **Table 1**). These measures are critical for research and monitoring response to therapy because of the standardized assessment of questions clinicians ask every day in clinical practice and inclusion of HRQoL measures.

The Qualiveen was the first instrument specifically created for the evaluation of urinary difficulties, specifically SCI and MS, in the early 2000s.[21,22] It primarily addresses the impact of bladder dysfunction on patients' feelings, fears, and constraints. The questionnaire was developed in French and consists of 30 items that examine 4 domains: bother with limitations, frequency of limitations, fears, and feeling. Each item is scored on a Likert scale with a total overall score calculated from answers to each domain. A lower scores denotes a poorer QoL. One advantage of the Qualiveen is its translation into 26 different languages.[23–29] An 8-item short form of the Qualiveen also has been developed more recently, although it has not been evaluated as rigorously as the long form.[30] The short form consists of 8 of the 30 questions in the full Qualiveen. One recent small single-institution study examining QoL in patients with SCI and used the short form of the Qualiveen.[26] The investigators were able to establish differences in the QoL of patients with indwelling catheters, performing intermittent catheterization, and those having undergone urologic reconstructive surgery.

Despite the questionnaire's availability over the past 15 years, the Qualiveen has been used in very few clinical studies. This is not a reflection on the quality of the questionnaire, but likely several factors, including the overall lack of patient-centered studies over the past decade and required royalty/distribution fees for most researchers. The Qualiveen was also developed with industry support (Coloplast, Lyon, France).

Welk and colleagues[31] recently developed another NGB-specific PROM entitled the Neurogenic Bladder Symptom Score (NBSS). The 24-item instrument was validated in a cohort of patients with SCI, MS, and congenital NGB and covers domains of incontinence, storage and voiding symptoms, urinary complications, and QoL. This instrument uniquely incorporates self-reported urinary complications, such as urinary tract infections, kidney and bladder stones, and pain, with an assessment of urinary symptoms. There is also identification of specific bladder management method, storage, and voiding symptoms, whereas previous applications of PROMs in NGB have focused on only incontinence. In contrast to the Qualiveen, the NBSS is much less about the impact of bladder dysfunction on feelings and perceptions but does have one global bladder-specific HRQoL question: "If you had to live the rest of your life with the way your bladder (or urinary reservoir) currently works, how would you feel?" The tool is available for research use without royalty fees. The NBSS has not been used in clinical outcome studies published to date, but is administered in several registered ongoing clinical trials.[32]

A very comprehensive PROM for patients with SCI is the Spinal Cord Injury Quality-of-Life Measurement System (SCI-QOL), which is a panel of different questionnaires assessing all aspects of a patient's experience with SCI.[33] SCI-QOL was developed from a framework established by the National Institutes of Health–initiated Patient-Reported Outcome Measurement Information System (PROMIS) and the Quality of Life In Neurologic Disorders (Neuro-QOL) instruments. These 2 instruments are validated in neurologically intact and neurologically injured populations, respectively. SCI-QOL used the Neuro-QOL item banks to include more SCI-relevant content not addressed by Neuro-QOL. SCI-QOL uses item response theory and computer adaptive testing, which allows the computer to statistically adjust to a patient's responses throughout the test. Computer adaptive testing has been used previously for graduate record examinations, but adaption for patient-reported outcomes is novel.[34] A set of individualized questions is drawn from larger item banks based on initial responses using computer adaptive testing. For example, in a general physical function questionnaire, if a participant responds that he or she cannot get out of bed in the morning, then the participant is next asked if he or she can complete other

basic activities of daily living, such as brushing his or her hair rather than if the participant can run a mile. A final calibrated score is produced for each health domain to provide a comprehensive assessment of an individual's QoL. In addition to providing more precise measurements, the adaptive nature of the questionnaire decreases the burden on the respondent, because irrelevant questions are eliminated and the questionnaire is shortened. Item banks in SCI-QOL produce a composite score (referred to as a T-score), which is on a scale of 1 to 100 with the mean score in the validated SCI population of 50. Thus, subjects can be compared with the mean of the validated population, and T-scores can be compared before and after interventions. The disadvantage of the SCI-QOL item banks is they require computer administration to use the computer adaptive testing and calculate summary T-scores. SCI-QOL is currently only available on Northwestern University's "Assessment Center" Web site[35] and is planned to be available in Research Electronic Data Capture (REDCap) in the future.[36]

There are 22 SCI-QOL item banks depending on desired measurements. Two of these instruments, Bladder Management Difficulties and Bladder Complications, assess patients' feelings and consequences of bladder dysfunction, combining certain aspects of both the Qualiveen and the NBSS.[37] Application of these 2 item banks in an external SCI patient population has yet to be published but is currently being used in several registered clinical trials.[32]

NEUROLOGIC PATIENT-REPORTED OUTCOME MEASURES FOR SPECIFIC NEUROGENIC POPULATIONS

There are several PROMs developed and validated for specific neurogenic populations, but they are not designed to assess bladder-related symptoms or bladder-specific QoL. Some of these instruments may have a few items to assess the impact of genitourinary dysfunction on HRQoL, but are not specifically designed for this purpose. In most cases, if these general PROMs are used exclusively, no insight may be gained about the impact of NGB.

Spinal Cord Injury

Spinal cord injury quality of life
As detailed previously, SCI-QOL is comprehensive QoL assessment instrument that uses 22 item banks.[33] Item response theory is used to create fixed-length short forms and computerized adaptive tests using this platform. As mentioned

previously, there are 2 item banks specifically on Bladder Management Difficulties and Bladder Complications.[37] There is also an item bank on Bowel Management Difficulties, which most urologists would find useful as an adjunct assessment.

Spinal cord injury–functional index
The spinal cord injury–functional index (SCI-FI) is a comprehensive instrument with 5 scales, including basic mobility, fine motor function, self-care, ambulation, and wheelchair mobility, which also uses computerized adaptive testing to minimize assessment burden.[38] The instrument was initially validated in a large sample of patients with traumatic SCI from several SCI Model Systems in the United States.

Spinal cord injury secondary conditions scale
The spinal cord injury secondary conditions scale (SCI-SCS) is a 16-item scale based on the Seekins Secondary Conditions Scale that allows comparisons of functional, medical, and psychosocial factors in patients with SCI.[39] The instrument assesses the impact of various secondary conditions over the past 3 months on activities and independence. In the validation study, the most common secondary conditions reported were chronic pain, joint and muscle pain, and sexual dysfunction.

Craig handicap assessment and reporting technique
The Craig handicap assessment and reporting technique (CHART) was initially validated in a cohort of stroke survivors, and also has been validated to assess rehabilitation outcome in patients after acute traumatic brain injury or SCI.[40] Although this instrument does not provide information regarding HRQoL, it is used for assessment of handicap after SCI and facilitates comparisons in HRQoL in combination with other instruments with varying levels of handicap.

Multiple Sclerosis

Multiple sclerosis quality of life-65
The multiple sclerosis quality of life-65 (MSQOL-54) is a multidimension instrument that combines generic HRQoL measures with additional 18 items to captures MS-specific issues.[41] There are 52 items that provide 12 subscale scores and 2 summary scores for physical health and mental health. There are additional 2 single-item measures regarding sexual function and changes in health. The MSQOL-54 has been translated and validated in several languages and more recently a short form has been developed using item response theory to reduce assessment burden.[42]

Multiple sclerosis impact scale-29
The MS impact scale-29 (MSIS-29) is an instrument with 20 items on physical health and 9 items on psychological health in patients with MS.[43]

Functional assessment of multiple sclerosis
The functional assessment of MS (FAMS) is a 59-item English language instrument that includes the following subscales: mobility, symptoms, emotional well-being, general contentment, fatigue, and social well-being.[44] Unlike other instruments that have derived their assessment of generic QoL based on the SF-36, the FAMS assesses generic QoL as derived from the Functional Assessment of Cancer Therapy (FACT) scale.[45]

Multiple sclerosis quality-of-life inventory
The MS quality-of-life inventory (MSQLI) is a battery of 10 scales that provide both generic and MS-specific HRQoL information.[46] Short forms are also available for several of the item banks, which reduce assessment burden. Individual scores for each subscale are reported separately and there is no composite score. The Bladder Control Scale (BLCS) is a 4-item instrument that is a component of MSQLI that specifically assesses urinary-specific–related HRQoL in patients with MS.

Spina Bifida

Quality of life in spina bifida
The quality of life in spina bifida (QoL-SB) is a combination of 2 instruments, 1 completed by the child or adolescent with spina bifida and 1 to be completed by the parents.[47] Validity of this instrument was assessed against the Piers-Harris Children's Self-Concept Scale.

Overall Quality of Life

Health status questionnaire of the medical outcomes study short form
The SF-36 and SF-12 are generic QoL instruments that are the most widely used in the study of neurogenic populations and other chronic conditions.[9,10] There is considerable population-level normative data from various countries using the SF-36 and SF-12 that is available for comparison with study populations of interests. The SF-36 has 8 subscales, including physical functioning, role limitations due to physical problems, bodily pain, general health perceptions, vitality, social functioning, role limitations due to emotional problems, and mental health, and 2 summary scores, including the physical component summary and the mental component summary. Newer neurogenic population–specific instruments, such as the SCI-QOL, SCI-FI, SCI-SCS, MSQOL-54, and

MSQLI, are derived from the SF-36 and SF-12. The SF-36 and SF-12 do not include any specific domains regarding urinary dysfunction and, therefore, may overlook specific patient-reported outcomes and satisfaction with urinary management strategies.

INTEGRATION OF PATIENT-REPORTED OUTCOME MEASURES IN NEUROGENIC BLADDER RESEARCH

The role of PROMs in NGB research is evolving, as the focus on clinical interventions has shifted from placebo or nontreatment to comparative interventions. Comparative effectiveness research (CER) evaluates the risks, benefits, and harms of a specific intervention for a clinical condition and comprehensively involves the patient perspective.[48] Data from CER can help guide informed decisions by patients, caregivers, providers, and policy makers. Since passage of the 2009 Patient-Centered Outcomes Research Act, an initial $1.1 billion established the Patient-Centered Outcomes Research Institute (PCORI) and annual funding of approximately $500 million funds independent CER.[48]

It is helpful to use existing frameworks to conceptualize how PROMs fit into research on NGB. For example, Wilson and Cleary[49] developed a model to map the various relationships between clinical outcomes and variables with outcomes that would matter to patients and impact overall QoL. There are symptom-specific variables of interest for research in NGB, including assessment of urinary incontinence, bladder filling/emptying, and urinary-specific complications. Additionally, urinary-specific QoL and health-related QoL must be considered together as a comprehensive assessment of how NGB impacts QoL. Although there is not a single instrument currently available to comprehensively assess various self-reported clinical and patient-reported outcomes, a combination of the validated instruments detailed previously provides a strong conceptual framework for use of PROMs in NGB research.

There are several unique considerations for the interpretation of PROM data that should be considered before initiation of collection of PROM. Often PROMs are collected longitudinally to assess changes in response to natural disease course or specific intervention. Missing data points can significantly impact the estimated effect of disease or intervention on PROMs leading to systematic biases.[50,51] Considerations should be made before initiation of collection of PROMs to minimize missing data and appropriate statistical tests should be used to assess and correct for its impact on the PROMs of interest. There must also be a consideration of what is a minimal important difference or traditionally what is thought of a statistically significant change. With patient-reported outcomes research, a patient-reported minimal important difference may be much lower than what may be traditionally thought of as a clinically significant difference. An attempt to estimate the minimal important difference must be done before initiation of PROM collection, with a consideration from various stakeholders, including patients, caregivers, clinicians, and rehabilitation providers.[52]

Method of administration is another consideration when collecting PROM data. The increasing use of electronic, Internet-based personal health records (PHRs) whereby patients have online access to their individual health records and are able to securely message providers, will likely facilitate the use of patient-reported outcomes research in NGB. In the Kaiser Permanente system, PHR has enhanced patient health care management and quality of care.[53] Integration of patient-reported outcomes with PHR allows for timely collection of data points and allows patients to choose the environment they would like to complete instruments, whether it be during their clinic visit or within their home. This will enable longitudinal collection of simultaneous clinical and PROMs. As described for the SCI-QOL item banks, some PROMs require electronic administration because of computer adaptive testing methods. Others are available electronically and on paper forms. In patients with an underlying neurologic condition, disability associated with limited hand function must be considered in collection of PROM. Additionally, many of these instruments are validated for self-administration and the impact of assistance by a caregiver or clinical/research assistant is unknown.

SUMMARY

PROMs are gaining a larger role in the assessment of clinical outcomes and HRQoL in those with NGB. These self-reported data are highly applicable to a specific patient and provide an accurate assessment of the patient's perception of their symptoms. Obtaining HRQoL measures initially can help trend the longitudinal impact of various treatment modalities. This is particularly of interest when there is a discordance between clinical and patient-reported outcomes in the evaluation of interventions. As a profession, we are just starting to recognize the need for understanding the degree of bother caused by NGB and the correlation

Long-Term Complications of the Neurogenic Bladder

Unwanaobong Nseyo, MD, Yahir Santiago-Lastra, MD*

KEYWORDS

- Neurogenic bladder • Urinary diversion • Spina bifida • Neurogenic lower urinary tract dysfunction
- Urinary incontinence • Low bladder compliance • Spinal cord injury • Multiple sclerosis

KEY POINTS

- Patients with neurogenic bladder are at highest risk for long-term complications, particularly upper urinary tract deterioration, including spinal cord injury, myelomeningocele, transverse myelitis, and other conditions in which there is a high burden of spinal disease.
- The greatest underlying contributing factor is the loss of coordinated bladder storage and emptying function, typically mediated by the pontine micturition center.
- Evaluation of the patient with neurogenic lower urinary tract dysfunction should involve an assessment of their upper urinary tract, their bladder safety, their continence status, and quality-of-life concerns.

INTRODUCTION

Mere decades ago, urologic sequelae were primarily responsible for the high mortality rates among patients with neurogenic bladder (NGB). As recently as the 1950s, upper urinary tract (UUT) damage was the number one cause of mortality in patients with spinal cord injury (SCI). Renal failure and urinary tract infections (UTIs) were the major culprits.[1] Children born with spina bifida (SB) were rarely expected to reach adulthood, often because of the severity of urologic complications. Since then, advancements in UTI treatment, implementation of regimented bladder management strategies, and the use of diagnostic tools such as urodynamics have brought about a dramatic reduction in previously high rates of mortality due to NGB complications: 80% of patients with SCI in the 1940s to 3% of renal-related mortality in this population nearly 4 decades later.[2]

Although the successful reduction in mortality for this population has now been observed, NGB management still confers a high degree of morbidity and greatly impacts psychosocial well-being. Recently, the conversation has transitioned from mortality reduction to improving quality of life. These concerns are less binary and require a more nuanced approach. The goal for the urologist caring for the NGB population continues to be the prevention and management of long-term complications, with the added responsibility of balancing this goal with a compassionate focus on preserving quality of life. Successfully reconciling these 2 goals requires an understanding of the long-term urologic complications of NGB, particularly in the high-risk patient.

Disclosure Statement: None.
Department of Urology, UC San Diego Health, University of California–San Diego, 200 West Arbor Drive, San Diego, CA 92103-8897, USA
* Corresponding author.
E-mail address: ysantiagolastra@ucsd.edu

Urol Clin N Am 44 (2017) 355–366
http://dx.doi.org/10.1016/j.ucl.2017.04.003
0094-0143/17/© 2017 Elsevier Inc. All rights reserved.

Within the NGB population, certain patients will have higher risk of complications secondary to their underlying disease neurophysiology. The American Urological Association (AUA) Guidelines statement on urodynamics outline those individuals who have a higher likelihood of lower urinary tract dysfunction resulting in complications: SB, SCI, high burden of spinal cord disease (a de facto SCI due to demyelinating disease, tumor burden, infarction, or other causes), transverse myelitis, and men with multiple sclerosis (MS).[3]

The pathophysiology of the neurologic injury and its interaction with coordinated micturition creates the background for lower urinary tract dysfunction. First, the injury or deficit disrupts communication between the bladder and brain, specifically disrupting the pontine micturition center (PMC). The severity of this interruption correlates directly with how the lower urinary tract can execute a coordinated storage and voiding mechanism. The PMCs role in bladder emptying, via urethral sphincter relaxation and detrusor contraction, is well known and often reviewed. However, the PMC also has a pivotal role in the bladder's storage function. Without direct PMC feed-forward inhibition of detrusor contractility, the bladder loses its ability to maintain low pressures during filling. Over time, its normal elasticity is lost, leading to decreased compliance manifested at gradually lower filling volumes. The presence of poor compliance is likely the single greatest risk factor for devastating long-term complications, although no study has linearly correlated poor compliance with incidence of long-term UUT complications. However, it is the incidence of low compliance that separates the high- and low-risk NGB categories. For high-risk patients, long-term complications may be an added source of morbidity if not adequately anticipated or treated.

Specifically, the complications found in greater incidence in high-risk patients with NGB are upper tract disease, urinary incontinence, stones, and UTIs. UUT deterioration occurs as a direct result of decreased bladder compliance. The relationship between impaired compliance, detrusor leak point pressure, and renal dysfunction was first reported by McGuire and colleagues[4] in 1981. It was further described in the late 1980s, when Gormley[2] noted that poor compliance on urodynamics (UDS) predicted poor renal outcomes in children with myelodysplasia. The sum of the findings of this era suggested a close association between elevated outlet pressures, via either the fixed sphincter activity or the detrusor sphincter dyssynergia, and the incremental loss of detrusor compliance resulting in the "high-pressure bladder." In turn, increased detrusor pressure impairs delivery of urine from the kidneys. In addition, vesicoureteral reflux (VUR) can develop as a "pop-off" mechanism, ultimately resulting in UUT impairment. The validity of this connection was bolstered by several studies that demonstrated stabilization or improvement in upper tract deterioration when outlet pressures were pharmacologically or surgically lessened. In addition to UUT deterioration, other complications can occur concomitantly, especially in the long-term period. Urinary incontinence is multifactorial but can often occur in the setting of detrusor overactivity.[2]

Although this longer-term impact makes vigilance imperative to the provider, quality-of-life data also affirm additional psychosocial impact to the patient. Patient-reported outcome measures among individuals with NGB consistently demonstrate that nonfatal conditions, such as lack of social continence, presence of an indwelling catheter, frequent hospitalizations, and recurrent UTIs, can have profoundly devastating effects on a patient's satisfaction with their life.[5,6] Extending life expectancy without also working to ensure that those years of life are considered of substantial quality to the patient can potentially downplay any mortality reduction.

The goal of this article is to introduce the reader to the pathophysiology that informs lower urinary tract dysfunction among patients with NGB, specifically focusing on those at highest risk for complications; characterize the complications associated with lower urinary tract dysfunction in these patients; and evaluate the evidence in support of interventions aimed at curtailing the long-term urologic manifestations of NGB.

GOALS OF MANAGEMENT IN THE NEUROGENIC BLADDER PATIENT

At the authors' institution, a fundamental premise is that management recommendations for the patient with NGB should balance the patient's own social goals and desires with the provider's assessment of their specific risk of complications. Balancing these priorities results in management strategies that are often patient specific and dependent on a wide set of variables. Even so, the driving principles rest on a foundation of balancing the patient's quality-of-life goals with their health and safety. Preserving renal function, promoting urinary continence, minimizing risks for associated sequelae such as UTIs and bladder stones, and enhancing the patient's quality of life are primary concerns from both a clinician and a patient perspective and form backbone of the primary "checklist" used when evaluating these patients (Box 1). Addressing the first 2 goals requires knowledge

Box 1
Sample outpatient neurogenic bladder patient evaluation checklist

Essential intake questions:

Underlying neurologic diagnosis

Level (if applicable)

Mobility status

Current catheterization regimen if used

Size/type of catheter and complications with catheterization if present

Continence status (dry, pads, diapers)

Bladder medications

Accidental bowel leakage

Bowel regimen

Febrile versus nonfebrile UTI in past year

Occurrence of hematuria

Prior bladder/upper urinary tract surgery

Recent upper tract imaging

Previous urodynamics results

Assessment should include the following plans to address:

1. Baseline evaluation and preservation of renal function

2. Bladder safety evaluation (with urodynamics if indicated)

3. Continence plan

4. Quality-of-life concerns

Information is obtained during the history and physical and uploaded into the chart as part of their initial consultation.

Box 2
Principles of neurogenic bladder management

- Management in line with patient's goals
- Absence or control of infection
- Preservation of upper urinary tract function
- Maintenance of low-pressure continent bladder that empties well
- Avoidance of indwelling catheter

attention placed on those individuals at highest risk for long-term complications. Appropriate prevention and treatment are addressed in subsequent sections.

RENAL INJURY AND DETERIORATION

Specific populations with NGB are at higher risk for UUT deterioration as sequelae of their lower urinary tract dysfunction. As identified above, individuals with SB, SCI, high burden of spinal cord disease, transverse myelitis, and men with MS make up this group. **Fig. 1** illustrates the relationships between neurologic injury and lower urinary tract function. The degree of uninterrupted input from the PMC dictates the likelihood of a neurologic injury resulting in possible upper tract damage. The PMC is responsible for mediating a coordinated mechanism of bladder storage and bladder emptying through organizing the interaction between the PMC, the sacral micturition center, and the cerebral cortex. When the PMC is interrupted, the normal opposing relationship between the detrusor and the internal/external sphincter is lost.[8]

An examination of the pathophysiology of neurologic injury in the lower-risk patient with NGB highlights the role of PMC in maintaining coordinated bladder function. In contrast to the high-risk patient with NGB, an individual with a cerebrovascular accident (CVA), for example, has preserved feedback from the PMC and therefore maintains a low-pressure, normal compliance bladder. Similarly, an individual with peripheral neuropathy secondary to diabetes mellitus may have reduced bladder sensation and therefore some degree of lower urinary tract dysfunction. However, the incidence of diminished bladder compliance is rare, although a significant caveat exists for patients managed with a chronic indwelling catheter. Patients whose bladders are primarily managed with indwelling catheters, either suprapubic tube or urethral Foley, are at increased risk of loss of compliance over time when compared with those managed with clean intermittent catheterization (CIC) or voiding. Current data suggest that alternative methods of

of the storage and emptying capacity of the patient. In addition, data by Spindel and colleagues[7] have shown that bladder function will vary over a single patient's natural history if they are followed longitudinally. Therefore, periodic assessments have been recommended by many experts, although individualized recommendations for specific NGB populations have not yet been published. Stratification of patients should be based on their lower urinary tract abnormality, symptom severity, and the risk of developing UUT damage.

LONG-TERM COMPLICATIONS IN THE NEUROGENIC BLADDER PATIENT

This section focuses on defining the scope of the problem with respect to long-term complications among patients with NGB (**Box 2**), with special

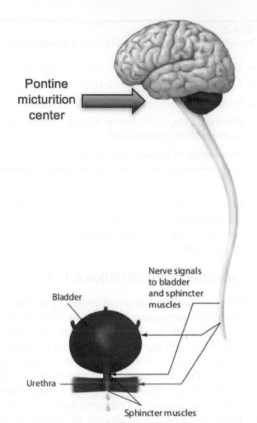

Pontine
micturition
center

Nerve signals
to bladder
and sphincter
muscles

Bladder

Urethra

Sphincter muscles

Fig. 1. Neurologic coordination of lower urinary tract function. Why is UUT deterioration more likely in certain NGB conditions? The most at risk are patients with significant spinal lesions, such as traumatic SCI and SB, for example, disrupted transmission between the PMC and neurons in the sacral spinal cord prevent the PMC from resulting detrusor compliance during storage and coordinating bladder and sphincter activity during voiding. Over the long term, this can result in permanent changes to detrusor function and elasticity, leading to upper tract damage.

bladder drainage should be pursued when possible, and increased frequency of UDS should be performed if long-term catheter drainage is necessary.[6]

A comparison of renal failure rates among the high-risk group to those who are not considered high risk highlights the impact of the loss of coordinated pons control on lower urinary tract function.[9] Similarly, individuals with MS, whose neurologic disease process in comparison is slowly progressive and nontraumatic, have much lower rates of UUT deterioration compared with those with SB and SCI.[9] The AUA Guidelines make a point to categorize men with MS as higher risk for upper tract deterioration. In their systematic review, De Sèze and colleagues[10] identified several risk factors for UUT deterioration among individuals with MS, of which male gender was a factor as well as

the duration of MS, high-amplitude detrusor contractions, and similarly to other NGB populations, presence of a chronic indwelling catheter. Ultimately, a determination of whether the PMC is impacted by the neurologic disease as well as the presence of a long-term indwelling catheter are both reasonable litmus tests for identifying patients that are at highest risk for complications and therefore warrant closer follow-up and evaluation.

The declines in mortality related to UUT deterioration among patients with NGB have come as the result of early identification with close follow-up and assessment. Among children with occult spinal dysraphism, 15% developed UUT deterioration and 7.5% ultimately developed renal failure.[11] Work by Zhang and Liao[12] found that lumbosacral SCI and chronic indwelling urethral and suprapubic catheterizations were predictors of UUT deterioration. Part of this higher risk with respect to chronic catheterization is attributable to the association between these characteristics and bladder compliance with catheterization serving as a proxy for decreased bladder function. Overall, patients with SB and SCI have a substantially higher risk of developing renal failure compared with the general adult population, in comparison to patients with slowly progressive disorders such as Parkinson disease and MS, in which the risk is significantly lower.[9] McGuire and colleagues[4] linked the risk of UUT deterioration to detrusor leak point pressure of greater than 40 cm H_2O in patients with SB, although this figure may not be generalizable to the entire population of patients with NGB, and to date, no studies have extrapolated these results in other high-risk populations. In addition, exposure to repeated upper tract infections, often secondary to underlying VUR, is a significant risk factor for renal injury and scarring that is independent of lower urinary tract abnormality.[13]

Aside from being the direct result of loss of bladder compliance, UUT deterioration can occur when in the setting of a variety of other factors. A cross-sectional study of VA patients, including those with and without SCI, identified a statistically significant higher rate of chronic kidney disease (CKD) among those with SCI (35% vs 20%, respectively).[14] Recurrent upper tract infections, hydronephrosis, loss of bladder compliance, and stone disease have all been linked to increased risk of CKD among patients with SCI.[10]

URINARY INCONTINENCE

Urinary incontinence can stem from several causes—detrusor overactivity, stress urinary incontinence, and overflow incontinence, the first of which is the most common cause. Regardless, incontinence has a far-reaching impact on individuals with NGB and is a significant contributor to their quality of life, influencing their self-esteem and ability to successfully navigate the social sphere. Incontinence is also associated with significant psychosocial stress, with the potential downstream sequelae of reducing rehabilitation potential with respect to the patient's neurologic disease.[15] Therefore, the goal of continence is a primary concern with respect to the quality of life of patients with NGB. Detrusor sphincter dyssynergia, detrusor overactivity, and intrinsic sphincter deficiency present obstacles to achieving continence in the NGB patient. The root cause of the incontinence provides insight as to possible treatment modalities; however, ultimately, the goal of continence is a long-term pursuit for individuals with NGB, and its devastating effects on the patient's psychosocial well-being place it at the top of the priority list for many patients. Throughout their adult life, approximately 50% of patients with SCI, when questioned, will report some degree of bothersome urinary incontinence.[15] In studies focused on the MS population, up to 21% to 50% of patients experience frequent episodes of urinary incontinence.[16] For adult patients with SB, incontinence rates are even higher, with approximately 45% to 70% of patients reporting some degree of urinary leakage,[11] making it the most widely prevalent of the long-term sequelae.

URINARY TRACT INFECTIONS

UTIs represent a significant burden of disease for individuals with NGB. Overall rate of UTI estimated within an NGB cohort has been 2.5 episodes per year.[16] In addition, due to several patient-related factors, increased susceptibility to upper tract infections, delay in diagnosis due to atypical symptoms, each episode can be relatively morbid with notable health care expenditures. In a prospective cohort study of patients with SCI, one-fifth of the hospital readmissions were due to UTI with an average hospital stay 15.5 days.[17] Within the SB population, review of national data has demonstrated that high proportions of hospital admissions for these patients were related to symptomatic UTIs. For example, Kinsman and Doehring[18] noted that nearly 50% of admissions for patients with SB were attributed to UTIs as well as to urolithiasis, the 2 of which often coexist in these patients.[18] For individuals with MS, UTI poses a risk to their overall disease state as retrospective data have highlighted UTIs as a trigger for MS exacerbations, with recurrent UTIs being linked to neurologic progression.[19]

Patients with NGB are at risk for chronic UTIs stemming from several factors, including their bladder management, potential for poor bladder emptying resulting in urinary stasis, chronic bacteriuria and potential for reflux, and subsequent upper UTIs, all of which introduce or help to maintain sources of bacteria in the urinary tract. Because of the baseline bacteriuria of this patient population, triggers for treatment are different and are based on symptoms, such as change in urine odor or color, fever, change in voiding habits. Similarly, given the propensity for bacteriuria resulting from many of the factors mentioned above, UTI among those with NGB has been strictly defined. The National Institute on Disability and Rehabilitation Research consensus conference recommended a standard definition of UTI in the patient with SCI using urine culture data, urinalysis, and clinical symptoms including fever.[20] With respect to urine culture data, the cutoff was based on bladder management, including individuals with indwelling catheters, whom perform CIC, and patients with condom catheter and ranged from $\geq 10^2$ to $\geq 10^4$ colony forming units (CFU).[20] The Infectious Disease Society of America used the data to propose $\geq 10^3$ as the cutoff because it balances sensitivity with meaningful detection.[21]

Because of the possibility for atypical presentations especially given the degree to which the patient is able to communicate regarding their symptoms, a high index of suspicion is needed in addressing UTI in this patient population because many can be plagued by recurrent infections, and many more can be plagued by overtreatment of bacteriuria. Routine imaging and cystoscopy in those with recurrent, febrile, symptomatic infections can help potentially identify any structural abnormalities or possible nidus of infection. Although there are no guidelines for treating bacteriuria in patients with SD, Elliott and colleagues[22] found in their survey of 59 SB clinics that greater than 100 CFU/mL paired with symptoms was used to guide treatment for a positive urine culture in the SB patient. To date, there is no consensus on the diagnosis and prevention of recurrent UTI or bacteriuria in the NGB population. Recent evidence by Cox and colleagues[23] suggests that intravesical instillation of antibiotic such as gentamicin can reduce the incidence of for-cause treatment of bacteriuria in the NGB population. The vigilance for UTI within the NGB population must also be balanced with a tendency toward overtreatment. Retrospective data have demonstrated that the sometimes-reflexive treatment of bacteriuria in the ambulatory setting has driven resistance patterns toward more multi-drug-resistant strains. A fine balance must be struck between addressing bouts of UTI with its associated downstream sequelae and downsides to overtreatment.

UROLITHIASIS

Urinary stasis and chronic bacteriuria place many patients with NGB at high risk for urinary stone formation, although no difference in bacteriuria rates has been found among stone-formers and non-stone-formers in the NGB population. In addition, UTI has been noted as an independent risk factor for stone disease among these patients.[24] The increased prevalence of urease-producing bacteria among patients with SCI suggests a direct link between infection and stone formation. Risk factors for upper tract calculi include bladder catheterization, bladder calculi, VUR, and environmental factors. Overall, this patient population is at a higher risk for stone disease, bilateral stone formation, and staghorn calculi. The form of bladder management also influences the stone risk. Zhang and Liao[12] found that there was a much higher rate of bladder stone in patients with an indwelling Foley catheter (38.3% vs 81.5%, respectively). Similarly, Bartel and colleagues[25] found bladder stones more often associated with suprapubic catheter in 11%, transurethral catheter in 6.6%, with intermittent catheterization in 2% and with reflex micturition in 1.1%. A colinear association also exists between stone disease and upper tract deterioration. Of patients with SCI who had died of renal failure, these patients were 4 times more likely to have renal stones.[26] Some studies have observed rates as high as 28% to 32% of impaired renal function in patients with NGB with stone disease[26,27] but the causative mechanism has not been identified. Despite improvements in treatment and imaging, the rate of stone formation in this population has been relatively stable, likely because of ascertainment bias.

MALIGNANCY

The rationale for bladder cancer screening among patients with NGB is equal parts anecdotal and evidence based. Overall, the incidence of bladder cancer in patients with NGB is relatively rare. Studies looking at the incidence of bladder cancer among individuals with NGB range from 0.2% to 2% with many studies with an incidence of less than 0.5%.[28] For example, a recent retrospective study of more than 7000 patients using Medicare data quoted a rate of 0.21%.[29] These rates are even lower when compared with a non-SCI population. Lee and colleagues[30] looked at patients with SCI and found 33% lower risk of prostate

cancer in the SCI population as compared with age- and gender-matched controls and an equivalent risk for bladder cancer.

Although data suggest that bladder cancer is a rare occurrence among certain NGB populations, biology of their cancers when they do occur warrants early identification and routine surveillance. When individuals with NGB do develop bladder cancer, whether it is squamous cell carcinoma or urothelial cell carcinoma, they have significantly higher mortality rates; Groah and colleagues[31] found a 71-fold higher standardized mortality compared with the general population.[32] Case report series of patients with SB have also shown higher grade at presentation, earlier age at diagnosis, and high mortalities.[33] The exception to this relationship is among individuals with MS, where there is a lower the risk of cancer in this population, regardless of the state of disease-modulating treatment.[34,35]

The concern for malignancy among individuals with NGB is often attributed to the use of chronic indwelling catheters due to persistent inflammation. Within the NGB population, there are several risk factors for festering inflammation, including recurrent infections, urolithiasis, and chronic indwelling catheterization. The presence of bladder stones has been identified as a risk factor in retrospective review.[36] Data suggest that patients with SCI are at a higher risk for developing bladder malignancies at both a younger age and a higher stage at initial presentation. The risk factor identified in this cohort was chronic UTIs, which were seen in higher rates among those with bladder cancer.[37]

The need for bladder cancer surveillance among individuals with NGB is not based on the neurologic injury or neurologic disease itself but reflects the downstream effects of different aspects of NGB disease and disease management. Elements of bladder management such as chronic indwelling catheterization and sequelae of NGB such as bladder stones and recurrent UTIs all contribute to the chronic inflammation/irritation that is linked to bladder malignancy in NGB. In addition, although the rates of malignancy are not necessarily higher in this group, the poorer prognosis of disease at the time of presentation tips the balance in favor of close surveillance among this patient population. At the authors' institution, they do not perform routine screening for bladder malignancy in all patients with NGB. However, they recommend yearly screening cystoscopy for patients who have any of the following: gross hematuria, greater than 4 UTIs per year, chronic indwelling catheters, chronic perineal or pelvic pain, abnormal radiographic studies, or colon augments after the patient is older than 50 years (the suggested age of screening colonoscopy for colorectal cancer). This surveillance strategy has not yet been validated for cost-effectiveness, sensitivity, and specificity in its detection of bladder cancer.

THE ROLE OF EARLY EVALUATION IN ASSESSING LONG-TERM COMPLICATION RISK

The goal of the workup of the patient with known neurologic disease is to determine to what degree that disease has affected the function of the urinary tract, a lifelong dynamic process. The tools available to assess these patients include urinalysis, post-void residual, ultrasonography, uroflowmetry, blood chemistry, urine culture and urine cytology, urodynamics (including videourodynamics), pelvic floor neurophysiology, and renal scintigraphy. Each of these tests is valuable in answering specific questions regarding presence of infection, evidence of voiding dysfunction, and concern for upper tract deterioration.

The timing of using these tests and the relative weight that is placed on them in any given time is informed by the other components of the patient evaluation: history, symptoms, and physical examination findings. Retrospective data from Dik and colleagues[38] suggest that a strategy that optimizes treatment of the NGB from birth can improve outcomes with respect to renal function. As the guidelines regarding urologic surveillance are based mostly on expert opinion and retrospective data, there is no consensus as to what components of these tests should constitute routine screening.[39] In the systematic review by Cameron and colleagues,[40] as compared with IVP and renal scan, renal ultrasound was found to be cost-effective and with better sensitivity for identifying anatomic abnormalities. The authors' institutional practice in the high-risk patient includes initial assessment with a full chemistry panel, baseline urodynamic evaluation for determination of bladder safety, and renal ultrasonography. From there, they recommend a yearly urologic evaluation with assessment of renal function. In addition, UUT imaging is obtained with renal ultrasound being the most commonly used imaging modality. The inclusion of urodynamic testing is determined based on change in symptoms, increase in number of UTIs in the past year, or significant changes on ultrasound and are typically ordered *for cause* with a specific clinical question in mind and not for screening after the patient's baseline urodynamic evaluation.

Based on their systematic review of long-term urologic follow-up among patients with MS, SCI, and SB, Averbeck and Madersbacher[39] proposed a risk-adaptive model for determining the approach to screening among patients with NGB. Overall, recommendations are determined based on the risk categorization of the patient. It is recommended that in high-risk patients, individuals with SB, SCI, high burden of spinal cord disease, transverse myelitis, and men with MS, renal ultrasonography be performed as often as every 6 months.[41] The higher frequency of upper tract surveillance is especially pertinent among individuals with a history of lower urinary tract reconstruction.[42] Although routinely used as a proxy for renal deterioration, serum creatinine has not been found to be a reliable tool in this population as compared with creatinine clearance when the appropriate correction factors are used. Notably, these correction factors are based on patients with SCI and cannot be extended to the variability of patients in the NGB population.[43] Renal scintigraphy can serve to make up for the shortcomings of creatinine by offering a reliable estimate of glomerular filtration rate particularly in patients with poor muscle mass or with poor renal function.[41] In addition, although creatinine itself can be an inaccurate measure in this patient population, the measurement of creatinine over time has been shown to be a reliable estimate of overall renal function as the baseline creatinine serves as an internal control.

Of these tests, urodynamics is central to the continued evaluation of the patient with NGB. Although the review by Cameron and colleagues[40] addressed the usefulness of renal ultrasound as an assessment tool in the NGB population, not enough evidence was present in the 11 studies examined to recommend an optimal frequency of UDS. Videourodynamics has also been shown to be useful in obtaining baseline assessments of adult patients with NGB because it allows for comparison of bladder abnormality with bladder function; for example, to rcompare the elationship between compliance and the development of bladder diverticula. Videourodynamics can be an instrumental tool in the assessment of the patient with NGB, offering information not only on bladder function but also on the relationship between the external urinary sphincter and bladder contraction as well as the presence of VUR.

Evidence supports the role of surveillance in reducing the risk of long-term complications in those with NGB. Serial examination has been shown by Waites and colleagues[44] to assist in the preservation in long-term renal function in patients with SCI when continued after initial evaluation. In this matched-pairs design, individuals with close follow-up (annual) were compared with those who had not undergone any follow-up for a period of 3 to 15 years before study enrollment. No statistical differences were noted with respect to the demographics and injury-associated variables of the 2 populations. One of their major conclusions was that after several years of stability, the screening interval can be lengthened.

Although there are obvious benefits to close follow-up in this population, a review of Medicare data demonstrates that even basic evaluations are not routinely being performed among these patients. In a retrospective cohort study using a sampling of Medicare data, 7162 patients with SCI were identified and were evaluated with respect to their compliance with urologic surveillance: urologist visit, serum creatinine, and upper tract imaging within a 2-year period. Only 24.6% of the patients received adequate screening during the study period.[29] The study provided key insight into the current surveillance practices among this patient population. With evidence suggesting a positive link between urologic surveillance and improved urinary tract outcomes among patients with NGB, more emphasis must be placed on, as well as better defining, the timelines and elements that should constitute routine follow-up.

SITE OF NEUROLOGIC DISEASE AND THE RISK FACTORS FOR LONG-TERM COMPLICATIONS

The level of neurologic injury can be useful in predicting the observed urinary tract dysfunction. Certain categories of patients may be at higher risk for long-term complications. The level of the lesion in the nervous system can influence patterns of lower urinary tract dysfunction. The lesion can occur in the central or peripheral nervous system.

Suprapontine lesions, above the PMC, which coordinates synergistic voiding, are typically seen in individuals with CVA, Parkinson disease, multiple system atrophy (MSA), MS, and dementia. In these situations, primarily the storage function of the urinary bladder is impacted. The resultant action is decreased bladder capacity and overactivity of the detrusor muscle. These patients are primarily bothered by incontinence, which is the downstream effect of their lesion. Those with dementia may suffer incontinence driven by their neurologic insult, further exacerbated by their behavioral problems and possibly immobility. The same concerns are true for individuals with Parkinson disease or MSA or who have suffered a CVA. In addition to their limitations with mobility, urodynamics will typically demonstrate detrusor overactivity, although there are reports of detrusor underactivity and urinary retention following a hemorrhagic stroke.[45] In Parkinson disease, the degree of neurologic disability strongly correlates with the degree of lower urinary tract dysfunction, suggesting a relationship between the 2 disease states on the level of pathophysiology and dopaminergic neurons.[46] Similarly, in MSA, disease progression and the function of the genitourinary tract are covariate with lower urinary tract symptoms often preceding a diagnosis, further characterized by the presence of an open bladder neck in men on videourodynamics.[47]

For individuals with MS, urinary symptoms develop several years into the disease, and once they begin, increase with severity the longer the patient has MS, especially among individuals with progressive subtypes of the disease. Moreover, those with an earlier onset of symptoms are likely to have a worse disease outcome with respect to their MS.[48,49] However, even in the absence of changing urinary symptoms, changes could develop in those patients' urodynamics and detrusor compliance during follow-up.[50] In those where urodynamic abnormality was found, factors such as being in a wheelchair, an MS-type other than relapsing-remitting, and use of more than one incontinence pad per day were identified.[51] Also among individuals with MS, both storage and voiding can be affected with a predominance of detrusor overactivity, and less frequently, an elevated post-void residual.[10] Detrusor-sphincter dyssynergia has been associated with pyelonephritis in patients with MS, more so than in other NGB populations. Even with the possibility of incomplete bladder emptying, the likelihood of upper tract damage is lower in patients with MS, although recent data suggest an increased prevalence in men, likely secondary to concomitant benign prostatic hyperplasia.[10,52]

Spinal cord abnormality can present with variable symptoms, depending on the level and completeness of injury. The variability in symptoms applies to SCI and myelomeningocele populations. With respect to the risk of long-term complications, several factors have been identified within this group of patients with NGB. Lawrenson and colleagues[9] found a significantly increased risk of renal failure as compared with the general population among those with paraplegia or neural tube defects.[53] According to Bellucci and colleagues,[54] when looking at patients with SCI, ambulatory patients were as likely as their wheelchair-bound counterparts to have abnormal urodynamic findings. The similarity in urodynamic parameters suggests that regardless of mobility or level of injury, patients with SCI should undergo the same type of screening.[55] Although early evaluation is standard for all children born with SB, continued surveillance is necessary because changes can occur throughout the first years of life and in adolescence with the potential onset of spinal cord tethering.[39,56] These patients are often at high risk for long-term complications because they are less likely to have close follow-up because of their baseline level of functioning. Even in the absence of cord tethering, the transition to adulthood for SB is associated with increased mortality given the impact of hormonally driven changes on the urinary tract. The adult SB patient is faced with increased risk: Combined with potentially detrimental changes to the lower urinary tract, decreased access to urologic care likely impacts the morbidity and mortality associated with transition care for these patients.[57] Adequate transition programs are key to addressing the risk factors that translate into poor health outcomes for this patient population, and studies are ongoing to demonstrate the value of transition care programs in preventing long-term complications in the underserved SB population.[58]

BLADDER MANAGEMENT OPTIONS FOR THE HIGH-RISK NEUROGENIC BLADDER

There are several management strategies available for the lower tract in patients with NGB. The type of bladder management is key to achieving the patient's continence goals in addition to being an integral part in prevention of detrimental outcomes for the patient with NGB. Certain bladder management options carry higher risks for infection, stone formation, malignancy, and renal deterioration. According to prospective cohort by Zhang and Liao,[12] bladder management played a critical role in eventual UUT damage. UUT abnormalities, such as VUR, elevated serum creatinine, and hydronephrosis, all of which were considered risk factors for UUT deterioration, were more often present in those patients with indwelling (78.9%) and suprapubic (87.5%) catheters as compared with those performing CIC (20%). Given the nature of this study, it was only possible to evaluate associations. Although catheter management is associated with UUT deterioration, it may be more suggestive of the fact that patients with those abnormalities were then managed with a chronic indwelling catheter because they had failed another alternative method of bladder management, such as CIC, condom catheter, reflex voiding. Although there is no consensus given the specific nature of patient-driven factors, each option aims to achieve the goal of continence and low-pressure voiding/maintaining low bladder pressure while emptying.

CIC is recommended as first line for individuals with NGB. Although CIC has been cited as conferring a significant burden to the caregivers of those individuals with NGB, if it can be performed consistently and appropriately, or better yet by the patient themselves, this approach to bladder management can be a worthwhile investment. As opposed to other forms of bladder management, such as chronic indwelling Foley catheters, suprapubic catheters, and continent diversions, CIC carries a significantly lower risk of infection and stone formation. In addition, when performed in a timely fashion, and often paired with an anticholinergic, CIC avoids many of the urologic complications, such as infections, calculi, renal scarring, and VUR.[59] CIC induced fewer UTI episodes than did the chronic indwelling catheter. Notwithstanding, patients with NGB consistently report that their bladder management strategy negatively impacts their quality of life, reaffirming the need for innovation that balances the risk of long-term complications with a bladder-emptying solution that can be easily implemented with lower burden to the patient.

Recent reports from Feifer and Corcos[60] have shown that suprapubic tubes can be a safe option in select patients with the appropriate surveillance. These patients were well managed with frequent catheter changes, bladder irrigation, and maintenance of a low bladder volume, all of which resulted in a morbidity similar to those performing CIC. Although the long-term complications of indwelling catheterization have been well documented, bladder management method can considerably change over an NGB patient's lifetime, with most patients alternating between different bladder management methods.[38–40]

Urethral or suprapubic catheter management is used by about a third of patients with SCI. Many female patients with SCI rely on indwelling catheterization because they are unable, unwilling, or unsuitable for CIC.[61] Female patients with adductor spasms or with poor manual dexterity are unsuitable for CIC. The drawbacks associated with indwelling catheter use stem from the development of bacteriuria. From the moment the urethral catheter is introduced, the incidence of bacteriuria is 5% to 10% per day.[19] The resultant bacteriuria is responsible for many the complications associated with the indwelling catheter.

Previously, bladder augmentation and urinary diversion were performed early on for children born with NGB. Enterocystoplasty is still routinely performed in patients with NGB but is reserved for those individuals with impaired bladder compliance, diminished capacity, and upper tract deterioration. Today, botulinum toxin has greatly reduced the utilization of bladder augmentation and urinary diversion, although both have a significant role, particularly in patients with a poorly compliant "end-stage" bladder. A review of patients with SB at Children's Hospitals nationwide found a small percentage had undergone bladder augmentation.[29] Despite difficulties in cross-comparison, populations of children who underwent bladder augmentation had long-term preservation of their renal function. Therefore, although the surgery itself is not without attendant risks, bladder augmentation can be a reasonable option for patients whose upper tracts are at risk for deterioration due to their baseline bladder abnormality.[30] Cystectomy with urinary diversion can be the last treatment option for patients with NGB and severe lower urinary tract symptoms who have not responded to less-invasive forms of treatment. Because the primary goal of a cystectomy performed for this indication is to decrease the patient's morbidity, understanding the outcomes and potential complications are essential to ensure proper patient selection for the intervention.

There are considerable data in the literature regarding radical cystectomy and urinary diversion in patients with bladder cancer demonstrating high morbidity and readmission rates associated with the procedure. Even with improvements in outcomes, the mortality of cystectomy today is between 1% and 2%, and the perioperative morbidity of this procedure remains high.[62] However, there are limited data on the perioperative morbidities and mortalities for cystectomies performed for nonmalignant indications.[62] Most data are retrospective and pooled among patients with varying benign urologic conditions in addition to NGB. There are also no long-term survival data on patients who undergo cystectomy and urinary diversion for nonmalignant indications. Despite this lack of data, patients with NGB are the largest population that undergoes cystectomy and urinary diversion for benign indications, emphasizing the need for further investigation of the outcomes for patients requiring urinary diversion.

SUMMARY

The term neurogenic bladder refers to a population with diverse urologic needs. The baseline assessment tools traditionally used in this population, renal ultrasound, basic laboratory studies, urodynamics/videourodynamics, can aid in appropriate risk stratification. The highest-yield dividends stem from the ability to identify those at the highest risk for upper tract deterioration. The 4-tiered goal of avoiding upper tract complications, maintaining

social continence, avoiding UTI, and preserving quality of life should be practiced in each patient, often in an individualized manner. Although there are no strict guidelines, data have consistently shown that routine surveillance, especially in high-risk groups, is key to lowering long-term sequelae. More dedicated research is needed to determine specific, patient-centered strategies by which to limit the risk of complications in this unique patient population.

REFERENCES

1. Capoor J, Stein AB. Aging with spinal cord injury. Phys Med Rehabil Clin N Am 2005;16(1):129–61.
2. Gormley EA. Urologic complications of the neurogenic bladder. Urol Clin North Am 2010;37(4): 601–7.
3. Collins CW, Winters JC. AUA/SUFU adult urodynamics guideline: a clinical review. Urol Clin North Am 2014;41(3):353–62.
4. McGuire EJ, Woodside JR, Borden TA, et al. Prognostic value of urodynamic testing in myelodysplastic patients. J Urol 2002;167(2):1049–53.
5. Ku JH. The management of neurogenic bladder and quality of life in spinal cord injury. BJU Int 2006; 98(4):739–45.
6. Weld KJ, Graney MJ, Dmochowski RR. Differences in bladder compliance with time and associations of bladder management with compliance in spinal cord injured patients. J Urol 2000;163(4):1228–33.
7. Spindel MR, Bauer SB, Dyro FM, et al. The changing neurourologic lesion in myelodysplasia. JAMA 1987; 258(12):1630–3.
8. Dorsher PT, McIntosh PM. Neurogenic bladder. Adv Urol 2012;2012:816274.
9. Lawrenson R, Wyndaele JJ, Vlachonikolis I, et al. Renal failure in patients with neurogenic lower urinary tract dysfunction. Neuroepidemiology 2001; 20(2):138–43.
10. De Sèze M, Ruffion A, Denys P, et al. The neurogenic bladder in multiple sclerosis: review of the literature and proposal of management guidelines. Mult Scler J 2007;13(7):915–28.
11. Capitanucci ML, Iacobelli BD, Silveri M, et al. Long-term urological follow-up of occult spinal dysraphism in children. Eur J Pediatr Surg 1996;6(Suppl 1):25–6.
12. Zhang Z, Liao L. Risk factors predicting upper urinary tract deterioration in patients with spinal cord injury: a prospective study. Spinal cord 2014;52(6): 468–71.
13. Soygür T, Arikan N, Yeşilli C, et al. Relationship among pediatric voiding dysfunction and vesicoureteral reflux and renal scars. Urology 1999; 54(5):905–8.
14. Fischer MJ, Krishnamoorthi VR, Smith BM, et al. Prevalence of chronic kidney disease in patients

with spinal cord injuries/disorders. Am J Nephrol 2012;36(6):542–8.

15. Pellatt GC. Neurogenic continence. Part 1: pathophysiology and quality of life. Br J Nurs 2008; 17(13):836–41.

16. Siroky MB. Pathogenesis of bacteriuria and infection in the spinal cord injured patient. Am J Med 2002; 113(1):67–79.

17. DeJong G, Tian W, Hsieh CH, et al. Rehospitalization in the first year of traumatic spinal cord injury after discharge from medical rehabilitation. Arch Phys Med Rehabil 2013;94(4):S87–97.

18. Kinsman SL, Doehring MC. The cost of preventable conditions in adults with spina bifida. Eur J Pediatr Surg 1996;6(Suppl 1):17–20.

19. Rapp NS, Gilroy J, Lerner AM. Role of bacterial infection in exacerbation of multiple sclerosis. Am J Phys Med Rehabil 1995;74(6):415–8.

20. The prevention and management of urinary tract infections among people with spinal cord injuries. National Institute on Disability and Rehabilitation Research consensus statement. January 27-29, 1992. J Am Paraplegia Soc 1992;15(3):194–204.

21. Hooton TM, Bradley SF, Cardenas DD, et al. Diagnosis, prevention, and treatment of catheter-associated urinary tract infection in adults: 2009 International Clinical Practice Guidelines from the Infectious Diseases Society of America. Clin Infect Dis 2010;50(5):625–63.

22. Elliott SP, Villar R, Duncan B. Bacteriuria management and urological evaluation of patients with spina bifida and neurogenic bladder: a multicenter survey. J Urol 2005;173(1):217–20.

23. Cox L, He C, Bevins J, et al. Gentamicin bladder instillations decrease symptomatic urinary tract infections and oral antibiotic use in patients on intermittent catheterization. Hoboken (NJ): Wiley-Blackwell; 2015.

24. Chen Y, DeVivo MJ, Roseman JM. Current trend and risk factors for kidney stones in persons with spinal cord injury: a longitudinal study. Spinal Cord 2000; 38(6):346.

25. Bartel P, Krebs J, Wöllner J, et al. Bladder stones in patients with spinal cord injury: a long-term study. Spinal Cord 2014;52(4):295–7.

26. Welk B, Fuller A, Razvi H, et al. Renal stone disease in spinal-cord–injured patients. J Endourol 2012; 26(8):954–9.

27. Ramsey S, McIlhenny C. Evidence-based management of upper tract urolithiasis in the spinal cord-injured patient. Spinal Cord 2011;49(9):948–54.

28. Welk B, McIntyre A, Teasell R, et al. Bladder cancer in individuals with spinal cord injuries. Spinal Cord 2013;51(7):516–21.

29. Cameron AP, Lai J, Saigal CS, et al. Urological surveillance and medical complications after spinal cord injury in the United States. Urology 2015; 86(3):506–10.

30. Lee WY, Sun LM, Lin CL, et al. Risk of prostate and bladder cancers in patients with spinal cord injury: a population-based cohort study. Urol Oncol 2014; 32(1):51.e1-7.

31. Groah SL, Weitzenkamp DA, Lammertse DP, et al. Excess risk of bladder cancer in spinal cord injury: evidence for an association between indwelling catheter use and bladder cancer. Arch Phys Med Rehabil 2002;83(3):346–51.

32. Nahm LS, Chen Y, DeVivo MJ, et al. Bladder cancer mortality after spinal cord injury over 4 decades. J Urol 2015;193(6):1923–8.

33. Austin JC, Elliott S, Cooper CS. Patients with spina bifida and bladder cancer: atypical presentation, advanced stage and poor survival. J Urol 2007; 178(3):798–801.

34. Lebrun C, Debouverie M, Vermersch P, et al. Cancer risk and impact of disease-modifying treatments in patients with multiple sclerosis. Mult Scler J 2008; 14(3):399–405.

35. De Ridder D, van Poppel H, Demonty L, et al. Bladder cancer in patients with multiple sclerosis treated with cyclophosphamide. J Urol 1998; 159(6):1881–4.

36. Stonehill WH, Dmochowski RR, Patterson AL, et al. Risk factors for bladder tumors in spinal cord injury patients. J Urol 1996;155(4):1248–50.

37. Pannek J. Transitional cell carcinoma in patients with spinal cord injury: a high-risk malignancy? Urology 2002;59(2):240–4.

38. Dik P, Klijn AJ, van Gool JD, et al. Early start to therapy preserves kidney function in spina bifida patients. Eur Urol 2006;49(5):908–13.

39. Averbeck MA, Madersbacher H. Follow-up of the neuro-urological patient: a systematic review. BJU Int 2015;115(S6):39–46.

40. Cameron AP, Rodriguez GM, Schomer KG. Systematic review of urological followup after spinal cord injury. J Urol 2012;187(2):391–7.

41. Pannek J, Blok B, Castro-Diaz D, et al. Guidelines on neuro-urology, European Association of Urology. In: Abrams P, Cardozo L, Khoury S, et al, editors. Lncontinence. 5th edition. International Consultation on Urological Diseases and European Association of Urology; 2014. p. 827–1000.

42. Blok BF, Karsenty G, Corcos J. Urological surveillance and management of patients with neurogenic bladder: results of a survey among practicing urologists in Canada. Can J Urol 2006; 13(5):3239–43.

43. Chikkalingaiah KBM, Grant ND, Mangold TM, et al. Performance of simplified modification of diet in renal disease and Cockcroft-Gault equations in patients with chronic spinal cord injury and chronic kidney disease. Am J Med Sci 2010;339(2):108–16.

44. Waites KB, Canupp KC, DeVivo MJ, et al. Compliance with annual urologic evaluations and

preservation of renal function in persons with spinal cord injury. J Spinal Cord Med 1995;18(4): 251–4.

45. Han KS, Heo SH, Lee SJ, et al. Comparison of urodynamics between ischemic and hemorrhagic stroke patients; can we suggest the category of urinary dysfunction in patients with cerebrovascular accident according to type of stroke? Neurourol Urodyn 2010;29(3):387–90.

46. Uchiyama T, Sakakibara R, Yamamoto T, et al. Urinary dysfunction in early and untreated Parkinson's disease. J Neurol Neurosurg Psychiatry 2011; 82(12):1382–6.

47. Sakakibara R, Hattori T, Uchiyama T, et al. Videourodynamic and sphincter motor unit potential analyses in Parkinson's disease and multiple system atrophy. J Neurol Neurosurg Psychiatry 2001; 71(5):600–6.

48. Stoffel JT. Contemporary management of the neurogenic bladder for multiple sclerosis patients. Urol Clin North Am 2010;37(4):547–57.

49. Myhr KM. Diagnosis and treatment of multiple sclerosis. Acta Neurol Scand 2008;117(s188):12–21.

50. Ciancio SJ, Mutchnik SE, Rivera VM, et al. Urodynamic pattern changes in multiple sclerosis. Urology 2001;57(2):239–45.

51. Wiedemann A, Kaeder M, Greulich W, et al. Which clinical risk factors determine a pathological urodynamic evaluation in patients with multiple sclerosis? An analysis of 100 prospective cases. World J Urol 2013;31(1):229–33.

52. Betts CD, D'Mellow MT, Fowler CJ. Urinary symptoms and the neurological features of bladder dysfunction in multiple sclerosis. J Neurol Neurosurg Psychiatry 1993;56(3):245–50, 18.

53. De Jong TP, Chrzan R, Klijn AJ, et al. Treatment of the neurogenic bladder in spina bifida. Pediatr Nephrol 2008;23(6):889–96.

54. Bellucci CS, et al. 1650 Repeatability of urodynamic investigations in patients with neurogenic lower urinary tract dysfunction results of same setting repeated studies. J Urol 2012;187(4):e666–7.

55. Schöps TF, Schneider MP, Steffen F, et al. Neurogenic lower urinary tract dysfunction (NLUTD) in patients with spinal cord injury: long-term urodynamic findings. BJU Int 2015;115(S6):33–8.

56. Cardenas DD, Mayo ME, Turner LR. Lower urinary changes over time in suprasacral spinal cord injury. Paraplegia 1995;33(6):326–9.

57. Le JT, Mukherjee S. Transition to adult care for patients with spina bifida. Phys Med Rehabil Clin N Am 2015;26(1):29–38.

58. Mourtzinos A, Stoffel JT. Management goals for the spina bifida neurogenic bladder: a review from infancy to adulthood. Urol Clin North Am 2010;37(4):527–35.

59. Weld KJ, Dmochowski RR. Effect of bladder management on urological complications in spinal cord injured patients. J Urol 2000;163(3):768–72.

60. Feifer A, Corcos J. Contemporary role of suprapubic cystostomy in treatment of neuropathic bladder dysfunction in spinal cord injured patients. Neurourol Urodyn 2008;27(6):475–9.

61. Jamil F. Towards a catheter free status in neurogenic bladder dysfunction: a review of bladder management options in spinal cord injury (SCI). Spinal Cord 2001;39(7):355.

62. Osborn DJ, Dmochowski RR, Kaufman MR, et al. Cystectomy with urinary diversion for benign disease: indications and outcomes. Urology 2014; 83(6):1433–7.

Surveillance Strategies for Neurogenic Lower Urinary Tract Dysfunction

Randy A. Vince Jr, MD[a], Adam P. Klausner, MD[b],*

KEYWORDS

- Neurogenic bladder • Neurogenic lower urinary tract dysfunction (NLUTD) • Surveillance
- Spinal cord injury • Urodynamics

KEY POINTS

- Individuals with neurogenic lower urinary tract dysfunction (NLUTD) are at high risk for complications, including upper tract/renal deterioration and bladder cancer.
- Surveillance for individuals with NLUTD using diagnostic tests, such as urine analysis, renal laboratory tests, imaging, urodynamics, and cystoscopy, may help prevent serious complications.
- Guidelines for NLUTD from multiple organizations review the evidence for available surveillance strategies and make wide-ranging recommendations.
- Guideline recommendations for surveillance in NLUTD are supported by limited evidence suggesting the need for development and testing of standardized protocols.

INTRODUCTION

According to the International Continence Society, the definition of neurogenic lower urinary tract dysfunction (NLUTD) is: "lower urinary tract dysfunction due to disturbance of the neurologic control mechanisms. Neurogenic lower urinary tract dysfunction thus can be diagnosed in presence of neurological pathology only."[1] The broad nature of this definition, which includes bladder or urethral dysfunction resulting from insults to the brain, spinal cord, ganglia, or peripheral nerves is, in part, what makes the establishment of evidence-based surveillance strategies so challenging. Add to this the fact that the causes of neurologic injury can be equally wide ranging and include medical conditions, neurologic disease, trauma, cancer, infection, inflammation, and ischemia, and the complexity inherent in the term NLUTD becomes quite daunting. Perhaps we are in an era of understanding of NLUTD that is like the time, in the middle of the 20th century when "Cancer" was considered a mysterious, single entity, and not a myriad of conditions that we now know to be defined by very specific genetic mutations. As an eerie reflection of our own limited understanding of NLUTD, we may remember that the overwhelming majority of clinicians in the early 1960s reported that they would not tell their patients about the diagnosis of a cancer for fear of irreparable psychological harm.[2]

WHY PERFORM SURVEILLANCE?

NLUTD is associated with a wide range of complications,[3,4] including recurrent UTIs, stones, fistulae,

Disclosure Statement: No authors of this work have any direct or indirect conflicts of interest associated with this article. The work was not funded. Dr A.P. Klausner is funded by the National Institutes of Health (R01-DK101719).
[a] Division of Urology, Department of Surgery, Virginia Commonwealth University School of Medicine, Richmond, VA, USA; [b] Division of Urology, Department of Surgery, Virginia Commonwealth University School of Medicine, PO Box 980118, Richmond, VA 23298-0118, USA
* Corresponding author.
E-mail address: adam.klausner@vcuhealth.org

Urol Clin N Am 44 (2017) 367–375
http://dx.doi.org/10.1016/j.ucl.2017.04.004
0094-0143/17/

incontinence, skin breakdown, traumatic hypospadias, urethral erosion, and autonomic dysreflexia. However, the 2 complications that have been most widely studied and that lead to significant morbidity and mortality have been upper tract deterioration and increased risk of bladder malignancy. Most of the data about these complications in individuals with NLUTD is obtained from the population with spinal cord injury and disorders (SCI&D).

Bladder Cancer

Bladder cancer is a main cause of increased morbidity and mortality in individuals with NLUTD. Major risk factors for bladder cancer include smoking, chronic urinary tract infections (UTI) and/or inflammation, bladder calculi, and exposure to toxins.[5] Indwelling catheters cause chronic inflammation, which, in turn, may lead to an increased risk of bladder cancer.[6]

Welk and colleagues[7] performed a literature review looking at the incidence of bladder cancer, age at the time of bladder cancer diagnosis, disease invasiveness, and cancer-specific mortality in 21 separate studies of individuals with SCI&D. The investigators concluded that the incidence of bladder cancer in SCI&D was 16 times higher than in individuals without SCI&D (0.32% vs 0.02%), equivalent to 32 patients per 100,000 in SCI&D and 2 per 100,000 in the general population. Likewise, they found that the mean age of bladder cancer was more than a decade earlier in SCI&D (48–61 years of age) compared with non-SCI (60–70 years of age). Across the studies reviewed, the investigators identified that 58% to 100% of individuals with SCI&D presented with muscle invasive disease at the time of diagnosis, compared with only 25% of the general population.[7] Importantly, the gold standard for treatment of muscle-invasive bladder cancer is a radical cystectomy and urinary diversion using an intestinal segment, a treatment associated with high complication rates in this population.[8] In addition, the overall 5-year survival rate for all patients with muscle invasive bladder cancer is only 50%.[9] Finally, cancer-specific mortality was found to be much higher in SCI&D, ranging from 12% to 57%. This cancer-specific mortality rate was 71% greater compared with individuals without SCI&D.[7]

In a large study of US Veterans, West and colleagues[10] reviewed data from 33,500 Veterans with SCI&D and identified 130 with a diagnosis of bladder cancer. These investigators found that the 1-year survival was 61% and the 5-year survival was only 31%. This poor survival data speaks to the very lethal nature of bladder cancer in this specific population. Unfortunately, the type of bladder management was only available in 42 of these 130 Veterans (32%), limiting understanding of potential risk factors.[10]

Risk factors for bladder cancer in SCI&D have been investigated and include indwelling Foley catheters, chronic UTIs, smoking, bladder calculi, increased urine contact, and immune dysregulation. In the Veterans Affairs study discussed above,[10] 62% of SCI&D individuals with bladder cancer used indwelling Foley or suprapubic catheters and 38% used other means for bladder management. This suggests that indwelling catheters increase the risk for patients with NLUTD, but that indwelling catheter use is not the ONLY significant risk factor.

Upper Tract Deterioration

The other major urologic complication of NLUTD leading to increased morbidity and mortality is upper tract deterioration. Upper tract changes can manifest as new onset hydronephrosis or acute kidney injury (AKI). Although the exact pathophysiology of how NLUT directly leads to upper tract deterioration and AKI has not been elucidated, 2 urodynamic risk factors have been identified. These risk factors include poor detrusor compliance and increased intravesical pressures.

Detrusor compliance is defined as the change in detrusor volume divided by the change in detrusor pressure ($\Delta V/\Delta P$) during the urodynamic filling phase.[11] Reduced (poor) compliance can occur when there are structural changes in the detrusor, mediated by replacement of the detrusor smooth muscle with collagen and fibrosis.[12,13] This increase in stiffness is associated with reduced capacity, vesicoureteral reflux, and elevated intravesical pressures. Poor compliance often occurs with longstanding obstruction as in NLUTD in which there is obstruction due to detrusor sphincter dyssynergia.

Although exact values for poor compliance have not been explicitly defined, several researchers have examined the question. Hackler and colleagues[14] examined compliance measurements in SCI&D and found that 69% with compliance values less than 20 mL/cmH$_2$O had signs of upper tract deterioration on renal imaging (mainly hydronephrosis) as compared with only 21% with compliance values greater than 20. Based on this, they proposed that a cutoff value for poor compliance should be 20 mL/cmH$_2$O. Weld and colleagues[15] found that the highest rates of renal damage were seen with compliance values less than 12.5 mL/cmH$_2$O. The lack of specificity of these cutoff values for poor compliance is one of many reasons that lifelong surveillance of individuals with NLUTD may be necessary. More research is needed to identify subgroups with the diagnosis of neurogenic bladder to identify which patients are, and under what circumstances place them, at risk for developing low bladder compliance.

The other proposed urodynamic risk factor for upper tract deterioration is the presence of elevated intravesical pressures. Sentinel work by McGuire and colleagues[16] demonstrated that greater than 80% of individuals with NLUTD due to myelodysplasia and bladder pressures greater than 40 cmH_2O had associated ureteral/renal dilatation. Thus, the value of greater than 40 cmH_2O has been widely accepted in the urologic literature. Other neurogenic bladder subgroups have also demonstrated risk for elevated detrusor leak point pressures. Kim and colleagues[17] attempted to evaluate the elevated pressure question in SCI&D individuals with at least one sphincterotomy. These investigators found, similarly, that bladder pressures greater than 40 cmH_2O were associated with the greatest risk of renal damage. Similarly, Shingleton and Bodner[18] showed sustained bladder pressures greater than 40 cmH_2O were found to be associated with greater risk of upper tract deterioration. Thus, until more detailed and prospective studies can be performed, urodynamically identified detrusor pressures of greater than 40 cmH_2O should continue to be considered a risk factor for upper tract deterioration on surveillance urodynamics for individuals with NLUTD.

Which individuals with neurogenic lower urinary tract dysfunction require surveillance?

In general, all causes of NLUTD can lead to complications, but those with the highest risk, specifically for upper tract deterioration, include suprasacral spinal cord injury, adult spina bifida, and multiple sclerosis (MS). Lawrenson and colleagues[19] showed an increased age standardized risk of renal failure in patients with SCI and neural tube defects. For individuals with spina bifida, studies demonstrate that the risk of renal failure increases with age, and adult spina bifida patients have an 8-fold increase in age-adjusted risk for renal deterioration.[20] Finally, individuals with MS, especially those with spinal predominant lesions, can present with silent NLUTD and are also considered to be at high risk for upper tract deterioration.[21] Therefore, the most prudent strategy for surveillance would be to take the most aggressive approach for individuals with suprasacral SCI, adult spina bifida, and MS.

In the authors' own practice, which provides care for one of the largest SCI&D units in the Veterans Affairs hospital system, they ensure that all patients have a baseline videourodynamic study. This study is best obtained after the initial spinal cord injury when neurologic symptoms have stabilized (ie, after the period of spinal shock). Typically, the development of spontaneous voiding (called "kicking off" by the patients) is an easy way to ensure that the period of spinal shock has ended. However, even if a patient is years out from injury, establishing this baseline urodynamics test provides an excellent framework for bladder management and for evaluation of any future changes in lower urinary tract function. Subsequent urodynamics are only offered if changes in bladder function are suspected (ie, recurrent UTIs, autonomic dysreflexia of unknown origin, incontinence between catheterizations, or changes in renal function testing or upper tract imaging). All patients in the SCI&D system at the authors' institution receive an annual evaluation, which includes a KUB (kidneys, ureter, and bladder) study, renal/bladder ultrasound, basic metabolic panel, and 24-hour urine for creatinine clearance testing. Cystoscopy is only offered for clinical indications (ie, hematuria) and for individuals who have had indwelling catheters for greater than 5 years. In this subgroup, the authors offer repeat cystoscopic evaluations on an every 2-year basis.

GUIDELINES OVERVIEW

Based on the information presented about the prevalence and morbidity/mortality of bladder cancer in NLUTD as well as the risk of upper tract deterioration/AKI from NLUTD associated with poor compliance and elevated detrusor pressures, the rationale for lifelong surveillance in individuals with NLUTD is quite clear. However, the timing, frequency, and type of surveillance have not been well established through high-quality evidence-based research. Therefore, the best available information is published as "consensus statements" (in the form of guidelines) as well as select articles that were not discussed in the published guidelines. These articles are presented and summarized in the following sections. In the review of available guidelines, the authors have chosen to present only those that have been vetted by large stakeholder organizations (as opposed to those from single groups or centers). Based on these criteria, the published guidelines the authors have chosen to present have been authored by the European Association of Urology (EAU), the Veterans Health Administration (VHA), the Consortium for Spinal Cord Medicine (CSCM) sponsored by the Paralyzed Veterans of America (PVA), the United Kingdom's National Institute for Health Care and Excellence (NICE), and the American Urological Association/Society of Urodynamics Female Pelvic Medicine and Reconstructive Urology (AUA/SUFU).

European Association of Urology

The EAU guidelines entitled, "Guidelines on NLUTD,"[22] were initially published in 2009 and updated in 2013.[23] The document contains information on risk factors, diagnosis, and treatment. However, of the entire 64-page document, only one paragraph was devoted to "follow-up" in patients with NLUTD. The guidelines state, "Neurogenic lower urinary tract dysfunction is an unstable condition and can vary considerably, even within a relatively short period. Meticulous follow-up and regular checks are necessary."[23] Twenty references are cited, but none of the details and evidence within the publications are discussed or reviewed. The guidelines also state that "depending on the type of the underlying neurologic pathology and on the current stability of the NLUTD, the interval between the detailed investigations should not exceed 1 to 2 years."[23] The guidelines cover upper tract imaging, bladder function testing, and infection monitoring but do not address renal function testing or cystoscopic evaluation. A summary of EAU surveillance guidelines is listed in **Table 1**.

United Kingdom's National Institute for Health and Care Excellence

In 2012, the United Kingdom's NICE published guidelines entitled, "Urinary Incontinence in Neurologic Disease: Management of Lower Urinary Tract Dysfunction in Urologic Disease."[24] The follow-up/surveillance sections cover areas

Table 1 European Association of Urology guidelines for neurogenic lower urinary tract dysfunction surveillance	
Test	**Frequency (mo)**
Urine analysis	**2**
Blood chemistry and urine laboratory	**12**
Renal/bladder ultrasound	**6**
Urodynamics	**12–24**
Cystoscopy	Not addressed

Bold, recommended.

Table 2 National Institute for Health Care and Excellence guidelines for neurogenic lower urinary tract dysfunction surveillance	
Test	**Frequency (mo)**
Urine analysis	Not addressed
Blood chemistry and urine laboratory	Not recommended
Renal/bladder ultrasound[a]	**12–24**
Urodynamics	**12–24**
Cystoscopy	Not recommended

Bold, recommended.
[a] Recommended against plain films or renal scintigraphy.

including renal function testing, upper tract imaging, urodynamics, and cystoscopy. The summary recommendations from the NICE guidelines are listed in **Table 2**.

Consortium for Spinal Cord Medicine

The CSCM published guidelines for bladder management in adults with SCI&D in 2006.[25] These guidelines did not make surveillance recommendations on the type of imaging, and there were no recommendations on the timing and frequency of urodynamics or cystoscopy. The guidelines made recommendations based on the method of bladder management.

Veterans Health Administration Handbook

Section 1176.01 of the VHA Handbook addresses SCI&D Systems of Care.[26] In this section, specific recommendations for follow-up are provided, including infection monitoring, renal function testing, imaging, urodynamics, and cystoscopy with bladder biopsy. However, the VHA Handbook does not provide or cite references in support of the recommendations. VHA guidelines are listed in **Table 3**.

American Urological Association/Society of Urodynamics Female Pelvic Medicine and Reconstructive Urology

In 2012, the AUA and the SUFU published joint guidelines on the use of urodynamics.[27] The guidelines addressed the indications for urodynamics for a wide range of conditions and included a section devoted to NLUTD. However, these organizations have not published broader guidelines on follow-up for NLUTD using other types of testing modalities.

Table 3
Veterans Health Administration guidelines for neurogenic lower urinary tract dysfunction surveillance

Test	Frequency (mo)
Urine analysis[a]	**12**
Blood chemistry and urine laboratory[b]	**12**
Renal/bladder ultrasound	**12**
Urodynamics[c]	12–24
Cystoscopy[d]	Not specified

Bold, recommended.
[a] With culture and sensitivity.
[b] With renal function test (scintigraphy) or creatinine clearance test.
[c] When objective information on voiding function is needed.
[d] With cytology and bladder biopsy for indwelling catheterization.

RENAL FUNCTION TESTING
Serum Creatinine and Creatinine Clearance (24-hour Urine)

EAU guidelines recommend yearly "blood chemistry and urine laboratory"[23] for individuals with NLUTD but do not specify tests or discuss supporting evidence. Therefore, it appears that the EAU guidelines are meant to suggest that surveillance should be performed as frequently as possible in this high-risk population. Indeed, the final guideline statement in this section states, "all of the above should be more frequent if the neurologic pathology or NLUTD status demand this."[23]

NICE guidelines recommend against the use of serum creatinine and estimated glomerular filtration rate (GFR) as the sole means of monitoring renal function in NLUTD. Evidence supporting the limited utility of creatinine in populations with NLUTD comes from studies demonstrating that individuals with SCI&D have reduced creatinine clearance despite normal serum creatinine levels.[28,29] In addition, studies suggest that there is poor correlation between serum creatinine and creatinine clearance calculated with the more definitive DPTA renal scintigraphy.[28] Although 24-hour creatinine clearance testing may be more accurate in normal individuals, studies suggest that even this test can be highly variable in individuals with SCI&D.[29] However, it is important to recognize the limited evidence quality of these retrospective studies.

The only other guideline that specifically addresses renal function testing is the Department of Veterans Affairs, which states that "BUN/creatinine" (blood urea nitrogen) testing should be performed on an annual basis in NLUTD[26] but does not provide supporting evidence.

Cystatin C

Not included in any of the guidelines are recent studies that show that cystatin C may represent an improved means to measure and monitor renal function. Cystatin C is a nonglycosylated low-molecular-weight protein that is produced by all nucleated cells. Production is constant, and cystatin C is freely filtered by the glomeruli. It is also reabsorbed and catabolized in the proximal tubules. Cystatin C levels are independent of gender, age, and muscle mass, allowing it to correlate better with creatinine clearance.[30] Erlandsen and colleagues[30] examined the use of cystatin C in estimating GFR in SCI&D and developed a novel equation to accurately estimate GFR in this population.

Imaging

NICE guidelines recommend against the use of plain films or renal scintigraphy for routine surveillance for NLUTD.[24] Rather, they recommend lifelong kidney ultrasound surveillance for individuals at high risk for renal complications.[24] Specific studies comparing ultrasound versus renal scintigraphy demonstrated that ultrasound had higher sensitivity, specificity, and positive and negative predictive values.[29] Likewise, studies comparing ultrasound versus plain films found that ultrasound had improved ability to identify renal and bladder abnormalities, but plain films were better only at the identification of kidney stones.[31] Based on this, the guidelines state, "offer lifelong ultrasound surveillance of the kidneys to the people who are judged to be at high risk of renal complications (for example, consider surveillance ultrasound scanning at annual or 2 year intervals)."[24]

The EAU guidelines recommend the use of ultrasound imaging to assess the "upper urinary tract, bladder morphology, and residual urine every 6 months."[23] However, these consensus statements are based on the high rate of complications in NLUTD and not on the efficacy or data from specific studies. The VHA guidelines recommend annual imaging with ultrasound in order to assess the anatomy of the upper urinary tracts.[26] Other guidelines do not specifically address the need or frequency for surveillance imaging in NLUTD.

Urodynamics

Of the 17 studies used to provide evidence for recommendations in the monitoring section of the NICE guidelines, none specifically address the need for urodynamics. Despite the lack of cited evidence, the NICE guidelines state, "consider urodynamic investigations as part of a surveillance regimen for people at high risk of urinary tract complications."[24] EAU guidelines recommend that specialized evaluation for NLUTD should be performed every 1 to 2 years and should include a "videourodyamics investigation and should be performed in a leading neurourologic centre."[23] The CSCM recommends urodynamics specifically for individuals with NLUTD who use reflex voiding for bladder management. For these individuals, the guidelines state, "conduct a thorough urodynamic evaluation to determine whether reflex voiding is a suitable method for a particular individual."[25] However, no frequency of the investigation or supporting evidence is included.

The AUA/SUFU urodynamics (UDS) guidelines recommend that "clinicians should perform pressure flow analysis during the initial urological evaluation of patients with relevant neurological conditions with or without symptoms and as part of ongoing follow-up when appropriate, in patients with other neurologic disease and elevated PVR or in patients with persistent symptoms."[27] The text is clear about the UDS for "initial" evaluation but the frequency and indications for follow-up are quite vague.

The VHA handbook states, "a standard medical history and physical examination (evaluating symptoms and signs) is not sensitive in screening for high intravesical pressures"[26] in individuals with NLUTD. Therefore, UDS is recommended, "when objective information on voiding function and intravesical pressures is needed."[26] Listed indications include recent onset of SCI&D, deterioration in renal function, anatomic changes in the upper tracts, recurrent autonomic dysreflexia of unknown causes, and urinary incontinence in the absence of UTI.[26] Again, evidence in support of the recommendations as well as frequency of testing is not included.

Despite recommendations in all 5 major guidelines, no specific studies are cited in support of UDS surveillance for NLUTD. Therefore, some more recent studies are included in the current review. Schops and colleagues[32] studied the use of regular follow-up urodynamics in SCI&D. These investigators performed a prospective evaluation of the first and the most recent UDS study on 246 individuals with SCI&D with greater than 5 years since injury. The key finding of the study was an increased detrusor pressure during storage (25 cmH_2O vs 34 cmH_2O). This provides evidence that serial (yearly) UDS studies may be required to evaluate for changes in detrusor pressure in NLUTD.

Cystoscopy

The use of cystoscopy in routine surveillance was not recommended in the NICE guidelines.[24] In support of this recommendation, the guidelines cite a single study in which annual cystoscopy was performed in 59 individuals with SCI&D with greater than 6 years since injury.[33] Participants either had indwelling catheters greater than 10 years or were smokers with an indwelling catheter for greater than 5 years. Ninety-three biopsies were performed, all of which were negative. In addition, 18 urine cytologies were performed, all of which were negative, and the 4 participants who developed bladder cancer were all outside of the study protocol. Based on this evidence, cystoscopy was not recommended.

The guidelines of the CSCM recommend more frequent *cystoscopic* evaluation for individuals with NLUTD using indwelling catheters compared with those patients who use other bladder management options.[25] The VHA guidelines recommend that any individual using indwelling catheters for bladder management should have surveillance cystoscopy, cytology, and random bladder biopsy if warranted on a regular basis.[26] However, the exact definition of "regular basis" is not specified.

The EAU guidelines and AUA/SUFU guidelines do not address the need for cystoscopic surveillance.[23,27] However, other studies have been performed that were not cited in any of the published guidelines. Sammer and colleagues[34] examined 129 individuals with NLUTD over a 34-month period. In the study, the investigators prospectively examined individuals with at least a 5-year history of NLUTD. As part of their management protocol, all participants underwent both routine cystoscopy and bladder washings regardless of bladder management. Any patient with suspicious cystoscopy or bladder washings underwent either transurethral resection of bladder tumor (TURBT) or random bladder biopsy. They report that 10% had suspicious findings and underwent TURBT and/or bladder biopsy. Of all participants, 5% were found to have relevant histologic changes, including one individual with muscle invasive adenocarcinoma. Based on this, the investigators recommend that "surveillance cystourethroscopy might be warranted, although the ideal starting point and frequency remain to be determined."[34] However, the use of the term "relevant" in the study is somewhat questionable as the premalignant nature of the identified conditions (melanosis, intestinal metaplasia, nephrogenic adenoma) has not been well established, and the single cancer would likely have been detected using routine surveillance ultrasound.

El Masri y and colleagues[35] performed a systematic literature review regarding the need for surveillance cystoscopy in individuals with NLUTD. Only individuals with traumatic SCI&D using indwelling catheters were included. They identified 79 studies, of which only 6 met criteria for inclusion. In total, they evaluated 419 cystoscopies performed on a total of 262 individuals over 5 years. They also stratified patients based on having indications for the cystoscopy (ie, recurrent UTIs, catheter blockage, autonomic dysreflexia, radiographic findings of bladder calculi) or being asymptomatic. In the asymptomatic group, high rates of positive findings were identified in most cystoscopic studies including metaplasia, inflammation, bladder stones, and thick proteinaceous debris. However, no cancers were detected. The investigators acknowledge the need for additional study but recommend cystoscopy 2 years after indwelling catheter placement and repeating every 1 to 2 years thereafter.[35]

McPartlin and colleagues[36] studied whether incidental bladder wall thickening identified on computed tomographic (CT) imaging for nonurologic indications was a justified indication to perform cystoscopy. The investigators performed a retrospective review of 3000 consecutive cystoscopies at a Veterans Administration medical center with a large SCI&D center and identified 22/3000 cystoscopies performed purely for incidental bladder wall thickening on CT. Of the

22 patients, 11 had focal thickening, 8 had diffuse thickening, and 3 had a focal bladder mass. None of the patients with focal thickening or diffuse thickening had cancer. However, 2 of the 3 patients with focal bladder masses had cancer. This demonstrates that in the absence of a focal bladder mass, incidental bladder wall thickening may not warrant cystoscopic evaluation. As many individuals with NLUTD will have bladder wall thickening, this data, although limited, should be considered in the workup.

GUIDELINE IMPLEMENTATION

Cameron and colleagues[37] performed a Medicare database study and identified greater than 7000 individuals with SCI&D with greater than 2 years of follow-up based on International Classification of Diseases-9 codes. Using the PVA guidelines (yearly urology visit, creatinine testing, and renal ultrasound) as a standard, they found that 25% of patients received complete (recommended) surveillance, 70% received some surveillance, and 5% received no surveillance. Although this type of surveillance seems to be an acceptable minimum, the PVA (CSCM) guidelines do not actually include these recommendations, which appear to derive from the VHA handbook. However, the take-home point is that surveillance practices for NLUDT in the United States are highly variable and nonstandardized.

Table 4
Recommended neurogenic lower urinary tract dysfunction surveillance by organizations with published guidelines

Evaluation	Frequency (mo)	Organization	Bladder Management	Total Recommending (No., %)	Ave. (mo)
Renal function testing	12	EAU[a]	ND	2/5 (40)	12
	12	VHA[b]	ND		
Imaging	6	EAU	ND	3/5 (60)	12
	1–2	NICE	ND		
	12	VHA	ND		
Urodynamics	12–24	EAU	ND	5/5 (100)	18
	ND	NICE	ND		
	ND	CSCM	Reflex voiding		
	ND	AUA/SUFU	ND		
	ND	VHA[c]	ND		
Cystoscopy	ND	CSCM	Indwelling catheter	2/5 (40)	ND
	ND	VHA[d]	Indwelling catheter		
Infection monitoring	2	EAU	ND	2/5 (40)	7
	12	VHA	ND		

Abbreviation: ND, not discussed.
[a] BUN/Creatinine.
[b] BUN/Creatinine and 24-h creatinine clearance or renal scan.
[c] Various indications.
[d] With random biopsy and urine cytology.

In another study, active SUFU members were surveyed regarding surveillance practices for NLUTD.[38] Of 269 members surveyed, 60% responded. Of the respondents, 80% preferred ultrasound, 20% preferred nuclear renal scan, and 3% preferred CT as the main method of yearly imaging surveillance. In the study, 65% preferred annual or biannual video urodynamics, and 25% (40/160) preferred performing annual cystoscopy.

SUMMARY

Multiple stakeholder organizations have established guidelines for surveillance protocols for NLUTD with positive recommendations summarized in **Table 4**. The creation of these documents speaks to the importance of surveillance in this population at risk for upper tract deterioration and bladder cancer; however, there is limited high-quality evidence in support of any of the guideline recommendations, and there has been no attempt to develop consensus protocols between different organizations. A recent meta-analysis of follow-up strategies for NLUTD found that "there is a lack of high level evidence studies to support an optimal long-term follow-up protocol."[3] At this point, the decision for NLUTD surveillance with laboratory work, imaging, urodynamics, or cystoscopy should be based on individual needs, institutional resources, and cost. Regardless, the next logical step should consist of developing standardized protocols with clearly defined outcome measures that can be tested with high-quality randomized controlled trials. These types of studies will no doubt be difficult to coordinate, require multi-institutional participation, and will come at a significant financial cost. However, the benefits to individuals with NLUTD and to society in general should provide the rationale to move forward.

REFERENCES

1. Stohrer M, Goepel M, Kondo A, et al. The standardization of terminology in neurogenic lower urinary tract dysfunction: with suggestions for diagnostic procedures. International Continence Society Standardization Committee. Neurourol Urodyn 1999; 18(2):139–58.
2. Oken D. What to tell cancer patients. A study of medical attitudes. JAMA 1961;175:1120–8.
3. Averbeck MA, Madersbacher H. Follow-up of the neuro-urological patient: a systematic review. BJU Int 2015;115(Suppl 6):39–46.
4. Wyndaele JJ. The management of neurogenic lower urinary tract dysfunction after spinal cord injury. Nat Rev Urol 2016;13(12):705–14.
5. Burger M, Catto JW, Dalbagni G, et al. Epidemiology and risk factors of urothelial bladder cancer. Eur Urol 2013;63(2):234–41.
6. Gui-Zhong L, Li-Bo M. Bladder cancer in individuals with spinal cord injuries: a meta-analysis. Spinal Cord 2016;55(4):341–5.
7. Welk B, McIntyre A, Teasell R, et al. Bladder cancer in individuals with spinal cord injuries. Spinal Cord 2013;51(7):516–21.
8. Chong JT, Dolat MT, Klausner AP, et al. The role of cystectomy for non-malignant bladder conditions: a review. Can J Urol 2014;21(5):7433–41.
9. May M, Helke C, Nitzke T, et al. Survival rates after radical cystectomy according to tumor stage of bladder carcinoma at first presentation. Urol Int 2004;72(2):103–11.
10. West DA, Cummings JM, Longo WE, et al. Role of chronic catheterization in the development of bladder cancer in patients with spinal cord injury. Urology 1999;53(2):292–7.
11. Abrams P, Cardozo L, Fall M, et al. The standardisation of terminology of lower urinary tract function: report from the Standardisation Sub-committee of the International Continence Society. Neurourol Urodyn 2002;21(2):167–78.
12. Landau EH, Jayanthi VR, Churchill BM, et al. Loss of elasticity in dysfunctional bladders: urodynamic and histochemical correlation. J Urol 1994;152(2 Pt 2): 702–5.
13. Metcalfe PD, Wang J, Jiao H, et al. Bladder outlet obstruction: progression from inflammation to fibrosis. BJU Int 2010;106(11):1686–94.
14. Hackler RH, Hall MK, Zampieri TA. Bladder hypocompliance in the spinal cord injury population. J Urol 1989;141(6):1390–3.
15. Weld KJ, Graney MJ, Dmochowski RR. Differences in bladder compliance with time and associations of bladder management with compliance in spinal cord injured patients. J Urol 2000;163(4):1228–33.
16. McGuire EJ, Woodside JR, Borden TA, et al. Prognostic value of urodynamic testing in myelodysplastic patients. J Urol 1981;126(2):205–9.
17. Kim YH, Kattan MW, Boone TB. Bladder leak point pressure: the measure for sphincterotomy success in spinal cord injured patients with external detrusor-sphincter dyssynergia. J Urol 1998;159(2): 493–6 [discussion: 496–7].
18. Shingleton WB, Bodner DR. The development of urologic complications in relationship to bladder pressure in spinal cord injured patients. J Am Paraplegia Soc 1993;16(1):14–7.
19. Lawrenson R, Wyndaele JJ, Vlachonikolis I, et al. Renal failure in patients with neurogenic lower urinary tract dysfunction. Neuroepidemiology 2001; 20(2):138–43.
20. Lewis MA, Webb NJ, Stellman-Ward GR, et al. Investigative techniques and renal parenchymal damage

in children with spina bifida. Eur J Pediatr Surg 1994;4(Suppl 1):29–31.

21. de Seze M, Ruffion A, Denys P, et al, GENULF. The neurogenic bladder in multiple sclerosis: review of the literature and proposal of management guidelines. Mult Scler 2007;13(7):915–28.

22. Stohrer M, Blok B, Castro-Diaz D, et al. EAU guidelines on neurogenic lower urinary tract dysfunction. Eur Urol 2009;56(1):81–8.

23. Pannek J, Blok B, Castro-Diaz D, et al. EAU Guidelines on Neurogenic Lower Urinary Tract Dysfunction. 2013. Available at: https://uroweb.org/wp-content/uploads/20_Neurogenic-LUTD_LR.pdf. Accessed December 1, 2016.

24. NCGC. (National Cliical Guideline Center). Urinary incontinence in neurologic disease: management of lower urinary tract dysfunction in urologic disease. 2012. Available at: https://www.nice.org.uk/guidance/cg148/evidence/full-guideline-188123437. Accessed December 1, 2016.

25. CFSCM. (Consortium for Spinal Cord Medicine). Bladder Management for Adults with Spinal Cord Injury) A Clinical Practice Guideline for Healthcare Providers. 2006. Available at: http://www.pva.org/atf/cf/%7BCA2A0FFB-6859-4BC1-BC96-6B57F57F0391%7D/CPGBladderManageme_1AC7B4.pdf. Accessed December 1, 2016.

26. VHA. (Veterans Health Administration). Handbook Section 1176.01. Spinal Cord Injury and Disorders Systems of Care. 2010. Available at: http://www1.va.gov/vhapublications/ViewPublication.asp?pub_ID=2299. Accessed December 1, 2016.

27. Winters JC, Dmochowski RR, Goldman HB, et al. AUA/SUFU Guidelines: Urodynamics. 2012. Available at: http://www.auanet.org/education/guidelines/adult-urodynamics.cfm. Accessed December 1, 2016.

28. MacDiarmid SA, McIntyre WJ, Anthony A, et al. Monitoring of renal function in patients with spinal cord injury. BJU Int 2000;85(9):1014–8.

29. Sepahpanah F, Burns SP, McKnight B, et al. Role of creatinine clearance as a screening test in persons with spinal cord injury. Arch Phys Med Rehabil 2006;87(4):524–8.

30. Erlandsen EJ, Hansen RM, Randers E, et al. Estimating the glomerular filtration rate using serum cystatin C levels in patients with spinal cord injuries. Spinal Cord 2012;50(10):778–83.

31. Tins B, Teo HG, Popuri R, et al. Follow-up imaging of the urinary tract in spinal injury patients: is a KUB necessary with every ultrasound? Spinal Cord 2005;43(4):219–22.

32. Schops TF, Schneider MP, Steffen F, et al. Neurogenic lower urinary tract dysfunction (NLUTD) in patients with spinal cord injury: long-term urodynamic findings. BJU Int 2015;115(Suppl 6):33–8.

33. Yang CC, Clowers DE. Screening cystoscopy in chronically catheterized spinal cord injury patients. Spinal Cord 1999;37(3):204–7.

34. Sammer U, Walter M, Knupfer SC, et al. Do we need surveillance urethro-cystoscopy in patients with neurogenic lower urinary tract dysfunction? PLoS One 2015;10(10):e0140970.

35. El Masri y WS, Patil S, Prasanna KV, et al. To cystoscope or not to cystoscope patients with traumatic spinal cord injuries managed with indwelling urethral or suprapubic catheters? That is the question! Spinal Cord 2014;52(6):500.

36. McPartlin DS, Klausner AP, Nottingham CU, et al. Is cystoscopy indicated for incidentally identified bladder wall thickening? Can J Urol 2013;20(1):6615–9.

37. Cameron AP, Lai J, Saigal CS, et al, NIDDK Urological Diseases in America Project. Urological surveillance and medical complications after spinal cord injury in the United States. Urology 2015;86(3):506–10.

38. Razdan S, Leboeuf L, Meinbach DS, et al. Current practice patterns in the urologic surveillance and management of patients with spinal cord injury. Urology 2003;61(5):893–6.

Establishing a Multidisciplinary Approach to the Management of Neurologic Disease Affecting the Urinary Tract

Shree Agrawal, BS[a],*, Ravi R. Agrawal, BA[b],
Hadley M. Wood, MD[c]

KEYWORDS

• Neurogenic bladder • Multidisciplinary care • Neurologic diseases

KEY POINTS

• Patients with neuropathic bladder often demonstrate multisystem disease that requires interdisciplinary management to minimize polypharmacy and side effects.

• A complete urologic history includes operative procedures, urologic management, bowel management, neurologic management, and a clear understanding of what the patient's goals are.

• Preoperative and perioperative management necessitates neurologic assessment to assess ventriculoperitoneal shunt status, cardiopulmonary evaluation, or gastroenterologic evaluation.

• Decubitus ulcers and skin breakdown occur in conjunction with urologic demise, and plastic surgery, physiatry and others may help prevent and treat this outcome.

• Coordination with nephrology to monitor and treat preventable causes of renal deterioration and navigate the complexities of progression to end-stage renal disease and transplantation can be important.

INTRODUCTION

Neurogenic lower urinary tract dysfunction (NLUTD) can substantially impact quality of life in patients with neurologic diseases. Broadly categorized, NLUTD includes acquired, degenerative, and congenital conditions. The management of NLUTD aims to avoid or minimize complications such as recurrent urinary tract infections, urinary incontinence, urethral strictures, and renal deterioration.[1] Coordinated multidisciplinary care for the management of patients with neurologic conditions and secondary NLUTD can optimize long-term patient quality of life and urologic outcomes. Examples of acquired neurologic conditions include cerebrovascular injury and traumatic spinal cord injury (SCI). Degenerative conditions associated with NLUTD include mostly primary neurologic diseases (multiple sclerosis, myasthenia gravis, and Parkinson's disease) and common congenital neurologic diseases causing NLUTD are spina bifida and cerebral palsy.

Disclosures: All authors have no conflicts of interest to disclose.
Sources of Funding: None.
[a] Case Western Reserve University School of Medicine, 2109 Adelbert Road, Cleveland, OH 44106, USA;
[b] Boston University, One Silber Way, Boston, MA 02215, USA; [c] Glickman Urological and Kidney Institute, Cleveland Clinic, 9500 Euclid Avenue, Q10-1, Cleveland, OH 44195, USA
* Corresponding author.
E-mail address: shree.agrawal@case.edu

Urol Clin N Am 44 (2017) 377–389
http://dx.doi.org/10.1016/j.ucl.2017.04.005
0094-0143/17/

Patients with NLUTD, depending on their underlying predisposing etiology, have a greater risk of recurrent urinary tract infection, upper urinary tract and lower urinary tract deterioration and calculi, and skin and wound breakdown with their associated complications.[2] Symptoms of NLUTD, and potentially sexual dysfunction, may develop many years after diagnosis owing to deterioration of neuromuscular function.[3,4] For patients with childhood-onset and congenital forms of NLUTD, obstacles transitioning patients between pediatric and adult providers can result in a lapse of preventative services and secondary severe complications, such as advanced renal failure, decubitus ulcers, and sacral osteomyelitis.[5,6]

There are no guidelines established in North America for multidisciplinary care of NLUTD, especially over the lifespan of patients with neurologic conditions. This article reviews considerations for a multidisciplinary approach to care of patients with congenital and acquired NLUTD.

UROLOGIC ASSESSMENT

Patients presenting with any neurologic disease to a urologist should be assessed at minimum with a thorough history and physical examination—additional testing may include urodynamic testing, voiding cystogram, retrograde urethrogram, renal scan, cystoscopy, and/or select other diagnostic testing depending on the patient's presenting symptoms and prior history. Important factors to elicit in a history include past and present sexual, bowel, neurologic, and urologic histories at the time of consultation. **Box 1** demonstrates a typical history, not including a review of systems, in the subjective assessment of a patient presenting with NLUTD.

A physical examination should include a pelvic examination in female patients, digital rectal examination in male patients, perineal and S2 to S5 sensations, anal sphincter tone, and neurologic examination for upper and lower motor neuron deficits of the lower lumbar and sacral nerves.[7]

Urodynamic testing with warm fluid (contrast or saline, depending on whether video imaging is used) is frequently used to assess lower urinary tract dysfunction often after a voiding diary, postvoid residual urine volume, and urinalysis have been completed and suggest NLUTD. Bladder compliance, detrusor overactivity, bladder sensation, detrusor function, leak point pressures, and sphincter function are all quantified on urodynamic testing.[8] Fluoroscopic analysis may also be performed to visualize both the bladder and urethra during urodynamic testing to assess bladder capacity and shape, as well as the presence of

vesicoureteral reflux or detrusor sphincter dysynergia.[9] Additional upper urinary tract imaging may be performed if the clinical history suggests a risk for upper urinary tract deterioration. For example, patients with high postvoid residuals, urodynamic evidence of poor compliance, suspicion of detrusor sphincter dyssynergia (eg, retention and stuttering stream), or declining renal function by serial serum creatinine all merit upper urinary tract evaluation, typically with renal ultrasound examination at a minimum. Retrograde urethrogram or cystoscopy can be used to evaluate urethral problems. Cystoscopy further can be used to examine the bladder neck and bladder, to evaluate for foreign objects, diverticuli, mucosal lesions, functional integrity of the bladder neck and external sphincter, and evaluate for anatomic variations.

APPROACHES TO MULTIDISCIPLINARY CARE

Patients with NLUTD often demonstrate multisystem conditions that require treatments that may impact other organ systems. Among a spinal cord injured population, up to 72% of patients experience urologic problems, 50% with bowel problems, 42% with skin problems, 66% complained of limb spasticity, and 55% did not have adequate pain control.[10] Specialty involvement in the management of NLUTD may include urology, nephrology, neurology, neurosurgery, gastroenterology, physiatry, physical and/or occupational therapy, wound care, plastic surgery, primary care, internal medicine, gynecology, cardiovascular medicine, and pulmonary care. The involvement of each specialty may vary to a degree, depending on the etiology of the primary condition and each individual's coexisting comorbidities and disease manifestations. Although an exhaustive review of all of these possibilities is not possible in this article, herein we highlight some specific examples where urologic decision making for patients with NLUTD is substantially impacted by other medical disciplines (**Fig. 1**).

Urology

Urologic management at the initial consultation should be performed as described elsewhere. In addition to a thorough history, a reliable estimate of glomerular filtration rate and upper tract imaging is prudent in any patient with a concern for NLUTD at baseline. Among patients with storage dysfunction or compliance problems, behavioral management, antimuscarinic agents, desmopressin, onabotulinumtoxin A injections to the detrusor muscle tissue, neuromodulation, bladder augmentation, and urinary diversion are potential therapeutic

Box 1
History for patient presenting with neurogenic lower urinary tract dysfunction

Past history

   Past medical history, including both those related to and independent of neurogenic lower urinary tract dysfunction

   Past surgical history, including trauma and procedures to the spinal cord, central nervous system, and/or urologic procedures

   Previous strictures or other abnormalities of the urethra, bladder, and ureters

   Obstetric history, age at menarche, age at menopause, contraceptive use

   Hereditary or family history, including vesicoureteral reflux and congenital renal, bladder, and gynecologic conditions

   Urologic history in childhood and adolescence

   Current and previous medications

Social history

   Lifestyle—smoking, alcohol, drugs, nutritional and fluid intake (especially caffeine and alcohol)

   Current quality of life

   Occupation and physical activity or limitations

   Housing environment and resources

   Caregiver status

Urologic history

   Onset of lower urinary tract dysfunction

   Daytime and nighttime frequency, including nocturnal enuresis episodes

   Voiding modality, type, volume, frequency, urge, and leakage episodes

   Bladder sensation

   Micturition initiation and interruption, including frequency and type of clean intermittent catheterization, if applicable

   Aggravating factors

   Urinary incontinence, including the nature of leakage events (stress, urge, sensate, nighttime)

   Previous urinary tract infections, including present and prior use of prophylactic antibiotics

   Hematuria

Bowel history

   Number and quality of stools on a daily or weekly basis

   Constipation history, including prior and present bowel management strategies

   Fecal incontinence

   Desire to defecate

   Defecation pattern

   Rectal sensation

   Initiation of defecation

   Mode of defecation—digital rectal stimulation, enema, etc

Sexual history

   Sexual function or dysfunction, onset, treatments past and current

   Sensation in genital area

   Genital dysfunction

   Male sexual function—arousal, erection, anorgasmia, ejaculation

   Female sexual function—dyspareunia, arousal, anorgasmia

Neurologic history

    Acquired, congenital, or neuromuscular condition

    Mental status and cognition

    Level of lesion, if present

    Spasticity or autonomic dysreflexia

    Manual dexterity

    Neurologic symptoms, onset, and evolution

options, depending on symptom severity and treatment responses.[11] Voiding dysfunction, in contrast, can be managed, depending on physiology, with intermittent self-catheterization or indwelling catheterization, alpha-adrenoceptor blockers, onabotulinumtoxin A injections to the sphincter, neuromodulation, external sphincter or bladder neck incision, transurethral resection of the prostate, and urinary diversion.[12,13] All treatment decisions are patient specific and must be made in coordination with patients and their respective caregivers.

In settings of poor bladder compliance (high pressure storage) and detrusor sphincter dyssynergia, upper urinary tract changes may occur, including development of hydronephrosis and/or secondary vesicoureteral reflux.[14] When upper urinary tract changes are noted, prompt urologic management is prudent to prevent further renal functional loses. Detrusor leak point pressures of greater than 40 cm H_2O have been reported to result in substantial risk for upper urinary tract damage.[15–18]

Neurology and Neurosurgery

Patients presenting with NLUTD may already be managed by a neurologist and/or neurosurgeon. Often, neurologic consultation may be required to determine whether a urologic treatment may impair the neurologic care plan. The following are common examples where interdisciplinary decision making may be of benefit.

1. Medical therapy
   a. Antimuscarinic medications often counteract neurologic medications or compound the side effects such that the medications cannot be tolerated (**Table 1**). Cognitive side effects, dry mouth, and constipation may worsen current symptoms experienced by patients when taking these medications.[19,20] Treatment with anticholinergic medication in older patients has been associated with delirium and cognitive decline, especially when used as a long-term therapy.[21,22]

   b. Treatment with dopamine-2 agonists has demonstrated an effect on the neuromuscular signaling of the bladder, reducing bladder capacity and worsening detrusor overactivity if already present.[23]
   c. Monoamine oxidase inhibitor treatments may also predispose patients to obstructive voiding symptoms in addition to preexisting NLUTD symptoms.[24]

2. Intradetrusor botulinum toxin A (Botox): Many patients in need of intravesical botulinum toxin A treatment with coexisting neurologic diseases may receive injections elsewhere as well (eg, lower and upper extremities). Current recommendations for botulinum toxin A dosing describe a maximum cumulative dose of 400 U at 3-month intervals when treating adults for 1 or more indications. Patients especially receiving treatments to upper and lower extremities and the bladder may inadvertently receive more than this recommended dose. This overuse may place patients at an additional risk of experiencing adverse side effects, most commonly weakness, dysphagia, ptosis, dry eyes, and/or urinary retention.[25,26] Reported adverse side events among cerebral palsy patients receiving botulinum toxin A have been 23% in children.[27] Studies of high-dose botulinum toxin A therapy did not reveal additional incidences of side effects.[28] Regardless, neurologic conditions related to NLUTD and their related symptoms may be further exacerbated with botulinum toxin A injections, warranting monitoring of total dose in all therapies.[29] Although these complication are rarely seen, patients should be monitored for respiratory difficulty and weakness (eg, inability to transfer out of chair) after treatments that exceed 400 U.

3. Intrathecal baclofen: Intrathecal baclofen is a viable option for patients with severe spasticity related to neurologic conditions. Before the placement of an intrathecal baclofen pump, potential urologic side effects (most commonly urinary retention) should be assessed. Placement of the intrathecal pump may alter bladder

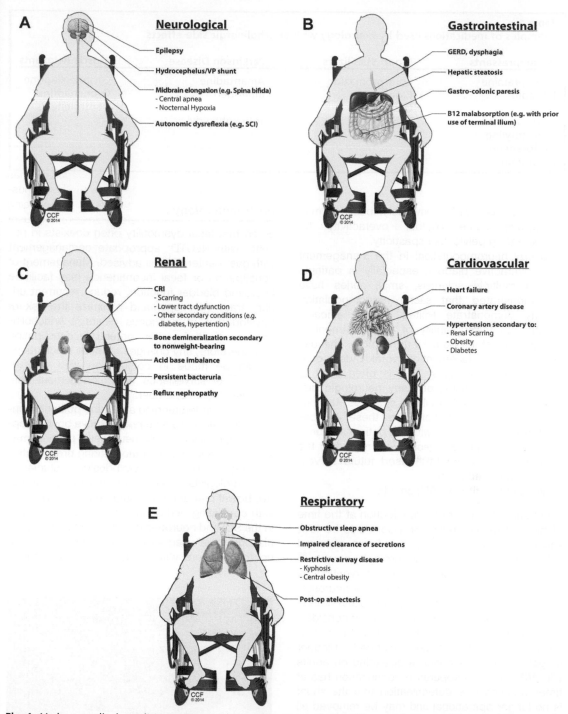

Fig. 1. Various medical conditions commonly found among patients with neurologic conditions and Neurogenic lower urinary tract dysfunction including neurologic (*A*), gastrointestinal (*B*), renal (*C*), cardiovascular (*D*), and respiratory (*E*) conditions. The presence of any of these issues should prompt a coordinated multidisciplinary care effort to optimize urologic management strategies and the overall health of the patient. CRI, chronic respiratory insufficiency; GERD, gastroesophageal reflux disease; SCI, spinal cord injury; VP, ventriculoperitoneal. (*Courtesy of* the Cleveland Clinic, Cleveland, OH; with permission.)

Table 1
Examples of medications used by neurology with anticholinergic side effects

Antidepressants	Mood Stabilizers	Parkinson Disease	Muscle Relaxants
Clomipramine	Chlorpromazine	Amantadine	Cyclobenzaprine
Doxepin	Clozapine	Biperiden	Orphenadrine
Paroxetine	Olanzapine	Benztropine	Dantrolene
Nortriptyline	Thioridazine	Trihexphenidyl	
Amitriptyline			
Desipramine			
Imipramine			

function as well.[30] Conversely, baclofen may improve some bladder overactivity by decreasing pelvic floor spasticity.

4. Sacral neuromodulation: In the management of overactive bladder, especially in patients with multiple sclerosis, small series have demonstrated that sacral neuromodulation may demonstrate limited clinical efficacy, although the durability of this treatment is not well-established.[31] Furthermore, the use of MRI after placement of sacral leads is contraindicated. Because MRI is often used to assess progression of many neurologic diseases, particularly multiple sclerosis, the potential urologic benefits to these devices should be discussed with the patient's neurologists and neurosurgeons with regard to the potential need for MRI-based future surveillance and treatment.

5. Ventriculoperitoneal (VP) shunts

Although the rate of shunt infection at the time of bladder reconstruction is reported to be low, shunt infection remains a significant potential risk to patients undergoing urologic surgery.[32] When an abdominal surgical intervention is planned, consultation with neurology or neurosurgery may be prudent if the patient has a VP shunt. Some investigators have advocated for consideration of conversion to ventriculopleural or ventriculoatrial shunts before planned bladder surgery.[33] In our experience operating on adults with VP shunts, preoperative consultation has at times resulted in a determination that the shunt is no longer operational and may be removed all together.

Patients presenting with unexplained abdominal pain, nausea, visual changes, or headaches after abdominal surgery, who also have VP shunts, should undergo immediate evaluation for pseudocyst formation or infection in conjunction with immediate neurosurgical consultation.[34] Abdominal ultrasound imaging is often diagnostic **(Fig. 2)**.

Gastroenterology

Given that fecal dysmotility often coexists in patients with NLUTD, appropriate comanagement with gastroenterology is advised. Management of constipation or fecal incontinence may facilitate improved bladder function, reduce recurrent urinary tract infections, and minimize the risk of development of decubitus ulcers.[35] Anticholinergic medications often potentiate constipation and, therefore, any changes to these medications should be made in conjunction with concurrent bowel surveillance and management with increased fluids and fiber.

Surgical understanding about the potential benefits and risks of routine preoperative bowel preparation is evolving.[36] and neurogenic patients may warrant special consideration during preoperative planning.[37] There are no well-designed studies to direct urologists in determining whether preoperative bowel preparation should be used in patients with coexisting neurogenic bowel. Some studies in the SCI and neurogenic bowel dysfunction populations have used extended bowel preparation up to 72 hours with a clear liquid diet and a

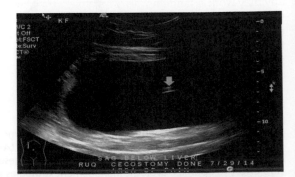

Fig. 2. Right upper quadrant (RUQ) ultrasound obtained 1 month after augmentation cystoplasty in a spina bifida patient complaining of acute RUQ pain and headaches. Image demonstrates a pseudocyst around the ventriculoperitoneal shunt tubing (*arrow*).

combination of magnesium citrate, polyethylene glycol electrolyte lavage solution, and NaP/biphosphate enemas to clear the bowel of any fecal matter before any procedures.[38–40] It is our practice to perform a KUB before surgery and use an extended (3-day) mechanical bowel preparation when the colon seems to be impacted, mainly to aid in visualization and access to the often-restricted pelvis at the time of surgery. This is particularly important if minimally invasive (laparoscopic or robotic) approaches are planned for pelvic surgery, because visualization may be substantially impaired with an impacted colon in this scenario. Special caution (and preferentially avoidance) needs to be taken with the use of magnesium-containing preparations in patients with coexisting severe renal impairment.

If bladder reconstruction or continent urostomy is planned using colon and the patient has not undergone his or her age- and risk-related surveillance colonoscopy screening, this should be done before the planned operation. Coordination of this may be challenging given that patients with advanced neurogenic bowel often require a 3-day bowel preparation before colonoscopy. If this procedure is needed, the bowel preparation can be conducted, colonoscopy performed the day before surgery. The patient can then be admitted for vigorous intravenous hydration and undergo elective bladder surgery the following day.

Physiatry, Physical Therapy, and Occupational Therapy

Physiatry services fulfill an important role in prescription of assistive devices for mobility, communication, and function as well as management of neuropathic pain. Physical and occupational therapy may work in tandem with physiatry.[41] The use of physical therapy has been shown to improve endurance and flexibility to improve upper body functions, and reduce complications with pressure ulcers, contractures, respiratory capacity, and poor posture.[42]

The urologist may serve as important touchpoint for and referral to physiatry and physical and occupational therapy, particularly for upper extremity functional needs for bladder management. The ability of patients to achieve manual dexterity required for self-catheterization or to implement a bowel routine may require initial and ongoing physical and occupational therapy.[43] In the preoperative setting for urinary diversion, consultation with physiatry, physical therapy, and/or occupation therapy may help to inform both the patient and the provider which operative diversion to

select to maximize the patient's ability to be independent in bowel and bladder management.

Additional physical and occupational therapy services may be required for patients with neurologic diseases during the postoperative period to maintain upper extremity strength for transfer, prevent pressure ulcers, and maintain range of motion and manual dexterity. Not only will this serve to promote early mobilization from bed, but these services may also may improve patients' abilities to manage their bladder, bowels, and wounds in the postoperative period.

Wound Care and Plastic Surgery

Patients with reduced sensation and those who rely on wheelchair support are at particularly high risk for pressure ulcers. Up to one-third of patients with SCI have been documented to develop pressure ulcers while transitioning from acute care to rehabilitation and/or the community.[44] There is an increased risk for developing wound ulcers after 10 years or more from the time of neurologic injury, as reported in a veteran population with traumatic spinal cord injuries.[45,46] Furthermore, wound problems are exacerbated when contaminated with urine and feces, as is common in urologic clinics. Appropriate wound care and timely debridement by plastic surgery is necessary to reduce wound exposure and tissue necrosis. Urologic and gastrointestinal management with a urinary and/or bowel diversion may also be needed before planned reconstruction by plastic surgery, so as to not unduly risk myocutaneous flap failure.[47] For complex perineal wounds, it is our practice to arrange for multispecialty office or intraoperative examinations with plastic surgery, colorectal surgery, and urology to determine what interventions are needed and how they will be staged.

Particularly when patients may be subject to prolonged recovery time after surgery, coordination with wound care teams for prevention of ulcers is imperative. Recommendations to manage pressure ulcers include frequent dressing changes and skin checks, pressure reducing mattresses, turning and repositioning the patients every 10 minutes to 2 hours, early mobilization, appropriate wheelchair materials and fitting, and the use of foam cushions.[48,49]

Nephrology

Some patients with NLUTD are at increased risk of upper urinary tract deterioration and progression to end-stage renal disease. When renal deterioration is evident, early involvement of nephrology is prudent.[50] This is especially true for patients who are non-weight bearing, and for whom creatinine-based estimates of the glomerular filtration rate are known to be inaccurate.[51] In this scenario, the nephrologist may assist in ascertaining a better estimate of the glomerular filtration rate using a non–creatinine-based technique, like cystatin C or iothalamate renal scan. This may prove useful in dosing potentially nephrotoxic drugs in the perioperative setting.

In urologic patients who have bowel in contact with their urinary system, particularly those who have baseline renal insufficiency, metabolic derangements may predominate. In addition to electrolyte imbalances, these patients are at increased risk for nephrolithiasis and bone malabsorption. Monitoring and treatment of urinary electrolytes, acid–base management, and blood pressure are critical contributions that the nephrologist may deliver as a patient develops progressive chronic kidney disease.

As patients with NLUTD near end-stage renal disease, the nephrologist plays a critical role in preparation of the patient for either dialysis or renal transplantation. The options available to patient at this time may require consultation between nephrology, urology, and transplant surgery.[52,53]

Transplant Surgery

Renal transplantation in patients with NLUTD comes with a high risk of morbidity, urinary tract infections, surgical complications, allograft dysfunction, and graft loss, necessitating appropriate preoperative urologic management and assessment of bladder function.[54] In addition to treatment strategies mentioned in the urologic management section, bladder augmentation, urinary diversion, and/or the need for native nephrectomies are surgical options that may be considered in preparation for renal transplantation. Bladder augmentation and urinary conduits have been reported to be performed within 3 to 9 months of renal transplantation to avoid calculi formation, infection, mucous production, and promote adequate wound healing.[55–58] Postoperative urologic monitoring of bladder emptying should be coordinated to maintain renal function postoperatively.[57,59] There is no literature guiding what a "safe" bladder filling pressure is for a transplanted kidney. Development of hydronephrosis in a graft without apparent reason should prompt video urodynamic testing in an upright position, so that the filling pressure at which reflux is seen can be assessed and treatment tailored to the individual patient (Fig. 3).

Cardiology and Pulmonary Medicine

Cardiovascular and pulmonary care should be incorporated into the perioperative evaluation of patients with NLUTD and must be evaluated periodically as patients with neurologic lesions demonstrate increased lifetime risk of venous thromboembolism and pneumonia. Asymptomatic deep vein thrombosis is a common finding, and can progress to emboli in 10% of patients in the acute setting, potentially leading to a fatal pulmonary embolism.[60–64] Perioperative prevention techniques are well-described and may include compression stockings, pneumatic compression devices, and pharmacologic treatments in the acute and outpatient settings.[65,66]

Pneumonia and substantial atelectasis are common concerns in SCI and spina bifida populations, because these patients may have an impaired

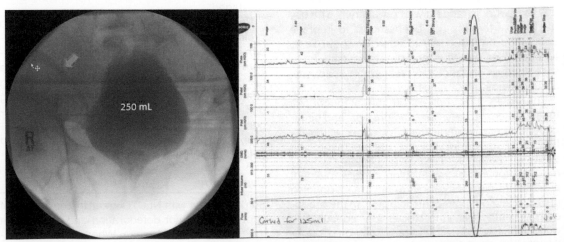

Fig. 3. Urodynamics demonstrate reflux at a volume of 250 mL, with pressure of detrusor (pdet) less than 10 mm Hg in a patient with a transplanted kidney, progressive hydronephrosis, and rising serum creatinine.

ability to clear secretions owing to abdominal muscular impairment. Patients with myelomeningocele and SCI often also have central apnea or obstructive sleep apnea.[67,68] Implementation of cough devices, continuous positive airway pressure, bilevel positive airway pressure, chest physiotherapy, bronchodilator medication, mucolytic medications, and vaccinations may be used to minimize such complications.[69] Assessment with pulmonary function testing or sleep testing in patients with suspected complex pulmonary diseases before a planned surgery may assist in postoperative and anesthesia planning.

As noted, patients with bowel in contact with their urinary tracts often demonstrate baseline acid–base imbalances. Preexisting respiratory conditions that promote respiratory acidosis may exacerbate the effects of metabolic acidosis, compounding the impact of both. Strong consideration of incontinent urinary diversion techniques may be prudent in the setting of a patient with preexisting respiratory acidosis and renal insufficiency to prevent severe metabolic derangements and their sequelae.[70,71]

Psychiatry and Psychology

Coexisting psychiatric conditions are well-described among patients with neurologic conditions of all types. A multiinstitutional study of 61 patients with spina bifida has reported high rates of up to 41% of depression and anxiety.[72,73] Estimates of major depression for patients with SCI range from 16% to 50%.[74,75] Patients with MS have been shown to experience a lifetime prevalence of depression of near 50%.[76,77] Coexisting psychiatric impairment may substantially influence a patient's ability to manage his or her bladder, including compliance with urologic medications and self-care, making coordination with psychiatry and psychology services imperative. Patients with chronic neurologic disease who undergo surgery are at risk for prolonged periods of isolation from their community support, particularly because many require rehabilitation services after their acute hospital admissions, putting them at particular risk of depression, anxiety, and other psychiatric conditions. Special attention and care should be focused on patients in the perioperative setting for signs of psychiatric distress and early consultation and treatment should be offered.

Specific examples of pharmacologic interventions that may bring psychiatric patients to a urologist's office include the following.

1. Mood stabilizers: Use of lithium as a mood stabilizer poses a risk for urologic symptoms of polydipsia with loss of bowel and/or bladder control, and potential impotence or low libido in addition to other side effects. Toxic lithium levels may result in additive renal deterioration in a patient who may already have baseline renal impairment from NLUTD.

2. Antidepressants: Selective serotonin reuptake inhibitors and selective norepinephrine reuptake inhibitors may cause low libido, anhedonia, erectile dysfunction, delayed ejaculation, and/or anorgasmia. Tricyclic antidepressants can have substantial anticholinergic effects, placing a patient at risk for urinary retention or compounding the side effects of anticholinergic medications.[78]

PROPOSED LONG-TERM MANAGEMENT

Patients who either are born with or develop NLUTD in pediatric life are often managed in highly coordinated, multidisciplinary settings in childhood. As these patients enter young adulthood, transition to adult care is often disjointed and can be hindered by a lack of access to multidisciplinary care. Navigation of the adult care environment in the United States, which has historically been provider by provider, is both complex and burdensome to patients with multisystem disease.

Transferring care whether from the acute to long-term settings or from pediatric to adult care prompts a comprehensive assessment of patient needs before referral for interdisciplinary care. The Royal College of Physicians have proposed a checklist for effective management of patients with SCI while transitioning, which is also applicable to NLUTD related conditions. Patient history of comorbid conditions are assessed with the following action items.[79]

- Bladder assessment and management plan in acute and long-term settings,
- Bowel assessment and management plan,
- Neurologic and musculoskeletal assessments,
- Establishment of a care plan for autonomic dysreflexia,
- Respiratory assessment for devices, therapy, and optimization,
- Thromboembolic prophylaxis management plan,
- Skin assessment and pressure sore prevention strategies, and
- Coordination with established primary care provider, community nursing, and/or additional care arrangements.

Coordination of care is often one of the major obstacles to maintaining multidisciplinary care. This is especially true when follow-up times vary between providers and there is an absence of any acute changes. In this environment, primary care providers can serve as an initial entry point to multidisciplinary care and may help to identify slowly progressive changes in patient status that may prompt appropriate evaluation by a specialty team. Primary care providers can manage patients overall with regular visits regarding health updates and physical evaluations and assessments. Monitoring of skin breakdown, urologic, bowel, pain control, and overall comorbid conditions and health status can be performed by primary care providers before referral. Communication by the specialist back to the primary care doctor's office is imperative, and may be facilitated by a portable or central electronic medical record. In an ideal system, case management support would be optimal in promoting receipt of appropriate care, care coordination, managing of financial limitations, and establishing home care services and/or transportation. However, these services are often limited in the current adult care environment in the United States.

Although there are no guidelines at present for NLUTD, the International Standards for Neurological Classification of SCI has proposed multisystem management by skilled nursing personnel as a part of a multidisciplinary coordinated effort. Skilled nursing can be used briefly from acute care to reintegrate patients into a home or community, especially to ensure environmental safety. Long-term skilled nursing may be incorporated into a long-term management plan depending on patient needs and caregiver resources. Responsibilities of skilled nursing in treating patients with NLUTD may require a combination of the following management areas:

- Neurologic assessment,
- Skin examination and maintenance of skin integrity,
- Compliance with a bladder and bowel management protocol,
- Supporting patient self-care,
- Monitoring nutritional intake,
- Assessing and managing any circulatory, respiratory, and musculoskeletal complications and regimens,
- Fostering compliance with medications and scheduling, and
- Assessment of pain management, especially related to neurologic disease.

Spinal cord guidelines suggest nursing providers with clinical experiences and knowledge specific to management practices for bowel and bladder benefit patients with SCI.[80] This system may permit greater access to provider resources for patients who have difficulty managing lower urinary tract symptoms despite intervention. Adapting to a system with skilled or community nursing ensures patients can be referred for urologic evaluations if NLUTD associated symptoms worsen.

Clinical practice guidelines on the management of neurogenic bowel were published in 2005 and were shown to provide clinical benefit to patients when enforced in a targeted approach by region.[81] Guideline preparation for multidisciplinary management of spina bifida patients is under development.[82]

SUMMARY

Neurologic diseases often affect the urinary tract and may be inborn or acquired. The progressive nature of many neurologic diseases mandates routine surveillance and treatment by urology in coordination with other providers. Urologic treatments may interfere substantially with pharmacologic or procedural interventions planned by other specialists, mandating close coordination of care and communication among providers. Primary care and nursing often can serve as the quarterback of the multidisciplinary team by identifying when a slowly progressive condition warrants investigation by specialists.

REFERENCES

1. Gormley EA. Urologic complications of the neurogenic bladder. Urol Clin North Am 2010;37(4):601–7.
2. Bycroft J, Hamid R, Bywater H, et al. Variation in urological practice amongst spinal injuries units in the UK and Eire. Neurourol Urodyn 2004;23(3):252–6 [discussion: 257].
3. de Seze M, Ruffion A, Denys P, et al, GENULF. The neurogenic bladder in multiple sclerosis: review of the literature and proposal of management guidelines. Mult Scler 2007;13(7):915–28.
4. DasGupta R, Fowler CJ. Sexual and urological dysfunction in multiple sclerosis: better understanding and improved therapies. Curr Opin Neurol 2002; 15(3):271–8.
5. Oskoui M, Coutinho F, Dykeman J, et al. An update on the prevalence of cerebral palsy: a systematic review and meta-analysis. Dev Med Child Neurol 2013;55(6):509–19.
6. Wood HM. Editorial comment. Urology 2014;84(2): 444.
7. Pannek J, Blok J, Castro-Diaz D, et al. Neurogenic lower urinary tract dysfunction. Eur Assoc Urol 2013;64(1):118–40. EAU Guidelines.
8. Reynard JM, Peters TJ, Lim C, et al. The value of multiple free-flow studies in men with lower urinary tract symptoms. Br J Urol 1996;77(6):813–8.

9. Fulgham PF, Bishoff JT. Urinary tract imaging: basic principles. In: Wein AJ, editor. Campbell-Walsh urology. 10th edition. Philadelphia: Elsevier Saunders; 2011. Chapter 4.

10. Glickman S, Kamm MA. Bowel dysfunction in spinal-cord-injury patients. Lancet 1996;347(9016):1651–3.

11. Gormley EA, Lightner DJ, Burgio KL, et al. Diagnosis and treatment of overactive bladder (non-neurogenic) in adults: AUA/SUFU guideline. J Urol 2015; 193(5):1572–80.

12. Gormley EA, Kaufman M. Urinary incontinence. American Urological Association Education and Research; 2016.

13. Urinary incontinence in neurological disease: assessment and management. National Institute for Health and Care Excellence; 2012. Available at: https://www.nice.org.uk/guidance/cg148/chapter/Introduction.

14. van Gool JD, Dik P, de Jong TP. Bladder-sphincter dysfunction in myelomeningocele. Eur J Pediatr 2001;160(7):414–20.

15. Madersbacher H, Wyndaele JJ, Igawa Y, et al. Conservative management in neuropathic urinary incontinence. In: Abrams P, Cardozo L, Khoury S, et al, editors. Incontinence. Plymouth (UK): Health Publication Ltd; 2002. p. 697–754.

16. Bruschini H, Almeida FG, Srougi M. Upper and lower urinary tract evaluation of 104 patients with myelomeningocele without adequate urological management. World J Urol 2006;24(2): 224–8.

17. Woodhouse CR. Myelomeningocele in young adults. BJU Int 2005;95(2):223–30.

18. McGuire EJ, Woodside JR, Borden TA, et al. Prognostic value of urodynamic testing in myelodysplastic patients. J Urol 1981;126(2):205–9.

19. Appell RA. Pharmacotherapy for overactive bladder: an evidence-based approach to selecting an antimuscarinic agent. Drugs 2006;66:1361.

20. Blackett H, Walker R, Wood B. Urinary dysfunction in Parkinson's disease: a review. Parkinsonism Relat Disord 2009;15(2):81–7.

21. Ehrt U, Broich K, Larsen JP, et al. Use of drugs with anticholinergic effect and impact on cognition in Parkinson's disease: a cohort study. J Neurol Neurosurg Psychiatry 2010;81(2):160–5.

22. Crispo JA, Willis AW, Thibault DP, et al. Associations between anticholinergic burden and adverse health outcomes in Parkinson disease. PLoS One 2016; 11(3):e0150621.

23. Brusa L, Petta F, Pisani A, et al. Central acute D2 stimulation worsens bladder function in patients with mild Parkinson's disease. J Urol 2006;175(1): 202–6 [discussion: 206–7].

24. Cardozo L. Voiding difficulties and retention: urogynecology. 1st edition. New York: Churchill Livingstone; 1997. p. 305–20.

25. Brashear A. The botulinum toxins in the treatment of cervical dystonia. Semin Neurol 2001; 21(1):85–90.

26. Jankovic J, Schwartz K. Botulinum toxin injections for cervical dystonia. Neurology 1990;40(2):277–80.

27. O'Flaherty SJ, Janakan V, Morrow AM, et al. Adverse events and health status following botulinum toxin type A injections in children with cerebral palsy. Dev Med Child Neurol 2011;53(2):125–30.

28. Goldstein EM. Safety of high-dose botulinum toxin type A therapy for the treatment of pediatric spasticity. J Child Neurol 2006;21(3):189–92.

29. Narayanan UG. Botulinum toxin: does the black box warning justify change in practice? Dev Med Child Neurol 2011;53(2):101–2.

30. Boster AL, Bennett SE, Bilsky GS, et al. Best practices for intrathecal baclofen therapy: screening test. Neuromodulation 2016;19(6):616–22.

31. Chartier-Kastler EJ, Ruud Bosch JL, Perrigot M, et al. Long-term results of sacral nerve stimulation (S3) for the treatment of neurogenic refractory urge incontinence related to detrusor hyperreflexia. J Urol 2000;164(5):1476–80.

32. Yerkes EB, Rink RC, Cain MP, et al. Shunt infection and malfunction after augmentation cystoplasty. J Urol 2001;165(6 Pt 2):2262–4.

33. Hayashi Y, Okazaki T, Kobayashi H, et al. Shunt conversion before bladder augmentation can prevent shunt infection. Asian J Surg 2008;31(4):207–10.

34. Rainov N, Schobess A, Heidecke V, et al. Abdominal CSF pseudocysts in patients with ventriculoperitoneal shunts. Report of fourteen cases and review of the literature. Acta Neurochir (Wien) 1994; 127(1–2):73–8.

35. Loftus CJ, Wood HM. Congenital causes of neurogenic bladder and the transition to adult care. Transl Androl Urol 2016;5(1):39–50.

36. Mariani P, Slim K. Enhanced recovery after gastrointestinal surgery: the scientific background. J Visc Surg 2016;153(6S):S19–25.

37. Gundeti MS, Godbole PP, Wilcox DT. Is bowel preparation required before cystoplasty in children? J Urol 2006;176(4 Pt 1):1574–6 [discussion: 1576–7].

38. Stiens SA, Bergman SB, Goetz LL. Neurogenic bowel dysfunction after spinal cord injury: clinical evaluation and rehabilitative management. Arch Phys Med Rehabil 1997;78(3 Suppl):S86–102.

39. Ancha HR, Spungen AM, Bauman WA, et al. Clinical trial: the efficacy and safety of routine bowel cleansing agents for elective colonoscopy in persons with spinal cord injury - a randomized prospective single-blind study. Aliment Pharmacol Ther 2009;30(11–12):1110–7.

40. Barber DB, Rogers SJ, Chen JT, et al. Pilot evaluation of a nurse-administered carepath for successful colonoscopy for persons with spinal cord injury. SCI Nurs 1999;16(1):14–5, 20.

41. Kubsik A, Klimkiewicz R, Klimkiewicz P, et al. Assessment of the pain patients with the multiple sclerosis after applying the physiotherapy treatment. Pol Merkur Lekarski 2016;40(238):230–4 [in Polish].

42. Emerich L, Parsons KC, Stein A. Competent care for persons with spinal cord injury and dysfunction in acute inpatient rehabilitation. Top Spinal Cord Inj Rehabil 2012;18(2):149–66.

43. Nakamura A, Osonoi T, Terauchi Y. Relationship between urinary sodium excretion and pioglitazone-induced edema. J Diabetes Investig 2010;1(5):208–11.

44. Fuhrer MJ, Garber SL, Rintala DH, et al. Pressure ulcers in community-resident persons with spinal cord injury: prevalence and risk factors. Arch Phys Med Rehabil 1993;74(11):1172–7.

45. Salzberg CA, Byrne DW, Cayten CG, et al. A new pressure ulcer risk assessment scale for individuals with spinal cord injury. Am J Phys Med Rehabil 1996;75(2):96–104.

46. Salzberg CA, Byrne DW, Cayten CG, et al. Predicting and preventing pressure ulcers in adults with paralysis. Adv Wound Care 1998;11(5):237–46.

47. Garber SL, Bryce TN, Gregorio-Torres TL, et al. Pressure ulcer prevention and treatment following spinal cord injury: a clinical practice guideline for health-care professionals. Spinal Cord Medicine. 2nd edition. 2014.

48. Benbow M. Working towards clinical excellence. Pressure ulcer prevention and management in primary and secondary care. J Wound Care 2012;21(9 Arjohuntleigh Suppl):S26–39.

49. National Pressure Ulcer Advisory Panel. Pressure ulcers: incidence, economics, risk assessment. Consensus development conference statement. Wes Dundee (IL): SN Publications; 1989.

50. Sullivan ME, Reynard JM, Cranston DW. Renal transplantation into the abnormal lower urinary tract. BJU Int 2003;92(5):510–5.

51. Quan A, Adams R, Ekmark E, et al. Serum creatinine is a poor marker of glomerular filtration rate in patients with spina bifida. Dev Med Child Neurol 1997;39(12):808–10.

52. Ercan Z, Yildirim T, Merhametsiz O, et al. Abdominal pseudocyst development in a peritoneal dialysis patient with a ventriculoperitoneal shunt: an indication for switch to hemodialysis? Perit Dial Int 2014;34(4):470–1.

53. Ram Prabahar M, Sivakumar M, Chandrasekaran V, et al. Peritoneal dialysis in a patient with neurogenic bladder and chronic kidney disease with ventriculoperitoneal shunt. Blood Purif 2008;26(3):274–8.

54. Nahas WC, Mazzucchi E, Antonopoulos I, et al. Kidney transplantation in patients with bladder augmentation: surgical outcome and urodynamic follow-up. Transplant Proc 1997;29(1–2):157–8.

55. Guimond J, Gonzalez R. Renal transplantation in children with reconstructed bladders. Transplantation 2004;77(7):1116–20.

56. Sheldon CA, Gonzalez R, Burns MW, et al. Renal transplantation into the dysfunctional bladder: the role of adjunctive bladder reconstruction. J Urol 1994;152(3):972–5.

57. Neild GH, Dakmish A, Wood S, et al. Renal transplantation in adults with abnormal bladders. Transplantation 2004;77(7):1123–7.

58. Fontaine E, Gagnadoux MF, Niaudet P, et al. Renal transplantation in children with augmentation cystoplasty: long-term results. J Urol 1998;159(6):2110–3.

59. Nahas WC, Antonopoulos IM, Piovesan AC, et al. Comparison of renal transplantation outcomes in children with and without bladder dysfunction. A customized approach equals the difference. J Urol 2008;179(2):712–6.

60. Geerts WH, Code KI, Jay RM, et al. A prospective study of venous thromboembolism after major trauma. N Engl J Med 1994;331(24):1601–6.

61. Spinal Cord Injury Thromboprophylaxis Investigators. Prevention of venous thromboembolism in the rehabilitation phase after spinal cord injury: prophylaxis with low-dose heparin or enoxaparin. J Trauma 2003;54(6):1111–5.

62. Chen D, Geerts WH, Lee MY, et al. Prevention of venous thromboembolism in individuals with spinal cord injury: a clinical practice guideline for health care providers. Spinal Cord Medicine. 3rd edition. 2016.

63. DeVivo MJ, Krause JS, Lammertse DP. Recent trends in mortality and causes of death among persons with spinal cord injury. Arch Phys Med Rehabil 1999;80(11):1411–9.

64. Aito S, Pieri A, D'Andrea M, et al. Primary prevention of deep venous thrombosis and pulmonary embolism in acute spinal cord injured patients. Spinal Cord 2002;40(6):300–3.

65. Sachdeva A, Dalton M, Amaragiri SV, et al. Graduated compression stockings for prevention of deep vein thrombosis. Cochrane Database Syst Rev 2014;(12):CD001484.

66. Morris RJ, Woodcock JP. Evidence-based compression: prevention of stasis and deep vein thrombosis. Ann Surg 2004;239(2):162–71.

67. Chiodo AE, Sitrin RG, Bauman KA. Sleep disordered breathing in spinal cord injury: a systematic review. J Spinal Cord Med 2016;39(4):374–82.

68. Patel DM, Rocque BG, Hopson B, et al. Sleep-disordered breathing in patients with myelomeningocele. J Neurosurg Pediatr 2015;16(1):30–5.

69. Parsons KC, Buhrer R, Burns SP. Respiratory management following spinal cord injury: a clinical practice guideline for health-care professionals. Spinal Cord Med 2005;28:259–93.

70. de Petriconi R. Metabolic aspects of bowel use in urologic surgery. Ann Urol (Paris) 2007;41(5):216–36 [in French].

71. Roosen A, Gerharz EW, Roth S, et al. Bladder, bowel and bones–skeletal changes after intestinal urinary diversion. World J Urol 2004;22(3):200–9.

72. Frohlich ED, Re RN. Introduction to the focussed section on molecular and cellular biology in hypertension. Cardiovasc Drugs Ther 1988;2(4):451–2.

73. Holmbeck GN, DeLucia C, Essner B, et al. Trajectories of psychosocial adjustment in adolescents with spina bifida: a 6-year, four-wave longitudinal follow-up. J Consult Clin Psychol 2010;78(4):511–25.

74. Khazaeipour Z, Taheri-Otaghsara SM, Naghdi M. Depression following spinal cord injury: its relationship to demographic and socioeconomic indicators. Top Spinal Cord Inj Rehabil 2015;21(2):149–55.

75. Saurí J, Chamarro A, Gilabert A, et al. Depression in individuals with traumatic and non-traumatic spinal cord injury living in the community. Arch Phys Med Rehabil 2016. [Epub ahead of print].

76. Stuke H, Hanken K, Hirsch J, et al. Cross-sectional and longitudinal relationships between depressive symptoms and brain atrophy in MS patients. Front Hum Neurosci 2016;10:622.

77. Feinstein A. Neuropsychiatric syndromes associated with multiple sclerosis. J Neurol 2007;254(Suppl 2):II73–6.

78. Sandson NB, Armstrong SC, Cozza KL. An overview of psychotropic drug-drug interactions. Psychosomatics 2005;46(5):464–94.

79. Gall A, Turner-Stokes L, Guideline Development Group. Chronic spinal cord injury: management of patients in acute hospital settings. Clin Med (Lond) 2008;8(1):70–4.

80. Linsenmeyer TA, Bodner DR, Creasey GH, et al. Bladder management for adults with spinal cord injury: a clinical practice guidelines for health-care providers. Spinal Cord Med 2006;29(5):527–73.

81. Goetz LL, Nelson AL, Guihan M, et al. Provider adherence to implementation of clinical practice guidelines for neurogenic bowel in adults with spinal cord injury. J Spinal Cord Med 2005;28(5):394–406.

82. Spina Bifida Association communication, 2017.

Evaluation and Lifetime Management of the Urinary Tract in Patients with Myelomeningocele

CrossMark

Diana Cardona-Grau, MD, George Chiang, MD*

KEYWORDS

- Spina bifida • Urology • Transitional care • Myelomeningocele • Neurogenic bladder

KEY POINTS

- Goals in the lifelong management center around renal preservation as a priority, achieving some degree of continence, and optimizing quality of life.
- Management is multimodal and can be complex; although management techniques may vary throughout a child's lifetime, the goals remain constant.
- Complex medical needs become more challenging as patients become older and need to transition to adult providers faced with incorporating these patients into their practice.
- Continued evaluation of development and implementation of transition plans is imperative to promote smooth and successful transitions in the future.
- Different phases in life offer new challenges and barriers that require vigilant health care interactions and patient dedication.

INTRODUCTION

Spina bifida (SB) is a neural tube defect that is one of the most common causes of congenital lower urinary tract dysfunction. Although disease manifestation can be variable from patient to patient, it commonly affects bladder and bowel function, cognition, and the neuromusculoskeletal system.[1] The most frequent form is myelomeningocele (MMC), characterized by the extrusion of the spinal cord into a sac filled with cerebrospinal fluid.[2]

Epidemiology

SB affects all racial and ethnic groups with an overall prevalence from 2004 to 2006 of 3.5 per 10,00 in the United States when adjusted for maternal race and ethnicity.[3] Using the Kids' Inpatient Database, Lloyd and colleagues[4] concluded that the prevalence of the disease has been stable from 1997 to 2009. The worldwide incidence of neural tube defects has been cited at 0.3 to 4.5 per 1000 births.[5]

According to data from the Centers for Disease Control and Prevention, the prevalence declined nearly 20% among infants born to non-Hispanic black mothers and remained constant in infants born to Hispanic mothers and mothers of non-Hispanic white ethnicity between 2000 and 2005.[6] In the analysis by Lloyd and colleagues[4] using the Kids' Inpatient Database, there was a higher prevalence of SB in the Hispanic cohort as well. Over the past, century survival rates for babies born with SB have improved drastically, and this can be attributed to improvements in

Disclosure Statement: The authors have nothing to disclose.
Pediatric Urology, University of California San Diego, Rady Children's Hospital, 3020 Children's Way MC 5120, San Diego, CA 92123, USA
* Corresponding author.
E-mail address: gchiang@rchsd.org

Urol Clin N Am 44 (2017) 391–401
http://dx.doi.org/10.1016/j.ucl.2017.04.006
0094-0143/17/© 2017 Elsevier Inc. All rights reserved.

medical and surgical management with the introduction of the ventriculoperitoneal shunt (VPS), antibiotics, and intermittent catheterization.[7] Today, 85% to 90% of children are surviving into adulthood and, compared with those born in 1975, twice as many newborns with SB survived in the United States in 1995.[7]

Management Goals

Primary goals in the lifelong management of SB patients centers around renal preservation as a priority, achieving some degree of continence, and optimizing quality of life. Although we can rely on specific markers of renal preservation, such as imaging and functional studies, continence measures can be more subjective and variably defined. Although the International Children's Continence Society guidelines define incontinence as "uncontrollable leakage of urine," this leaves room for a variable interpretation. Furthermore, no general consensus exists on specific measures of continence for research purposes. Lloyd and colleagues[8] reviewed the literature to assess the degree of standardization of urinary incontinence definitions in children with SB. They found that out of 105 articles that met inclusion criteria, only 57% of studies had a clear definition of continence. The most commonly used definition was "always dry," which was used in 24% of studies.

Other variables, including presence of a VPS, can also have a significant impact on quality of life. Ramachandra and colleagues[1] evaluated health status and demographic variables as potential factors in patient- and parent-reported health-related quality of life. The study found that patients with shunted hydrocephalus had worse perceptions of their physical health than those without; however, this perception seemed to improve in older patients. Other studies have found that spinal lesion level and the number of shunt revisions was associated with poorer quality of life.[9]

In the United States, there are currently an estimated 25,000 children ages 0 to 19 years and about 166,000 of all ages currently affected by SB.[10] The management of patients with SB is often multimodal and can be complex; although management techniques may vary throughout a child's lifetime, the goals remain the same. These goals center around the upper urinary tract, prevention of urinary tract infections (UTIs), and establishing some degree of acceptable continence. As noted by the International Children's Continence Society, continence is usually addressed as the child reaches school age; however, upper urinary tract damage secondary to elevated detrusor pressure and/or reflux, and chronic UTIs are continuously addressed and may evolve over time.[11] Additional considerations such as the development of urolithiasis and the associated burden are highlighted in the adolescent years and into adulthood. These complex medical needs become more challenging as pediatric patients become older and need to transition to adult providers who are faced with incorporating these patients into their adult practice.

PRENATAL DIAGNOSIS

SB can be diagnosed as early as the first trimester on prenatal ultrasound imaging. Antenatal ultrasound findings suggest that insults to both the central and peripheral nervous systems may be progressive and sequelae may worsen during gestation.[2] Damage to the spinal cord and peripheral nerves usually is evident at birth and is irreversible despite early postnatal surgical repair.[2] Given these findings and that long-term survivors usually have major disabilities, including paralysis and bowel and bladder dysfunction, the Management of Myelomeningocele Study (MOMS) sought to evaluate whether prenatal repair of MMC resulted in improved neurologic function.

Management of Myelomeningocele Study

The MOMS trial randomized eligible women to undergo either prenatal surgery before 26 weeks of gestation or standard postnatal repair. The study found the primary outcome (fetal or neonatal death or the need for a cerebrospinal fluid shunt) was reduced in the prenatal surgery group (relative risk, 0.7). In the prenatal group, 40% of patients still required shunting, however, this was compared with 82% in the postnatal intervention group. Prenatal surgery was associated with increased risk of preterm delivery and uterine dehiscence at delivery. Furthermore, although prenatal surgery decreased the need for VPS and improved lower extremity outcomes, the prenatal group required more procedures for delayed spinal cord tethering.[2] Based on these outcomes, it was concluded that prenatal closure seemed to improve neuromotor function and decrease the need for VPS. The long-term follow-up available on children who have undergone prenatal closure include those who underwent closure before the MOMS trial. Danzer and colleagues[12] reported on results in patients at a median age of 10 years supporting persistent improvement in neurofunctional outcome after fetal MMC repair (79% community ambulators; 9% household ambulators; and 14% wheelchair bound). Despite these improvements, behavioral abnormalities were common, with more deficits in executive function and behavioral adaptive skills in patients undergoing fetal MMC repair compared with the normal population. However, the authors acknowledge that these results are specific to specialized MOMS centers. More detailed reports from the full MOMS cohort addressing motor function and ambulatory status, maternal outcomes including psychological findings and maternal risk factors, and more detailed neonatal follow-up are expected.[13] It has been noted that these results are specific to the designated MOMS centers and may not be generalizable to less experiences centers. No set guidelines for prenatal versus postnatal closure have been established, but the criteria used for prenatal intervention by MOMS centers include vertebral defect at S1 or higher, hindbrain herniation on prenatal ultrasound imaging and MRI, normal karyotype, maternal age 18 years or older, gestational age from 19 to 25.6 weeks, and a singleton pregnancy.[13]

Urologic Outcomes After Prenatal Closure

Given the seemingly positive effect on neurologic outcomes, several follow-up studies have evaluated the effect of prenatal surgery on urologic outcomes. Early on, Holmes and colleagues[14] noted that patients undergoing prenatal surgery demonstrated the same changes on videourodynamics as children who underwent postnatal closure. In this cohort of 6 patients, videourodynamics was performed at 1 month and showed decreased bladder capacity for weight, increased detrusor storage pressures, and significant postvoid residuals in 4 patients. Four patients also demonstrated hydronephrosis and vesicoureteral reflux was seen in 3 patients.[14] The authors concluded that these patients seemed to have the same changes in urodynamic parameters as patients who underwent postnatal closure based on historical data.

Similarly, Vanderbilt analyzed urodynamic findings in their cohort of 23 patients after fetal closure. They showed that findings at age 6.5 months did not differ from historical data on postnatally closed newborns.[15] They found that 34% of patients had decreased capacity for age, 13% had detrusor overactivity and 82% had a detrusor leak point pressure of greater than 40 cm H_2O.[15] A follow-up study of this cohort included 28 patients who had undergone prenatal closure at the same MOMS center, which were followed to a mean age of 9.6 years. They noted that, on videourodynamics, 71% of patients had decreased bladder capacity, 35% demonstrated detrusor overactivity, and 25% showed increased detrusor pressure.[16] They concluded that there were no differences in bladder management, urinary tract surgery, or urodynamics in patients who underwent prenatal closure when compared with age- and sex-matched children who underwent postnatal closure.

Another study compared 11 patients who had undergone prenatal closure with a mean follow-up of 7.2 years with a matched (1:2) group of patients having undergone postnatal repair.[17] Similarly, this study found there was no difference in need for clean intermittent catheterization (CIC), incontinence between CIC, anticholinergic/antibiotic use, or in urodynamic parameters. Given the available literature, children who underwent prenatal closure still warrant close follow-up, similar to those who have undergone postnatal closure.

INITIAL NEONATAL MANAGEMENT AND SURVEILLANCE

As Dik and colleagues[18] point out, (1) ensuring safe intravesical pressures during urine storage and (2) establishing adequate emptying of the bladder at low pressures are key management principles to prevent renal damage. These factors must be recognized and addressed as early as possible in a child's life. However, challenges to evaluating the urinary tract soon after birth include the priority of spinal closure and neurologic status. Therefore, exact bladder function is difficult to establish for an individual patient in the neonatal period, especially before undergoing closure. Timing and use of urodynamic studies (UDS) and exact timing of interventions such as implementation of CIC is debated in the literature.[19] Despite these challenges, at the very least, renal ultrasound evaluation and determination of residual urine should be performed early on. Use of functional imaging early on can also help to detect silent damage to the upper tracts along the course of follow-up. In our practice, we rarely institute CIC at birth unless there is evidence of significant bilateral hydronephrosis. CIC is also instituted during the first year of life if there are recurrent UTIs or damage based on functional imaging.

Early Evaluation and Renal Preservation

Although some components for the initial evaluation in infants with SB remain controversial, key elements needed include renal ultrasound imaging, voiding cystourethrogram (VCUG), functional imaging such as a radionuclide scans, and UDS once feasible. The ultimate goal of the evaluation is to provide a baseline on the appearance of the upper and lower urinary tracts for future comparison with the ultimate goal being to detect early signs of upper tract deterioration to prevent significant renal damage. The timing of these studies during the first year of life can be controversial, especially urodynamics, but ideally a renal ultrasound examination should be performed soon after birth with a VCUG if findings such as hydronephrosis, ureteral dilation, renal size discrepancy, or increased bladder wall thickness are noted on ultrasound examination.[20] In our practice, a VCUG and renal ultrasound examination are performed in the neonatal period to determine the need for antibiotic prophylaxis in the context of vesicoureteral reflux or high-grade hydronephrosis. UDS and a dimercaptosuccinic acid (DMSA) scan are performed within the first 6 months of life. At that point, serial ultrasound examinations are performed every 3 to 6 months at our multidisciplinary clinic. Clinical changes or a change in the ultrasound parameters may necessitate a repeat UDS, VCUG, or DMSA. The use of radionuclide scans such as DMSA scans has been instrumental in providing a baseline during the first year of life as well as directing care based on actual renal functional loss or scarring.

Infants with SB have been found to exhibit a variety of urodynamic changes, including decreased capacity, decreased compliance, detrusor overactivity, bladder outlet obstruction, and complete denervation. In 1 study, urodynamics were performed in 40 neonates before spinal closure, within 7 days of closure, and at 3-month intervals thereafter. In this cohort, 3.3% of patients exhibited a change in neurologic status after spinal closure.[21] Most other studies include UDS performed after closure and serially thereafter. A study by Kaefer and colleagues[22] that included 36 infants with myelodysplasia showed that patients with detrusor external sphincter dyssynergia were at higher risk for renal deterioration than patients without detrusor external sphincter dyssynergia (72% vs 11%), although there was no use of radionuclide scans. However, in a study by Shiroyanagi and colleagues[23] of a cohort of 64 patients, 25% of which had abnormal DMSA scans, there was no significant difference in urodynamic findings (detrusor leak-point pressure and compliance) in those patients with normal and abnormal DMSA scans.

When it comes to management early on in life, 2 main themes prevail—expectant and proactive management.[19] In expectant management, patients are monitored clinically with renal ultrasound per International Children's Continence Society recommendations every 6 months until 2 years of age.[20] CIC or urodynamics are only performed if there is evidence of clinical deterioration (new or worsening hydronephrosis or reflux, increased postvoid residual volumes, changes in renal function, or development of a UTI) or renal ultrasound changes.[19] With this approach, Teichman and colleagues[24] found a 5% rate of renal deterioration, which was statistically associated with UTIs and vesicoureteral reflux. In this cohort, the renal deterioration that occurred was no different in patients with abnormal and normal UDS, implying that UDS did not predict renal deterioration. Proactive management entails early and regular UDS with CIC with or without anticholinergics initiated based on urodynamic findings. UDS have been performed once patients are medically stable and recovered from neurosurgical closure with repeat assessment yearly or if radiologic or clinical signs indicated increased outlet resistance.[25] The goal is to identify patients with poor compliance or high leak point pressures to intervene before causing upper tract damage. In rare cases, a vesicostomy may be required as a temporizing measure when there is evidence of high-grade vesicoureteral reflux with hydronephrosis and ongoing renal damage.

Part of the controversy between the management strategies stems from mixed results in the literature. For example, Woo and colleagues[26] found that early CIC was associated with an increased incidence in abnormalities in DMSA scans, suggesting that early CIC did not necessarily prevent renal damage. The authors acknowledged the inherent limitation of the retrospective nature of this study as well as the potential for selection bias, because patients at higher risk for renal damage may have been started on CIC earlier. Therefore, they did not imply causation but observed that in their cohort of patients CIC did not seem to prevent renal damage.[26] Other studies, including one by Edelstein and colleagues,[25] showed that children in whom CIC was started prophylactically had a decreased incidence of renal deterioration defined as worsening hydronephrosis, worsening vesicoureteral reflux, or increasing postvoid residuals. In this study, 80% of patients followed expectantly had upper tract changes and 14% went on to reconstructive surgery. In a retrospective study, Wu and colleagues[27] compared patients managed proactively (n = 46) and expectantly (n = 52) they found that although renal outcomes in terms of hydronephrosis were similar in both groups, there was a significant increase in augmentation rate (27% vs 11%) in the expectant management group. However, renal function or damage was not measured and the outcome was based on the need for surgical intervention. Given the mixed data and varying outcome measures from series to series, neither of these techniques has emerged as a gold standard. In our practice, we follow children with a baseline VCUG and ultrasound examination at birth and then a UDS and DMSA within the first 6 months of life. At that point, serial ultrasound examinations are performed every 3 to 6 months at our multidisciplinary spinal defects clinic. Clinical changes or a change in the ultrasound examination may necessitate a repeat UDS, VCUG, or DMSA scan.

Standardizing Management

Given the controversy surrounding expectant versus proactive management, there has been a call for the standardization of management. Recently, the Centers for Disease Control and Prevention has convened a working group of pediatric urologists, nephrologists, epidemiologists, methodologists, community advocates, and Centers for Disease Control and Prevention personnel to develop a protocol to optimize the urologic care of children with SB from the newborn period to 5 years of age.[28] This protocol aims to address the current inconsistencies in reporting of outcomes in the available literature by implementing a protocol to be followed at 9 different study sites (**Table 1**). Recruitment began in 2015 marking the beginning of the 5-year study period; therefore, the question is far from answered, but the results are eagerly awaited.

TODDLER YEARS AND SCHOOL AGE

As the child becomes older, some of the goals of care remain the same; however, with toilet training, continence becomes an added focus. Therefore, evaluation during this period of life should continue to focus on renal preservation, but begin to incorporate facilitation of bladder and bowel continence and begin to promote independence. Diagnostic studies such as renal and bladder ultrasound imaging and kidney, ureter, and bladder examinations are recommended on a yearly basis to assess the upper tracts and stool burden. Renal function may be followed with a yearly creatinine. Although in a recent study by Dangle and colleagues,[29] cystatin C-based glomerular filtration rate has been posed to be more sensitive than creatinine-based glomerular filtration rate for detecting early chronic kidney disease in MMC patients with poor muscle mass. Other studies including a VCUG, UDS, and DMSA scans may be considered at failure to toilet train and/or if there are changes on renal bladder ultrasound imaging, worsening incontinence, or UTIs.

Special attention to bladder function is required during the first 6 years of life and during puberty, because changes are most pronounced during these periods.[30] A study looking at the long-term follow-up of newborns with myelodysplasia but normal urodynamic findings in which 25 newborns were followed found that 32% showed neurologic deterioration owing to tethered cord during the first 6 years of life because these are years of rapid growth.[30] The mean follow-up was 9.1 years with the longest patient follow-up being 18 years.

Once toilet training begins, developing compliance with a CIC regimen is critically important. If the child had not been on started on CIC at an earlier age, a CIC regimen should be implemented once failure to toilet train is recognized. This can occur anywhere from 3 to 5 years of age. UDS may provide further information that can help to steer therapy and improve continence. After CIC is started, anticholinergics are also concomitantly used as a first step. Additional minimally invasive procedures may be used such as intravesical botulinum toxin or combined use of intravesical botulinum toxin with bulking agents for the bladder neck, depending on the physiology.[31]

Upon advancing the treatment ladder for individuals, surgical reconstruction can be performed during the school age years, but is usually performed during early adolescence. Attempts to minimize interventions must be taken into account while also assessing the risks of reconstruction with families and support structures that are integral for surgical reconstruction success. Many options exist within the realm of reconstruction, including methods to increase bladder capacity, creation of catheterizable channels, and increasing outlet resistance. A very brief summary of nonsurgical and surgical options is provided in **Table 2**.

ADOLESCENCE

As the child reaches adolescence, the goals of renal protection and safe bladder storage pressures continue to be important. In a study evaluating renal and functional outcome in a cohort of adolescents with congenital spinal malformations, patients were followed from birth over a 12- to 18-year period and went through the same follow-up and algorithm of intervention during childhood. In this algorithm, patients were risk stratified into no risk, low risk, and high risk at 6 to 9 months of age. Those without upper urinary tract dilatation, normal kidney function, normal cystometry, and no residual urine were classified as no risk and followed with annual ultrasound imaging and cystometry. Those in the low- and high-risk groups were started on antibiotic prophylaxis, anticholinergics, and CIC. Surveillance increased in the high-risk group to biannual ultrasound

Table 1
Protocol for urologic care of children with spina bifida

	Birth-NICU	1–3 mo	6–9 mo	Age 1–4	Age 5
Evaluation	• PVR assessment upon admission to NICU or after closure. • RBUS within 1 week or before discharge.	• Automated BP measurement, manually if abnormal. • DMSA scan • Serum Cr at same time as DMSA. • VUDS or VCUG (CM + VCUG if no video capability) • RBUS	6 mo: • Repeat RBUS • If hostile bladder, repeat VUDS or CMG. 9 mo: • RBUS	• Take BP manually at first visit each year. • VUDS or CMG + VCUG (ages 1 and 2). • RBUS • Serum Cr Ages 3 and 4: • VUDS or CMG (+VCUG only if VUR present on last study)	• Take BP manually at first visit. • GFR, serum Cr • RBUS • DMSA • VUDS or VCUG only if VUR present on last study.
Intervention	• Start CIC q6h or place indwelling catheter. • CIC teaching for family. • Adjust catheterization intervals based on volumes per cath. • Continue catheterizations at interval to maintain residuals ≤ 30 mL. May stop catheterizations if: • Residuals ≤ 30 mL at most checks for 3 and grade 2 or lower hydronephrosis. • If greater than grade 2 hydronephrosis, continue catheterization regardless of residuals.	VUR grades 1–4: • If hostile bladder, CIC q4h while awake and oxybutynin (0.2 mg/kg TID). Repeat VCUG or CMG at 6 mo. • If intermediate or low risk, no treatment. VUR grade 5: • Regardless of bladder characteristics: begin CIC, oxybutynin (0.2 mg/kg TID), and prophylactic antibiotics (MD preference).	Based on above findings.	Based on above findings.	Based on above findings.

Abbreviations: BP, blood pressure; Cath, catheterization; CIC, clean intermittent catheterization; CMG, cystometrogram; Cr, creatinine; DMSA, dimercaptosuccinic acid; GFR, glomerular filtration rate; NICU, neonatal intensive care unit; PVR, postvoid residual; RBUS, renal bladder ultrasound; TID, 3 times daily; VCUG, voiding cystourethrogram; VUDS, videourodynamics; VUR, vesicoureteral reflux.

Data from Routh JC, Cheng EY, Austin JC, et al. Design and methodological considerations of the Centers for Disease Control and Prevention urologic and renal protocol for the newborn and young child with spina bifida. J Urol 2016;196(6):1728–34.

Table 2
Summary of medical and surgical management options

	Non-surgical Management	Surgical Management
Bladder storage/emptying concerns (low capacity, low compliance)	CIC Antimuscarinics Overnight catheter drainage	Intravesical botulinum toxin Augmentation cystoplasty Urinary diversion
Low bladder outlet resistance		Bladder neck sling Bladder neck reconstruction Injection of bulking agents into bladder neck

Abbreviation: CIC, clean intermittent catheterization.
  Data from Wein AJ, Kavoussi LR, Partin AW, et al. Chapter 142. Neuromuscular dysfunction of the lower urinary tract in children. Campbell-Walsh urology. 11th edition. Philadelphia: Elsevier; 2016.

examinations and cystometry as well as annual DMSA scans and consideration for surgical intervention.[32] At adolescence, 81% of patients performed CIC, 50% used anticholinergics, and 62% were continent; the remainder had some form of leakage or incontinence, 19% had undergone augmentation, and none of the patients had developed end-stage renal disease. These rates are consistent with the existing literature.

Maintaining a successful bowel and bladder regimen to achieve social continence becomes even more important in this age group. This should be approached in a systematic fashion both for bowel and bladder issues. Although most patients may already be on CIC and anticholinergics, this regimen remains the first line in managing urinary incontinence. For incontinence refractory to these methods, intradetrusor botulinum toxin A injection is an option. In a systematic review of 12 published series, most studies reported a clinical and urodynamic improvement with resolution of incontinence in 32% to 100% of patients, a decrease in maximum detrusor pressure from 32% to 54%, an increase of maximum cystometric capacity from 27% to 162%, and an improvement in bladder compliance of 28% to 176%.[33] Although no randomized, controlled trials are available comparing botulinum toxin A with placebo in the pediatric or adult SB population, the available evidence suggest improvements in continence, detrusor pressure, cystometric capacity, and compliance in children with SB.

Once medical and minimally invasive procedures such as botulinum toxin A injections or bladder neck bulking agents have been exhausted, if incontinence persists, reconstructive surgery is often considered at this stage if it has not been performed at an earlier age. Augmentation cystoplasty is usually performed at age 9, but these are significant procedures with a high likelihood of morbidity and a 23% to 27%

readmission rate at 90 days.[34] Therefore, careful patient selection and extensive counseling is imperative before embarking on reconstructive surgery.

In addition to bladder and renal-specific goals, providers should be initiating sexual counseling. Although sexual counseling may be overshadowed by the importance of preservation of renal function and maintaining social continence, it should be discussed at this stage. One study exploring how young people with SB think about their disability in the context of sexuality found that patients can feel intense worry around when to have discussions and what exactly to say to partners about the impact of SB on their sexual or romantic relationships.[35] Therefore, issues such as sensation, masturbation, safer sex, and incontinence as it relates to sexuality and relationships should be discussed with adolescent and young adult patients.[35] However, although previous literature has noted that patients would have appreciated more guidance concerning issues like sensation and discussing the impact of SB with their sexual partners, this must be balanced with the patient readiness and openness to the discussion.[35]

TRANSITIONAL YEARS

Transitional care in the SB population has become a prominent topic of discussion now that 85% to 90% patients with SB are surviving into adulthood. The American Academy of Pediatrics recommends starting the discussion on transition at 14 years; however, this may take place at an earlier age if the child is developmentally appropriate.[36] According to the American Academy of Pediatrics, the goal of transitional care is to provide high-quality, developmentally appropriate health care services that continue uninterrupted as the individual moves from adolescence to adulthood.[37]

Moreover, as these children progress into adolescence and adulthood, an added focus of improving quality of life and promoting independence arises.

As evidenced by the literature, transitioning patients with SB is not always successful. A study from Riley Children's Hospital in Indiana found that only 40% of patients transitioned successfully from a multidisciplinary SB clinic to either a transitional urology clinic or adult urologist. Interestingly, the transitional clinic was established across the corridor from the existing multidisciplinary SB clinic. The patients who actually transitioned tended to have more active health issues than those who did not transition. However, those who did not transition were more likely to have emergency room visits.[38]

Much of the current literature centers around identifying barriers to transitional care and facilitating this transition for patients in the future. In general, one of the most prominent barriers to transition of care in patients with complex chronic conditions has been access to health care providers who take care of adults with special needs.[36] Another significant barrier seems to be insurance status, coverage of provider, and navigating the system. Grimsby and colleagues[39] tracked reasons for missed appointments for patients referred to the transitional urology clinic. In this cohort, 27% of patients referred to the transitional urology clinic did not make it to their appointment. The most common reason for missed appointments was related to health insurance coverage in 47% of patients.

In addition to overcoming the insurance hurdle, the importance of having a transition framework in place cannot be overemphasized. One transition clinic out of the University of Oklahoma has reported on the REACH transition program, which establishes a framework for transition that breaks up the process into stages (T0-T4) (**Table 3**).[7] The program starts at T0, which is before the patient is old enough to transition and typically includes 12- to 14-year-old patients who are categorized as eligible to transition once reaching adolescence.[7] The active transition phases are categorized as T1 to T4 and begins with introducing the program to patients from 12 to 15 years of age, depending on the individual patient's maturity and readiness (stage T1). Throughout this phase, readiness assessment is performed by the REACH team and the pediatric urologist remains the primary urologic provider. Next, the adult team is introduced when patients demonstrate advanced readiness, patients are typically greater than 16 years old (stage T2). In stage T3, the patient has been determined to be ready for transition and begins seeing the adult team in the pediatric clinic setting with the availability to the pediatric team. In the final phase of transition (stage T4), the patients are adult patients seen by adult providers in the adult setting.[7]

Dynamic assessment of the transition experience should be ongoing throughout the entire process. For example, it is important not only to gauge transition readiness, but also transition satisfaction once it is complete to improve the experience for future patients. Continued evaluation of development and implementation of transition plans is imperative to improve success rates of transitioning the care of these complex patients in the future.

ADULTHOOD

Because patients with SB are surviving into adulthood, characterizing and addressing their unique urologic needs has become the new challenge

Table 3
REACH transition program framework

Transition Phase	Description
T0	12- to 14-year-olds categorized as eligible to transition once reach adolescence.
T1	Program introduced to patients, typically 12–15 years old. Individual patient's maturity and readiness to transition assessed.
T2	Adult team is introduced when patients demonstrate advanced readiness, typically >16 years old.
T3	Patient determined to be ready for transition. Begins seeing adult team in the pediatric clinic setting. Pediatric team available.
T4	Adult patients seen by adult providers in the adult setting. Transition complete.

Data from Lewis J, Frimberger D, Haddad E, et al. A framework for transitioning patients from pediatric to adult health settings for patients with neurogenic bladder. Neurourol Urodyn 2016. http://dx.doi.org/10.1002/nau.23053.

for adult urologists managing these complex patients. In addition to the lifelong goals of care, adulthood presents new challenges of independence, sexuality, and access to health care.

The issue of appropriate transition recurs in the adult population because patients with SB have been found in the literature to present to adult clinics at a median age of 25 to 26 years indicating a coverage gap between pediatric and adult care.[40,41] As discussed, this can be secondary to lapse in insurance coverage, failure to establish a transition plan, or even the patient's readiness (or lack thereof) to transition. Transition becomes particularly important given that rates of outpatient physician visits and rates of admission were found to be 2.2 and 12.4 times higher, respectively, in adults with SB than for their age-matched peers in 1 study.[42]

The urologic evaluation and management for adults with SB remains complex well into adulthood. A retrospective review of 225 adult patients with a median age of 30 years noted that 70% of adult patients with SB used CIC, 50% were prescribed anticholinergics, and 65% had UDS performed at least once, but only 56% obtained appropriate upper tract imaging every other year.[40] In this cohort, 22% of patients had 1 or more comorbidities with the most common being hypertension (11%), gastroesophageal reflux (5%) and seizures (5%).[40] Of these patients, 45% underwent a urologic procedure during their lifetime. Sixty-three percent of procedures were performed after 18 years of age, indicating that these patients may need urologic continence or bladder procedures even in adulthood, emphasizing the importance of consistent urologic care.

The incidence of stone disease in individuals with neural tube defects is estimated to be 5% to 11%, significantly higher than the general population (1.0%).[43] It is also one of the most common causes for admission in this patient population.[44] Furthermore, in those undergoing interventions for stones, each episode was associated with significantly more stones and longer operative time compared with age-matched peers. These patients also had a higher complication rate (25% vs 16.8%) and there was a lower stone clearance rate (63% vs 86.6%).[45] Similarly, a study looking at ureteroscopy performed in patients with spinal abnormalities found a lower stone free rate and higher complication rate than in children with normal anatomy.[46]

Anywhere from 5% to 25% of patients with SB undergo augmentation cystoplasty and given that patients with SB are surviving into adulthood the potential for long-term complications arises.[47] It is difficult to definitively determine whether enterocystoplasty is an independent risk factor for bladder cancer. In 1 review of a prospective patient registry from the Mayo Clinic, patients treated with augmentation cystoplasty were matched (1:1) with a control group treated with intermittent catheterization.[47] In this cohort, there was no significant difference in the incidence of bladder cancer in patients with augmentation cystoplasty compared with the controls (4.6% vs 2.6%; $P = .54$).[47] However, there was a increased risk of cancer in both groups compared with the general population. Their data also supported the finding that bladder cancer in this population occurs at a younger age with more advanced disease on presentation.[47]

As in the adolescent years, sexual counseling is important and may be easily overshadowed by renal preservation and other chronic medical issues, but it should not be ignored. Compared with their peers, young people with SB reported no difference in sexual interests; however, 67% reported worries about intimate relationships.[35,48] Factors such as incontinence and erectile dysfunction can be obstacles to initiating a relationship; in fact, patients 15 to 35 years old with SB and urinary incontinence were significantly less likely to be sexually active compared with those without incontinence.[49] Furthermore, discussing their disability with peers and partners has been identified as a challenge by these patients, one that they have expressed interest in discussing with health care providers.[35]

SUMMARY

Patients with MMC represent complex patients who require intensive monitoring and treatments but are often underresourced and face additional challenges such as nonverbal learning disabilities and obesity. Although the urologic testing modalities are well-established, the timing and need for the studies is not defined but attempts are being made for standardized surveillance. Renal preservation is the primary goal and is achievable today, but continence, independence, and sexuality are more difficult to manage and achieving success or even stability can be a constant struggle. Each patient presents a unique situation in which treatments can not be standardized; different phases in life offer new challenges and barriers that require vigilant health care interactions and patient dedication. At Rady Children's Hospital, these children are followed in a multidisciplinary spinal defects clinic that includes physical medicine and rehabilitation, neurosurgery, orthopedic surgery, urology, occupational therapy, physical therapy, and social work. Patients are followed with renal bladder

Contemporary Evaluation and Treatment of Poststroke Lower Urinary Tract Dysfunction

CrossMark

Zachary Panfili, MD[a], Meredith Metcalf, MD[a],
Tomas L. Griebling, MD, MPH[a,b,*]

KEYWORDS

- Stroke • Overactive bladder (OAB) • Urinary incontinence • Underactive bladder (UAB)
- Lower urinary tract symptoms (LUTS) • Geriatrics

KEY POINTS

- A detailed clinical history and physical examination are key components to understanding lower urinary tract dysfunction in patients who have experienced stroke.
- The physiology and clinical function of the bladder depend on the location and severity of stroke, and can evolve over time.
- Urodynamic evaluation can be useful cases to evaluate bladder function and guide therapy, but should generally be delayed until the patient has reached a stable point.
- Many therapies can be used to treat poststroke lower urinary tract dysfunction; therapy should be tailored to each individual patient's unique clinical situation and goals of care.

INTRODUCTION

Strokes, sometimes referred to as cerebral vascular accidents, continue to be a leading cause of morbidity and mortality in the United States. Of the 800,000 strokes that occur annually in the United States, approximately 140,000 people die, leaving a substantial patient population with poststroke sequelae, such as urinary incontinence.[1] The prevalence of patients affected by urinary incontinence after a stroke ranges from 28% to 79%.[2] The odds of increased mortality are worse in patients with sustained incontinence at 1 year than those who regain normal function in the same time frame.[3] Poststroke urinary incontinence is a strong predictor of increased disability, greater institutionalization, and mortality.[4] These data suggest that poststroke urinary incontinence, when successfully treated, can improve the quality of life for patients. Additionally, when clinicians address and manage the specific urologic needs of stroke patients, such as urinary incontinence, evidence suggests better stroke outcomes.[5]

The literature for the specific management of lower urinary tract symptoms in stroke survivors is limited. The goal of this review is to evaluate the prevalence, risk factors, types, causes, and contemporary management of voiding dysfunction in stroke survivors. Studies were identified by performing an electronic database search of PubMed, Medline, and Cochrane Library using the following keywords: Stroke, Overactive Bladder (OAB),

[a] Department of Urology, The University of Kansas School of Medicine, 3901 Rainbow Boulevard, Kansas City, KS, USA; [b] The Landon Center on Aging, The University of Kansas School of Medicine, 3901 Rainbow Boulevard, Kansas City, KS, USA
* Corresponding author. Department of Urology, The Landon Center on Aging, Mailstop 3016, The University of Kansas School of Medicine, 3901 Rainbow Boulevard, Kansas City, KS 66160.
E-mail address: tgriebling@kumc.edu

Urol Clin N Am 44 (2017) 403–414
http://dx.doi.org/10.1016/j.ucl.2017.04.007
0094-0143/17/© 2017 Elsevier Inc. All rights reserved.

Urinary Incontinence, Underactive Bladder (UAB), Lower Urinary Tract Symptoms (LUTS), and Geriatrics. Articles reviewed included papers published before 2017 and in English or English translation.

PREVALENCE OF POSTSTROKE INCONTINENCE

Urinary incontinence is a well-described acute poststroke sequela, with reports of incidence at the time of initial hospitalization ranging from 28% to 79%.[6] Patel and colleagues[7] found that 40% of patients were incontinent 1 week after admission to the hospital after a cerebral vascular accident in a population-based study from 2001. Similarly, a community-based study by Kolominsky-Rabas and colleagues[8] spanning a 4-year period that included 699 patients reported incontinence rates of 35% 7 days after stroke in previously continent patients. Those patients with persistent incontinence at 12 months had worse morbidity from their stroke and a greater risk of being institutionalized (45% vs 5%). More recent data from 2012 by Williams and colleagues[4] found that nearly 44% of stroke survivors were incontinent at 3 months and 38% at 12 months with urge urinary incontinence being the most prevalent. If a patient has persistent urinary incontinence at 1 year, this is a predictor of greater mortality, poorer functional recovery, and institutionalization.[9] Importantly, many patients will show improvement in their voiding dysfunction within 1 year after cerebral vascular insult. This finding suggests the need for a dynamic and needs-specific treatment plan.

CAUSES OF POSTSTROKE URINARY INCONTINENCE

The causes of poststroke urinary incontinence seem to be multifactorial and distressing to both patients and their caregivers. It often negatively impacts a patient's well-being by creating social stigma, decreasing quality of life, and creating physical and emotional discomfort.[7] Jørgensen and colleagues[10] found an increased prevalence of urinary incontinence in stroke patients with impaired cognition, poor lower extremity motor function, and signs of depression. Tibaek and colleagues[11] demonstrated through questionnaires an association of poorer sense of well-being in stroke patients with lower urinary tract symptoms compared with stroke patients who did not develop urinary incontinence. Earlier data from Gelber and colleagues[12] prospectively studied 51 patients after a unilateral hemispheric stroke, of which 19 had urinary incontinence. Voiding dysfunction was associated with large infarcts, aphasia, cognitive impairment, and functional disability.

In many stroke patients, urinary incontinence is transient. Patel and colleagues[7] followed 235 patients over a 2-year period and found the prevalence rates of incontinence decreased with time: 19% at 3 months, 15% at 1 year, and 1% at 2 years. Rotar and colleagues[3] found that more than one-half of patients with first-ever stroke had urinary symptoms after vascular insult. Those patients who regained continence quickly after stroke, within 1 week, had a similar prognosis to those who did not have poststroke urinary incontinence. Sustained voiding dysfunction after stroke is a predictor of greater mortality and a poorer functional outcome.[7]

The relationship between infarct size and location with poststroke urinary incontinence remains controversial. An earlier study by Reding and colleagues[13] reported no correlation between infarct size and poststroke urinary incontinence. However, Feder and colleagues[14] did find a significant association between infarct size (>40 mm in diameter) and onset of urinary incontinence. Gelber and colleagues[12] elucidated that infarct size does matter, because it likely disrupts the neuromicturition pathway resulting in detrusor overactivity. More recent data from Patel and colleagues[5] found that patients who experienced total anterior circulatory infarctions were less likely to regain continence compared with patients with lacunar infarctions with an odds ratio of 3.65 (95% confidence interval, 1.1–12.2) at 3 months.

To date, these studies have linked poststroke urinary incontinence with depression, age, hemiparesis, motor weakness, and impaired cognition. There remains controversy about the relationship between infarct size and location, and their roles in poststroke urinary incontinence. This continues to be a fertile area for future research. It is clear, however, that those patients who have sustained incontinence do more poorly than their counterparts who regain continence quickly after a vascular insult.

NORMAL NEUROMICTURITION PATHWAY

Normal neural control of storage and voiding involves complex coordinated communication between the peripheral ganglia, spinal cord, and brain.[15] These pathways control smooth and striated muscles of the bladder, bladder neck, urethra, and sphincters that act in a coordinated manner to allow for bladder filling, or urine storage, and voiding at a socially acceptable time. The voiding reflex is mediated by the spinobulbospinal pathway that is either completely 'off' during the storage phase or 'on' during the emptying phase.[16]

Storage of urine requires the absence of involuntary bladder contraction. The ability of the bladder to accommodate urine is driven by a compliant bladder wall that allows for low pressure filling. This filling is driven by sympathetic stimulation to close the bladder neck through the hypogastric nerve and parasympathetic inhibition via low-intensity afferent signals from the pelvic nerves to decrease detrusor muscle tone. A closed bladder neck is accomplished with both voluntary and involuntary control. Voluntary or somatic stimulation via pudendal nerve outflow through Onuf's nucleus controls the striated or rhabdosphincter. Involuntary, sympathetic stimulation controls smooth muscle sphincter tone from the hypogastric nerve. The 'guarding reflex' is a collection of spinal reflexes that promote continence. Once a critical level of bladder distention is achieved, afferent signals from the pelvic nerves intensify, turning the spinobulbospinal pathway 'on.'[15,16]

Ascending afferent inputs from the pelvic nerves to the spinal cord are relayed to the periaqueductal gray region. After input from the limbic system and frontal lobe, information is relayed to the pontine micturition center (PMC), also called Barrington's nucleus. Stimulation of the PMC will promote urination if activated, whereas suppression will promote bladder filling.[17] Activation of the PMC leads to descending pathways back into the spinal cord that continues back to the bladder and sphincters and voiding (**Fig. 1**A).

Emptying requires the absence of bladder outlet obstruction. The first event in micturition is relaxation of the smooth and striated sphincters. This is accomplished by inhibition of both the sympathetic and somatic pathways respectively, both decreasing sphincter tone. Then, stimulation of the parasympathetic nervous system increases detrusor tone allowing for contraction, thus leading to increased bladder pressure and voiding.

Voluntary control over voiding is initiated in several areas in the suprapontine central nervous system including the cerebral cortex. The thalamus, insula, prefrontal cortex, anterior cingulate gyrus, periaqueductal gray, pons, and medulla are activated during urinary storage and play an important role in voluntary voiding based on functional brain MRI.[15,16] The periaqueductal gray seems to play an essential role in the voluntary storage of urine by relaying ascending signals from the bladder through the spinal cord to the higher control centers of the brain. Once the

information is interpreted, these signals are sent back to the PMC to sustain continued voluntary suppression of the micturition reflex or to allow for voiding if socially acceptable (see **Fig. 1**B).[18]

Tonic inhibition of the voiding reflex during urine storage is maintained by the higher brain centers. Damage to the white matter of the brain, as in stroke, can cause permanent incontinence by disrupting this pathway.[18] When the higher brain centers lose the ability to inhibit the PMC, such as in stroke patients, the voiding reflex cannot be inhibited, reflex voiding occurs, and patients will most commonly present with detrusor overactivity and urge incontinence (see **Fig. 1**C).

To better categorize various forms of lower urinary tract dysfunction based on etiologic factors, Powell[19] has proposed a neurogenic bladder classification system. He has suggested a new scheme to define neurogenic bladder in adults called the SALE system (Stratify by Anatomic Location and Etiology) that has 7 categories based on the anatomic level of neurologic dysfunction. These classification categories include suprapontine disorders (ie, stroke), pontine disorders, suprasacral spinal cord disorders, sacral spinal cord disorders, lower motor neuron disorders, demyelinating disorders, syndromes with no neurologic lesion, and biomarkers.[19] **Box 1** outlines the SALE system with its respective disease processes.

TYPES OF URINARY INCONTINENCE AFTER STROKE

The cause of poststroke urinary incontinence is multifactorial, and data are equivocal as to which cause is associated with the worst outcome. The different types of poststroke urinary incontinence that have been well-described include detrusor overactivity and urge incontinence, detrusor underactivity and overflow incontinence, functional incontinence, impaired awareness incontinence, and exacerbation of preexisting stress incontinence. The types of urinary incontinence are summarized in **Table 1**.

Poststroke Detrusor Overactivity and Urge Incontinence

As discussed in the section on the normal neuromicturition pathway, disruption of the white matter of the higher brain centers alters the tonic inhibition of the voiding reflex during urinary storage at the PMC. This disruption leads to uninhibited bladder contraction or detrusor overactivity and is often accompanied by urge incontinence.[12] Urodynamic testing in stroke patients can vary, but can reveal uninhibited detrusor overactivity in up to 90% of patients.[20] Involuntary urine leakage

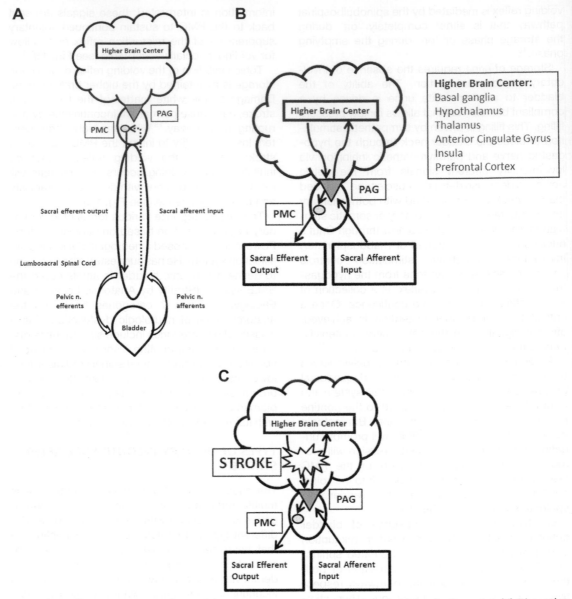

Fig. 1. (*A*) Reflex micturition pathway. (*B*) Voluntary control of micturition via higher brain center. (*C*) Disruption of voluntary micturition control after a stroke leading to uninhibited reflex pathway and detrusor overactivity and urge incontinence. PAG, periaqueductal gray; PMC, pontine micturition center.

accompanied or preceded by urgency are the symptoms most commonly seen by these patients. Questions remain regarding whether the general location or laterality of a hemispheric ischemic lesion plays a role in detrusor dysfunction.[21] Sakakibara and coworkers[22] answered this in some part by finding an association with detrusor hyperreflexia (68% of patients) with localized lesions to the frontal lobe and basal ganglia. Overall, detrusor overactivity is the most common urodynamic finding in stroke patients when higher centers of the brain are affected by an ischemic

event, which is consistent with the neuromicturition pathway.

Poststroke Detrusor Underactivity

The prevalence of detrusor underactivity is less common than overactivity in stroke patients, with rates in the literature of up to 35%.[23] Causes of detrusor underactivity in stroke patients remain unclear, but it has been suggested that existing comorbidities such as diabetic cystopathy or medications such as anticholinergics may be implicated.[12] The

Box 1
Stratify by anatomic location and etiology (SALE classification)

Suprapontine neurologic disorders

- Cerebrovascular accident
- Traumatic brain injury
- Normal pressure hydrocephalus

Pontine neurologic disorders

- Brain tumor
- Cerebellar ataxia syndromes

Suprasacral spinal cord/upper motor neuron disorders

- Spinal cord injury
- Degenerative disc disease
- Spina Bifida

Spinal cord disorders

- Cauda equina syndrome
- After radical pelvic surgery

Lower motor neuron/neuropathy disorder

- Diabetes mellitus
- Peripheral neuropathy
- Guillain-Barre syndrome

Demyelinization disorders

- Multiple sclerosis

Syndromes with no neurologic lesion

- Fowler syndrome
- Dementia

Stratify by biomarker

- Nerve growth factor
- Brain derived neurotrophic factor

prominent symptoms of detrusor underactivity are urinary retention and overflow incontinence, which may include occasional dribbling or continuous leakage.

Poststroke Functional Incontinence

Poststroke urinary incontinence is a strong predictor of increased disability, greater institutionalization, and higher mortality.[4] Jørgensen and colleagues[10] found an increased prevalence of urinary incontinence in stroke patients with impaired cognition, poor lower extremity motor function, and signs of depression. Cognitive and mobility difficulties may affect a patient's ability to maintain continence despite normal bladder function after

a stroke.[6] A report by Gelber and colleagues[12] found the presence of cognitive impairment and speaking difficulty was associated with development of poststroke urinary incontinence. A multivariate analysis by Patel and colleagues[7] found several factors associated with urinary incontinence immediately after stroke, including visual field defects, dysphagia, age greater than 75 years, and motor weakness. If patients are limited by immobility and an inability to communicate the need to void to caretakers after a stroke, it follows that incontinence, intentional or otherwise, would negatively impact their quality of life.

Poststroke Impaired Awareness Urinary Incontinence

Poststroke urinary incontinence also can occur with impaired awareness of the need to void. Pettersen and colleagues[24] followed a cohort of poststroke urinary incontinence patients prospectively and divided the group into 2 categories: urge urinary incontinence and urinary incontinence without awareness of bladder filling and with or without the ability to recognize leakage. The study concluded that incontinence with impaired awareness reflects greater cerebral damage than urge incontinence, involving structures for attention and recognition.

Another study investigated how stroke-related incontinence might be associated with various aspects of attention and mental processing speed and whether impaired awareness urinary incontinence would remain an independent risk factor after 1 year.[25] Of 65 patients with poststroke urinary incontinence, 27 had urge incontinence and 38 demonstrated impaired awareness urinary incontinence. Patients with impaired awareness urinary incontinence performed more poorly in all categories than continent patients and those with urge incontinence (all $P<.01$). The authors went on to explain that this probably reflects greater brain damage. Of the 38 patients with impaired awareness urinary incontinence, 16 were partially aware of leakage, but not of bladder fullness; the remaining 22 denied leakage. The patients with impaired awareness urinary incontinence were significantly more functionally and cognitively impaired and had more visible lesions on computed tomography scans and less frontal lobe involvement than those with urge urinary incontinence.[26]

Poststoke Stress Incontinence

Stress urinary incontinence is a prevalent condition among woman, affecting 10.2% of woman greater than 50 years of age in the general population.[27]

Table 1
Most common types of poststroke urinary incontinence

Type of Incontinence	Etiology	Signs and Symptoms
Detrusor overactivity and urge incontinence	Disruption of white matter of the higher brain centers, alters tonic inhibition of voiding reflex during urine storage at the pontine micturition center	Uninhibited bladder contraction often accompanied by urge incontinence
Detrusor underactivity and overflow incontinence	Etiology unclear, comorbidities and medications may be implicated	Urinary retention as seen with postvoid residual, which may include occasionally leakage or continuous leakage
Functional incontinence	Other systems affected by stroke: impaired cognition, poor motor function, depression	Inability to communicate or mobilize when there is a need to void, may have normal bladder function on urodynamics
Impaired awareness incontinence	Greater cerebral damage caused by stroke involving structures of attention and recognition	Typically more functionally and cognitively impaired without awareness of bladder filling or ability to recognize leakage

Poststroke stress urinary incontinence has been reported in up to 38% of patients.[28] Stress incontinence, although not caused directly by a stroke, may be intensified by weakened pelvic floor muscles and a new urge component.[29]

URODYNAMIC EVALUATION AFTER STROKE

As described, detrusor dysfunction after a stroke seems to be influenced by insult to the normal neuromicturition pathway at the higher brain centers leading to bladder overactivity and incontinence related to impaired awareness, language deficits, immobility, and medication use.[12]

Urodynamic testing is an important tool in assessing new-onset urgency and incontinence after a stroke because it may reveal conflicting results when compared with the clinical picture. Natsume[30] found that poststroke patients presented with various patterns of contractility. On urodynamic testing, 67% of men and 80% of women with symptoms of overactivity actually had underactivity. When comparing computed tomography and MRI studies in individuals who underwent urodynamic testing, Han and colleagues[31] found differences in bladder compliance and capacity and postvoid residuals based on stroke type (ischemic vs hemorrhagic). Ischemic stroke patients were more likely to have detrusor overactivity compared with underactivity in the hemorrhagic group. Similarly, Burney and colleagues[23] correlated urodynamic findings with stroke location. They identified 60 patients, of which two-thirds were ischemic

strokes and one-third hemorrhagic. Eighty-five percent of patients with hemorrhagic strokes presented with detrusor underactivity and 72.5% of those with ischemic strokes presented with detrusor overactivity. Kim and colleagues[21] looked to determine the effect of unilateral hemispheric lesions on lower urinary tract symptoms by comparing urodynamic findings based on dominant, nondominant, or bilateral hemispheric stroke. In the end, they found no differences in urodynamic findings of overactivity or underactivity based on stroke location, but did find that most patients would likely have detrusor overactivity (60.0%–66.7%) compared with underactivity (33.3%-40.0%) overall. Incontinent patients showed a worse functional outcome overall compared with continent stroke patients.

A study by Pizzi and colleagues[32] examined 106 patients with recent stroke in neurorehabilitation centers. Urodynamics were done on all patients at admission and repeated at 30 days in 63 patients. Many different urodynamic patterns were seen, with detrusor overactivity being the most common. This study showed that, over time, urodynamics results can change in a relatively short period of time in patients with ischemic stroke. With changing voiding symptoms over time, an adaptable treatment strategy is needed.

Urodynamics are a useful tool in identifying the underlying cause of voiding dysfunction after a stroke as the clinical picture and the objective findings of a properly completed test can vary. This study is a helpful adjunct that can help in the management and treatment of this complex patient group. A summary of the various urodynamic findings in stroke patients can be found in **Table 2**.

CONTEMPORARY TREATMENT OF POSTSTROKE URINARY INCONTINENCE

Implementing a treatment plan for this patient population is complex, multifactorial, and multidisciplinary. The importance of establishing an accurate picture of the voiding dysfunction after a stroke is essential to creating and implementing a tailored treatment plan.

There is limited stroke-specific research evaluating interventions for this population, but general principles used in the universal treatment of urinary incontinence and bladder overactivity can be adopted in many cases. There are several treatment strategies that can be applied and gleaned from well-established clinical principles and aspects of the American Urologic Associations guidelines for management of 'nonneurogenic' detrusor overactivity in the 'neurogenic' stroke population. A full assessment of a patient's degree and cause of poststroke urinary incontinence should be implemented before starting treatment.

A detailed voiding history before stroke can help clinicians to glean insight into a patient's poststroke voiding dysfunction. This insight may include comorbidities such as diabetes, a history of obstructive uropathy in men, stress urinary incontinence and prolapse in women, onset of symptoms, and bowel habits. In addition to a proper physical examination, a postvoid residual, uroflow test and voiding diary can also be considered.

If the history, physical examination, and noninvasive studies fail to characterize the urinary dysfunction fully, then urodynamics are indicated. For stroke patients who cannot undergo urodynamic testing, a patient's total bladder capacity and postvoid residual may provide useful information for treating patients, because these factors are correlated with urodynamic findings of detrusor overactivity and incontinence.[33] As discussed, urodynamics can unmask a confusing clinical picture; some patients with symptoms of detrusor overactivity actually can have underactivity, a different entity that is treated differently. The use of anticholinergics is effective in treating overactive bladder and is well-established, but should be used judiciously secondary to side effect profiles, which can lead to constipation and changes in cognition, which are of particular importance to the poststroke population.

For patients with detrusor overactivity and incontinence, bladder retraining has shown benefit in many patients in a relatively short period of time. Early treatment plans involved timed voiding, medications, and continence devices. These have been shown to improve long-term poststroke voiding dysfunction compared with those patients with delayed treatment.[34] Bladder retraining is labor intensive, and Booth and colleagues[35] described barriers to bladder retraining in rehabilitation nursing practice, likely owing to a lack of proven beneficial treatments. A recent Cochrane review by Thomas and colleagues[36] in 2008 concluded that the data from available trials are insufficient to guide continence care of poststroke patients, but did show that a multidisciplinary assessment and management of care may reduce incontinence in poststroke patients. If bladder retraining is not effective, then judicious use of anticholinergic medications should be considered.[37]

Level of cognition, mobility, mechanical deficiency, and level of independence should be considered when managing poststroke urinary incontinence. Timed voiding is an established treatment for the management of poststroke impaired awareness urinary incontinence. In a Cochrane Review by Ostaszkiewicz and colleagues[38] in 2004, the data supporting timed voiding as a mainstay in bladder retraining was found to be equivocal. Another Cochrane Review found the use of positive feedback, use of low-dose anticholinergics, staff support, and continence products found the intervention group dry 80% of the time versus 20% in the control group.[39]

In patients with detrusor underactivity and overflow incontinence, intermittent catheterization or an indwelling catheter should be considered.[37] Additionally, an aggressive bowel regimen to prevent constipation and discontinuing medications that may exacerbate symptoms may also be helpful.

It should be noted that men with a history of bladder outlet obstruction and poststroke urinary retention should be managed conservatively before considering surgical intervention. The urinary retention of men immediately after a stroke can typically be managed with clean intermittent catheterization or indwelling catheter until the retention resolves. Alpha-blockers such as tamsulosin or doxazosin can be used as adjunct therapy if not already prescribed.[40] The use of anticoagulation therapy for a period of months is common in the cerebral vascular accident population. This regimen severely limits surgical options in these patients. Several decades ago, Lum and colleagues[41] described the problems with surgical

Table 2
Studies examining poststoke UDS

Author	Purpose	Results	Conclusion
Kim et al,[21] 2010 (n = 69)	Determine effects of unilateral hemispheric stroke on voiding dysfunction using multiple UDS variables	Urodynamic variables did not vary based on laterality of hemispheric stroke patients ($P>.05$). Regardless of laterality, DO and DU was seen in (60.0-66.7%) and (33.3-40.0%) of patients respectively	No significant difference in LUTS between dominant, nondominant, and bilateral ischemic stroke patients
Burney et al,[23] 1996 (n = 60)	Effect of stroke on LUTS and correlated with findings on UDS	Cortical and internal capsule strokes resulted in DO; 85% of hemorrhagic infarcts had hypoactive compared with 10% with ischemic infarction	Confirmed previous data; hemorrhagic infarcts commonly have DU, whereas ischemic have DO
Natsume,[30] 2008 (n = 57)	Investigate detrusor contractility after stroke using UDS	35% of men had DU and 43% of women; 67% of men and 80% of women with DU had DO symptoms; DU was observed in 35% of men with DO symptoms and 42% of women	Patients with DO symptoms can actually be DU on UDS
Han et al,[31] 2010 (n = 84)	Compare bladder dysfunction on UDS in ischemic and hemorrhagic stroke patients	Total bladder capacity, postvoid residual urine volume and bladder compliance vary significantly based on stroke type; ischemic strokes have DO (70.7%), and DU (29.3%) vs and hemorrhagic strokes have DO (34.6%), DU (65.4%; $P = .003$)	Stroke type can be helpful in determining urinary dysfunction and bladder management
Pizzi et al,[32] 2014 (n = 106)	Investigate prognostic effect on functional status and UDS of institutionalized ischemic stroke patients	Incontinence was associated with age and functional disability ($P<.05$); UDS studies at admission showed normal studies in 15%, DO or impaired contractility in 70%, DU in 15%; after 30 days, repeat studies showed normal in 30, DO or impaired contractility in 52% and DU in 16%	Incontinent patients had worse functional outcomes; UDS patterns vary depending on timing of study poststroke and may lead to different treatment/ management strategies

Abbreviations: DO, detrusor overactivity; DU, detrusor underactivity; LUTS, lower urinary tract symptoms; UDS, urodynamics.

intervention in poststroke patients, such as transurethral resection of the prostate. These investigators specifically reported increased rates of incontinence and advocated for avoiding transurethral resection of the prostate after a stroke for 6 to 12 months. Avoiding this type of surgery in the poststroke population is an important concept, not only owing to anticoagulation, but, as discussed, voiding dysfunction can change dramatically over time as patients recover.

Although the American Urologic Association and Society for Urodynamics, Female Pelvic Medicine, and Urogenital Reconstruction guidelines, last modified in May 2014, are for 'nonneurogenic' overactive bladder diagnosis and treatment, many of the principles still apply to stroke 'neurogenic bladder' patients. In stroke patients, a careful history and physical examination are essential. Additional procedures may also be performed in carefully selected patients such as urine culture, postvoid residuals, voiding diaries, and questionnaires. Urodynamics should be considered in stroke patients with equivocal presentations. After the workup is complete, there are multiple lines of treatment available for detrusor overactivity after a stroke.

Behavioral therapies such as bladder training, urge suppression, pelvic floor muscle training, and fluid management can be applied to stroke patients with overactive bladder. Medications such as antimuscarinics and beta-3 agonists can be used as a second-line therapy. Patients should be counseled about the side effects of the medications, including dry mouth, constipation, and confusion for antimuscarinic anticholinergics and hypertension with beta-3 agonists. Importantly, more frequent adverse drug events can occur in frail elderly patients with mobility deficits, weakness, or cognitive decline, particularly with anticholinergic medications.[42] This factor is of particular importance when considering patients in the stroke population, because impaired awareness is a common problem. As of yet, the beta-3 agonists have not been well-studied in the frail elderly and stroke populations.

Neurogenic detrusor overactivity, as in stroke patients, and nonneurogenic detrusor overactivity part ways in management once behavioral modifications and oral medications have been exhausted. In patients refractory to behavioral retraining or oral medications there are third line treatments available to patients with nonneurogenic overactive bladder including intradetrusor injections of botulinum toxin A, percutaneous tibial nerve stimulation (PTNS), and sacral neuromodulation. However, patients with neurogenic detrusor overactivity, including those with stroke, spinal cord injury, multiple sclerosis, and Parkinson disease, represent a diverse patient population with very different and specific needs.

The literature for intradetrusor botulinum toxin injection in stroke patients is limited at this time. Kuo[43] injected 200 U of medication into the bladders of stroke patients. Approximately 50% of patients experienced complete or improved continence, but did experience increased voiding difficulty after treatment. Jiang and colleagues[44] studied the effects of injecting 100 U of medication into neurogenic bladders and found that it effectively improved urgency, but the patients who suffered a stroke had a higher rate of straining to urinate. A recent study by Leitner and colleagues[45] found that 60% of those with neurogenic bladders from all causes had good long-term therapeutic effects from botulinum toxin injections. However, only 10% of study participants were neurogenic from "other" causes, which included stroke, spinal stenosis, and inflammatory diseases other than multiple sclerosis. One of the challenges facing the stroke population is limited mobility and dexterity. With higher risks of urinary retention or incomplete voiding, a patient may require temporary intermittent catheterization. If a patient has limited dexterity secondary to neurologic insult such as stroke, botulinum toxin injections may not be a good treatment option.

PTNS is a minimally invasive therapy to treat overactive bladder symptoms. A recent review of PTNS in neurogenic bladder patients by Schneider and colleagues[46] included 16 studies and 496 patients, but only 25 of those included had suffered a stroke. Their findings suggest some benefit from PTNS as a therapy for overactive neurogenic bladder, but data were limited by poor numbers, confounders, and bias. A randomized, controlled trial by Monteiro and colleagues[47] examined the efficacy of PTNS in 24 stroke survivors. The patients were randomized to either a treatment or control arm. The PTNS cohort experienced effective and durable results at 12 months with no adverse effects. In a similar study comparing subjective symptoms as opposed to objective efficacy of PTNS treatment in stroke patients, Guo and colleagues[48] randomized 61 patients to either the treatment arm or control arm. They found significant improvement ($P<.05$) in frequency, nocturia, urgency, and urge incontinence. Definitive information regarding use of PTNS in stroke patients is limited; however, the preliminary data are promising. For stroke patients who fail more conservative therapy and oral medications, PTNS could be a viable noninvasive treatment that might offer relief.

Another therapy for nonneurogenic bladder overactivity includes sacral neuromodulation. This treatment has not been well-studied in the stroke population, however. Because the majority of stroke patients have significant improvement in continence with behavioral therapies within a relatively short period of time, sacral neuromodulation should not be used in this setting. Some patients with continued incontinence may benefit from subsequent sacral neuromodulation; however, the data on outcomes in this population are limited.

Indwelling urethral and suprapubic catheters are generally not recommended as a long-term management strategy for overactive bladder and are considered only as a last resort. Catheters are typically reserved for patients with progressing decubitus ulcers or patients in whom incontinence negatively affects activities of daily living or other disability that leaves them institutionalized. However, in stroke patients with neurogenic lower urinary tract dysfunction, multiple types of voiding dysfunction including detrusor overactivity, detrusor underactivity, impaired awareness incontinence, and functional incontinence that are refractory to more conservative measures can occur. These patients may be considered for an indwelling catheter more seriously than nonneurogenics. The risks of catheter-associated urinary tract infection, bladder stones, and urethral erosion should be deliberated carefully when choosing a catheter type. Suprapubic catheters are generally preferred over indwelling urethral catheters owing to ease of management and lower risks of tissue injury or erosion. Some patients prefer management with diapers or absorbent pads rather than using an indwelling catheter.

In summary (**Box 2**), current practical interventions for this population include bladder retraining, timed and scheduled voiding, intermittent catheterization, and judicious use of oral medications such as anticholinergics and beta-3 agonists. Mobility needs to be considered when caring for stroke patients, because they should have easy access to a commode, hand-held urinals, and nonrestrictive clothing. Abstinence from caffeine and exacerbating medications is good practice in poststroke voiding dysfunction. The literature is limited at this time on the use of intradetrusor botulinum toxin injections and tibial nerve stimulation. As a last resort, stroke patients with refractory incontinence may consider condom, indwelling, or suprapubic catheters or absorbent pads.

Unfortunately, in addition to voiding dysfunction, many stoke survivors also experience substantial other physical or cognitive impairments that can limit their functional status and quality of life. Embarrassment and depression are commonly associated with functional limitations after a stroke. Empathic care that focuses on specific needs and goals of treatment is crucial.[49]

Box 2
Key points: contemporary treatment of poststroke voiding dysfunction

- Obtain a detailed history including prestroke voiding habits, bowel behavior, obstructive uropathy, stress incontinence, prolapse, and so on.
- Perform a physical examination and obtain a postvoid residual to assess emptying ability.
  - Consider voiding diary, urine culture, and questionnaires.
- Urodynamics are indicated if the clinical picture equivocal.
- Bladder retraining, urge suppression, pelvic floor muscle training, fluid management, timed voiding, medications (anticholinergics,/beta-3 agonists), and continence devices for stroke patients with detrusor overactivity.
  - Judicious use of medications: consider side effects profile.
- Intermittent/indwelling catheterization for patients with detrusor underactivity.
  - Bowel regimen to prevent constipation.
- Timed/prompted voiding regimens for functional incontinence and impaired awareness patients.
- Avoid surgery (ie, transurethral resection of the prostate) for 6–12 mo after stroke because lower urinary tract symptoms may evolve and patients may be on anticoagulation.
- Data is limited on chemodenervation of the detrusor with botulinum toxin A, but may be a good option in carefully selected patients.
  - Avoid in patients unable to straight catheterize.
- Preliminary data for percutaneous tibial nerve stimulation is limited but promising and may be a good option for carefully selected stroke patients refractory to more conservative treatment.
- Sacral neuromodulation has not been well-studied in stroke patients.

SUMMARY

Stroke is an extremely common clinical entity, and poststroke incontinence is a major cause of morbidity for stroke survivors. Although patients can experience a wide variety of lower urinary tract symptoms, detrusor overactivity is one of the most common clinical findings after a stroke. All forms of LUTS can negatively impact physical and psychosocial function for affected patients and their caregivers and loved ones. Careful evaluation is critical for successful management of the condition. Treatment is tailored to the goals and needs of each individual patient. Improvements in continence status can help to enhance overall and health-related quality of life.

REFERENCES

1. Heron M, Hoyert DL, Murphy SL, et al. Deaths: final data for 2006. Natl Vital Stat Rep 2009;57(14):1–134.
2. Brittain KR, Perry SI, Peet SM, et al. Prevalence and impact of urinary symptoms among community-dwelling stroke survivors. Stroke 2000;31(4):886–91.
3. Rotar M, Blagus R, Jeromel M, et al. Stroke patients who regain urinary continence in the first week after acute first-ever stroke have better prognosis than patients with persistent lower urinary tract dysfunction. Neurourol Urodyn 2011;30(7):1315–8.
4. Williams MP, Shrikanth V, Bird M, et al. Urinary symptoms and natural history of urinary continence after first-ever stroke: a longitudinal population-based study. Age Ageing 2012;41(3):371–6.
5. Patel M, Coshall C, Lawrence E, et al. Recovery from poststroke urinary incontinence: associated factors and impact on outcome. J Am Geriatr Soc 2001; 49(9):1229–33.
6. Brittain KR, Peet SM, Castleden CM. Stroke and incontinence. Stroke 1998;29(2):524–8.
7. Patel M, Coshall C, Rudd A, et al. Natural history and effects on 2-year outcomes of urinary incontinence after stroke. Stroke 2001;32(1):122–7.
8. Kolominsky-Rabas PL, Hilz MJ, Neundorfer B, et al. Impact of urinary incontinence after stroke: results from a prospective population-based stroke register. Neurourol Urodyn 2003;22(4):322–7.
9. Turhan N, Atalay A, Atabek HK. Impact of stroke etiology, lesion location and aging on post-stroke urinary incontinence as a predictor of functional recovery. Int J Rehabil Res 2006;29(4):335–8.
10. Jørgensen L, Engstad T, Jacobsen BK. Self-reported urinary incontinence in noninstitutionalized long-term stroke survivors: a population-based study. Arch Phys Med Rehabil 2005;86(3):416–20.
11. Tibaek S, Dehlendorff C, Iversen HK, et al. Is well-being associated with lower urinary tract symptoms in patients with stroke? Scand J Urol Nephrol 2011; 45(2):134–42.
12. Gelber DA, Good DC, Laven LJ, et al. Causes of urinary incontinence after acute hemispheric stroke. Stroke 1993;24(3):378–82.
13. Reding MJ, Winter SW, Hochrein SA, et al. Urinary incontinence after unilateral hemispheric stroke: a neurologic-epidemiologic perspective. Neurorehabil Neural Repair 1987;1:25–30.
14. Feder M, Heller L, Tadmor R, et al. Urinary continence after stroke: association with cystometric profile and computerised tomography findings. Eur Neurol 1987;27(2):101–5.
15. Fowler CJ, Griffiths D, de Groat WC. The neural control of micturition. Nat Rev Neurosci 2008;9(6):453–66.
16. Griffiths D, Tadic SD, Schaefer W, et al. Cerebral control of the bladder in normal and urge-incontinent women. Neuroimage 2007;37(1):1–7.
17. Blok BF, Holstege G. Ultrastructural evidence for a direct pathway from the pontine micturition center to the parasympathetic preganglionic motoneurons of the bladder of the cat. Neurosci Lett 1997; 222(3):195–8.
18. Griffiths D, Tadic SD. Bladder control, urgency, and urge incontinence: evidence from functional brain imaging. Neurourol Urodyn 2008;27(6):466–74.
19. Powell CR. Not all neurogenic bladders are the same: a proposal for a new neurogenic bladder classification system. Transl Androl Urol 2016;5(1): 12–21. This study presents a recommended classification method to help conceptualize various forms of neurologic etiologies for voiding dysfunction. This can help to standardize terminology and comparison across patient groups in clinical practice or research.
20. Gupta A, Taly A, Srivastava A, et al. Urodynamics post stroke in patients with urinary incontinence: is there correlation between bladder type and site of lesion? Ann Indian Acad Neurol 2009;12(2):104–7.
21. Kim TG, Yoo KH, Jeon SH, et al. Effect of dominant hemispheric stroke on detrusor function in patients with lower urinary tract symptoms. Int J Urol 2010; 17(7):656–60.
22. Sakakibara R, Hattori T, Yasuda K, et al. Micturitional disturbance after acute hemispheric stroke: analysis of the lesion site by CT and MRI. J Neurol Sci 1996; 137(1):47–56.
23. Burney TL, Senapti M, Desai S, et al. Acute cerebrovascular accident and lower urinary tract dysfunction: a prospective correlation of the site of brain injury with urodynamic findings. J Urol 1996; 156(5):1748–50.
24. Pettersen R, Haig Y, Nakstad PH, et al. Subtypes of urinary incontinence after stroke: relation to size and location of cerebrovascular damage. Age Ageing 2008;37(3):324–7.
25. Pettersen R, Saxby BK, Wyller TB. Poststroke urinary incontinence: one-year outcome and relationships with measures of attentiveness. J Am Geriatr Soc 2007;55(10):1571–7.
26. Pettersen R, Stien R, Wyller TB. Post-stroke urinary incontinence with impaired awareness of the need to void: clinical and urodynamic features. BJU Int 2007;99(5):1073–7.

27. Komesu YM, Schrader RM, Rogers RG, et al. Urgency urinary incontinence in women 50 years or older: incidence, remission, and predictors of change. Female Pelvic Med Reconstr Surg 2011; 17(1):17–23.

28. Leandro TA, Araujo TL, Cavalcante TF, et al. Nursing diagnoses of urinary incontinence in patients with stroke. Rev Esc Enferm USP 2015;49(6):924–32 [in Portuguese].

29. Tibaek S, Gard G, Jensen R. Pelvic floor muscle training is effective in women with urinary incontinence after stroke: a randomised, controlled and blinded study. Neurourol Urodyn 2005;24(4): 348–57.

30. Natsume O. Detrusor contractility and overactive bladder in patients with cerebrovascular accident. Int J Urol 2008;15(6):505–10 [discussion: 510].

31. Han KS, Heo SK, Lee SJ, et al. Comparison of urodynamics between ischemic and hemorrhagic stroke patients; can we suggest the category of urinary dysfunction in patients with cerebrovascular accident according to type of stroke? Neurourol Urodyn 2010;29(3):387–90.

32. Pizzi A, Falsini C, Martini M, et al. Urinary incontinence after ischemic stroke: clinical and urodynamic studies. Neurourol Urodyn 2014;33(4):420–5.

33. Lee SH, Lee JG, Min GE, et al. Usefulness of total bladder capacity and post-void residual urine volume as a predictor of detrusor overactivity with impaired contractility in stroke patients. Exp Ther Med 2012;4(6):1112–6.

34. Wikander B, Ekelund P, Milsom I. An evaluation of multidisciplinary intervention governed by functional independence measure (FIMSM) in incontinent stroke patients. Scand J Rehabil Med 1998;30(1): 15–21.

35. Booth J, Kumilen S, Zang Y, et al. Rehabilitation nurses practices in relation to urinary incontinence following stroke: a cross-cultural comparison. J Clin Nurs 2009;18(7):1049–58.

36. Thomas LH, Cross S, Barrett J, et al. Treatment of urinary incontinence after stroke in adults. Cochrane Database Syst Rev 2008;(1):CD004462.

37. Roe B, Williams K, Palmer M. Bladder training for urinary incontinence in adults. Cochrane Database Syst Rev 2000;(2):CD001308.

38. Ostaszkiewicz J, Johnston L, Roe B. Timed voiding for the management of urinary incontinence in adults. Cochrane Database Syst Rev 2004;(1): CD002802.

39. Ostaszkiewicz J, Johnston L, Roe B. Habit retraining for the management of urinary incontinence in adults. Cochrane Database Syst Rev 2004;(2):CD002801.

40. Shamliyan TA, Wyman JF, Ping R, et al. Male urinary incontinence: prevalence, risk factors, and preventive interventions. Rev Urol 2009;11(3): 145–65.

41. Lum SK, Marshall VR. Results of prostatectomy in patients following a cerebrovascular accident. Br J Urol 1982;54(2):186–9.

42. Sternberg SA, Schwartz AW, Karurananthan S, et al. The identification of frailty: a systematic literature review. J Am Geriatr Soc 2011;59(11):2129–38.

43. Kuo HC. Therapeutic effects of suburothelial injection of botulinum a toxin for neurogenic detrusor overactivity due to chronic cerebrovascular accident and spinal cord lesions. Urology 2006;67(2):232–6.

44. Jiang YH, Liao CH, Tang DL, et al. Efficacy and safety of intravesical onabotulinumtoxinA injection on elderly patients with chronic central nervous system lesions and overactive bladder. PLoS One 2014; 9(8):e105989. This study examined the efficacy of botulinum toxin injection for bladder chemodenervation in patients with incontinence due to stroke, Parkinson disease or dementia compared to controls. It demonstrated good overall outcomes with improvement in symptoms for those with neurogenic OAB.

45. Leitner L, Guggenbühl-Roy S, Knüpfer SC, et al. More than 15 years of experience with intradetrusor onabotulinumtoxinA injections for treating refractory neurogenic detrusor overactivity: lessons to be learned. Eur Urol 2016;70(3):522–8. This study examined the long-term efficacy (> 10 years) of botulinum toxin injection for bladder chemodenervation in a cohort of patients with neurogenic voiding dysfunction. It showed that 60% of treated patients had good long-term outcomes and continue to pursue this therapy when symptoms recur.

46. Schneider MP, Gross T, Bachmann LM, et al. Tibial nerve stimulation for treating neurogenic lower urinary tract dysfunction: a systematic review. Eur Urol 2015;68(5):859–67. Percutaneous tibial nerve stimulation has been used extensively for nonneurogenic voiding dysfunction, but there has been relatively less research on use of this technology for treatment of neurogenic LUTS. This study reported results of a systematic literature review on the topic. Although the volume and quality of available data was not strong, the preliminary work from both randomized controlled trials and other research appears promising as a form of treatment for neurogenic voiding dysfunction.

47. Monteiro ÉS, de Carvalho LBC, Fukujima MM, et al. Electrical stimulation of the posterior tibialis nerve improves symptoms of poststroke neurogenic overactive bladder in men: a randomized controlled trial. Urology 2014;84(3):509–14.

48. Guo ZF, Liu Y, Hu GH, et al. Transcutaneous electrical nerve stimulation in the treatment of patients with poststroke urinary incontinence. Clin Interv Aging 2014;9:851–6.

49. Pilcher M, MacArthur J. Patient experiences of bladder problems following stroke. Nurs Stand 2012;26(36):39–46.

Parkinson's Disease and Its Effect on the Lower Urinary Tract
Evaluation of Complications and Treatment Strategies

Benjamin M. Brucker, MD[a,b,]*, Sidhartha Kalra, MD[a]

KEYWORDS

- Parkinson's disease • LUTS • Complications • Management

KEY POINTS

- Neurogenic lower urinary tract dysfunction is prevalent in patients with Parkinson's disease (PD) and has a great impact on quality of life, resulting in potentially debilitating sequelae.
- The key to diagnostic and therapeutic effectiveness lies in distinguishing centrally mediated lower urinary symptoms (LUTS) secondary to PD from LUTS that are merely coincidental.
- PD-associated bladder dysfunction is not significantly responsive to levodopa; add-on therapy for ameliorating lower urinary tract problems is often necessary; associated risk should be taken into consideration.
- Prostate reduction surgery for comorbid benign prostatic hyperplasia is no longer contraindicated in this population, assuming multiple system atrophy is excluded.
- We recommend a multidisciplinary approach, with health care providers focusing on motor and nonmotor symptoms and quality of life issues to maximize bladder-specific quality of life.

INTRODUCTION

Parkinsonian syndromes include Parkinson's disease (PD) and atypical Parkinsonism (multiple system atrophy [MSA], progressive supranuclear palsy, corticobasal degeneration, and Lewy body dementia). Differentiating these 2 clinical entities is challenging given the considerable overlap in their clinical profiles, especially early in the disease course.[1] However, careful understanding of the progression of symptomatology can help clinicians in establishing the correct diagnosis.[2] This is an integral aspect for adequate management of motor and nonmotor symptoms, estimating prognosis, and providing information to patients and their

caregivers. Differentiating among syndromes, however, is particularly important for lower urinary tract symptoms (LUTS), which evolve differently and with variable impact and prognoses. Although PD is the most common type of Parkinson's syndrome, 15% to 20% patients presenting with these conditions have an underlying atypical disease process progressing to primary atypical Parkinsonism syndrome or symptomatic Parkinsonism.[3]

PARKINSON'S DISEASE

PD is a progressive degenerative neurologic movement disorder, and motor symptoms are characterized by resting tremor, bradykinesia, (cogwheel)

[a] Department of Urology, New York University Langone Medical Center, 150 East 32nd street second floor, New York, NY 10016, USA; [b] Department of Obstetrics and Gynecology, New York University Langone Medical Center, 550 First Avenue, New York, NY 10016, USA
* Corresponding author. Department of Obstetrics and Gynecology, New York University Langone Medical Center, New York, NY.
E-mail address: Benjamin.Brucker@nyumc.org

Urol Clin N Am 44 (2017) 415–428
http://dx.doi.org/10.1016/j.ucl.2017.04.008
0094-0143/17/© 2017 Elsevier Inc. All rights reserved.

rigidity, and postural instability. PD is estimated to affect 100 to 180 per 100,000 of the population with an annual incidence of 4 to 20 per 100,000.[4] PD is associated with the degeneration of dopamine-producing cells in the substantia nigra of the midbrain and Lewy body formation. Braak and colleagues[5,6] proposed that the formation of intraneuronal Lewy bodies and Lewy neuritis begins at 2 sites and continues in 6 stages, during which components of other systems become progressively involved. In stages 1 to 2, the Lewy body pathology is confined to the medulla oblongata/pontinetegmentum and anterior olfactory structures. In stages 3 to 4, the substantia nigra, other nuclei of the basal midbrain and forebrain, and the mesocortex are affected; the illness usually becomes clinically manifest during this phase. Finally, lesions appear in the neocortex in stages 5 to 6. Lewy bodies and dopaminergic neuron degeneration are also observed in peripheral nerves innervating the gastrointestinal tract, even before the onset of motor symptoms (**Table 1**).[5] Over the last decade, there has been increasing interest in and understanding of nonmotor aspects of PD, which include dysphagia (30%–82% of patients), constipation (>50%), orthostatic hypotension (20%–58%), depression (>16%), cognitive decline and dementia (>6 times higher than healthy individuals), sexual dysfunction (43%–81%), and LUTS.[3]

Prevalence of Urinary Symptoms in Parkinson's Disease

Using validated questionnaires and that analyses that have included subtypes such as atypical

Parkinsonism, the prevalence of LUTS has been reported as urinary disturbances in 27% to 64% of PD patients.[7] Campos-Sousa and colleagues[7] studied 61 patients with PD and 74 control individuals using the International Prostate Symptoms Score. Thirty-nine percent of PD patients reported urinary symptoms on this questionnaire, whereas only 10.8% of control individuals had such symptoms. Nocturia was reported by 64% of PD patients and in 32% of control individuals; urgency was reported by 32% of PD patients and 9% of control individuals. Despite these findings, there is no clear consensus on the nature, severity, or temporal occurrence of LUTS among PD patients, although more data are becoming available as newer studies are using validated questionnaires to follow urinary symptoms. In a review on PD and urinary symptoms, Winge[3] noted that 2 study used the International Prostate Symptoms Score for assessing bladder symptoms and reported that urinary symptoms do not increase with disease severity, whereas another study using the Danish Prostate Symptoms Score questionnaire reported a positive correlation between urinary dysfunction and stage of PD. This seems to indicate that other symptoms, both motor and nonmotor, may affect the overall severity of urinary symptoms. Impaired mobility, tremor, gait, and balance deficits as well as attention span difficulties are thus postulated to exacerbate urinary urgency and other bladder symptoms.

PATHOPHYSIOLOGY OF BLADDER DYSFUNCTION IN PARKINSON'S DISEASE
Normal Neural Control of Micturition

The neurologic control of the bladder is a coordinated action between the somatic and autonomic nervous systems. During the urinary storage phase, the efferent sympathetic nervous system via hypogastric nerves originating in the lumbar spinal cord acts to relax the bladder muscle, as well as maintaining closure of the internal urethral sphincter, thereby helping in storage of urine. Efferent parasympathetic innervation to the bladder, originating in S2–S3–S4 segments of the spinal cord acting via pelvic splanchnic nerves, has the opposite effect of contraction of the detrusor muscle and facilitation of voiding. The central nervous system ensures that micturition occurs under voluntary control, at a time and place that is socially acceptable. Two micturition centers, namely the pontine micturition center and the pontine storage center, have been shown to control the micturition pathway centrally. The former is the more important of the 2 areas and

Table 1 Clinicopathologic correlation in Parkinson's disease		
Lewy Body Neuritis Stage	**Area of Brain Affected**	**Clinical Progression**
1–2	Medulla oblongata/ pontine tegmentum Anterior olfactory structures	Asymptomatic
3–4	Substantia nigra Nuclei of the mid and forebrain Mesocortex	Symptomatic
5–6	Mature neocortex	Advanced disease

Data from Braak H, Ghebremedhin E, Rub U, et al. Stages in the development of Parkinson's disease related pathology. Cell Tissue Res 2004;318:121–34.

facilitates the urinary reflex. Other area of the cortex, such as the periaqueductal gray area, receives afferent information from the bladder concerning degree of bladder fullness, as well as from the hypothalamus and other higher cortical centers. It may act as a relay center, facilitating voiding through connections with the pontine micturition center (**Fig. 1**).[8,9]

MICTURITION AND THE BRAIN–DOPAMINE RELATIONSHIP

Dopaminergic mechanisms have both inhibitory and stimulatory effects on micturition acting via the D1 and D2 receptors, respectively. These neurons are in abundance in the substantia nigra pars compacta and the ventral tegmental area of the midbrain. The substantia nigra pars compacta neuronal firing activates the dopamine D1-GABAergic direct pathway; this inhibits the basal ganglia output nuclei and the micturition reflex. High-frequency stimulation (leading to inhibition) in the subthalamic nucleus (STN) via an indirect pathway also results in bladder inhibition (see **Fig. 1**). Cell depletion in the substantia nigra pars compacta in PD results in loss of this D1-mediated inhibition and consequent detrusor

overactivity. There is also decreased integration of sensory input from the bladder to the periaqueductal gray and a defective ventral tegmental area, which prevents coordinated stimulation of the pontine micturition center at socially acceptable times. Patients with PD do not develop true detrusor–sphincter dyssynergia because the pontine micturition center is spared. In summary, the relationship between motor symptoms and bladder dysfunction in PD is complex and nonlinear. As a result of this complexity, the effects of dopaminergic treatment on bladder control and urodynamic parameters can be unpredictable.[7,10]

URINARY DISTURBANCES IN PARKINSON'S DISEASE

Neurogenic urinary tract dysfunction in PD generally follow the onset of motor disturbances by 4 to 6 years.[11] However, there is no clear consensus on the relationship between neurogenic urinary tract dysfunction and disease variables such as disease stage or duration. Some of the researchers have reported that the neurogenic urinary tract dysfunction may be more related to patients' age rather than the disease itself.[12]

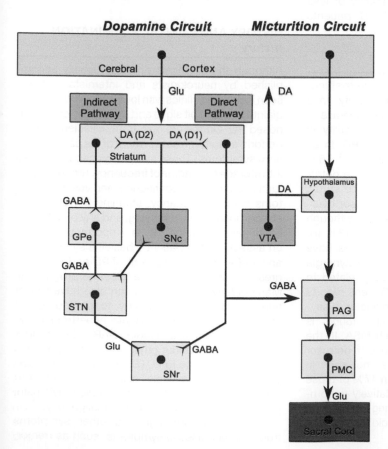

Fig. 1. Micturition and the brain–dopamine relationship. The micturition reflex (*right side pathway*) is under the influence of dopamine (DA; inhibitory D1 and facilitatory D2 receptors) and gamma-aminobutyric acid (GABA) (inhibitory). The substantia nigra pars compacta (SNc) dopaminergic neuronal firing activates the dopamine D1–GABAergic direct pathway, inhibits the basal ganglia output nuclei (eg, SNr), and also inhibit the micturition reflex through GABAergic collateral to the micturition circuit. High-frequency stimulation of the D2 receptor (indirect pathway) inhibits the subthalamic nuclei (STN) and also results in bladder inhibition. Glu, glutamate; GPe, globus pallidus externus; PAG, eriaqueductal gray matter; PMC, pontine micturition center; SNr, substantia nigra pars reticulate; VTA, ventral tegmental area. (*Adapted from* Sakakibara R, Tateno F, Kishi M, et al. Pathophysiology of bladder dysfunction in Parkinson's disease. Neurobiol Dis 2012;46:567; with permission.)

Storage Symptoms

Nocturia is the most common complaint, reported in 60% patients with PD. Urgency occurs in 33% to 54% of patients, and frequency is experienced by 16% to 36% of patients. Urinary incontinence was present in 26% of male and 28% of female patients with PD.[7]

Voiding Symptoms

Voiding symptoms are reported less commonly than storage symptoms in PD. Sakakibara and colleagues[13] reported hesitancy and poor stream to be a complaint in 44% and 70% of men, respectively; 28% of women reported straining to void compared with the control group.

URODYNAMICS, PRESSURE–FLOW ANALYSIS, AND SPHINCTER ELECTROMYOGRAPHY CHANGES IN PARKINSON'S DISEASE
Storage Phase

Reduced bladder capacity and detrusor overactivity are the primary storage phase abnormalities seen in PD. The rate of neurogenic detrusor overactivity in patients with PD is 45% to 93%. In 1 study, a bladder capacity of less than 200 mL was seen in 46% of patients with PD.[13]

Voiding Phase

One of the most common voiding phase dysfunctions seen in PD is detrusor underactivity. In a study of PD and MSA patients, Sakakibara and colleagues[13] found detrusor hypocontractility in 66% of women and 40% of men with PD. In an another study by Araki and colleagues,[14] 16% of 70 patients with PD were found to have detrusor hyporeflexia or areflexia. In the same study, 9% of PD patients had combined detrusor overactivity and detrusor underactivity, although another study reported an incidence of 18% for the same condition.[15] Some older studies have reported detrusor external sphincter dyssynergia or pseudodyssynergia in PD, possibly related to external sphincter bradykinesia. Recent reports comment that detrusor external sphincter dyssynergia is a very rare finding, and if found, is more likely is to be associated with MSA. In the study by Sakakibara and colleagues,[13] detrusor external sphincter dyssynergia was not seen in patients with PD but was present in 47% of those with MSA. Urinary retention is relatively uncommon in PD, irrespective of voiding symptoms, and the average volume of postvoid residuals in PD is less than 100 mL.[13–15]

DIAGNOSIS AND DIFFERENTIATION FROM OTHER CONDITIONS
When Diagnostic Workup Is Appropriate

LUTS are common as patients age, with a variety of causes contributing to this symptom complex. The important questions are: When to initiate a diagnostic workup, and how to perform the right workup? In our opinion, an individualized approach to the specific PD-related urinary problem is the key, and practitioners should consider deviating from a "standardized LUTS" approach when considering multisystem involvement of the disease. For example, practitioners should ask patients having profound motor dysfunction if they are having symptoms because they are unable to adhere to behavioral modifications. Additionally, PD patients with poor dexterity might not be suitable candidates for anticholinergic and botulinum toxin management for bladder overactivity because these treatments may result in the need to start clean intermittent catheterization. Patient's psychological strain (and at times the caregivers) also needs to be considered. Despite these limitations, most PD patients in our practice with mixed lower urinary tract dysfunction can be managed with behavioral modifications and anticholinergics.

HISTORY AND CLINICAL EXAMINATION
History

Although the diagnosis of PD is usually accomplished by neurologists and internists, patients seen in urologic clinics with lower urinary tract complaints may exhibit signs and symptoms of undiagnosed PD. On the urologic front, clinicians should perform a thorough assessment of the patient's urinary symptoms. These symptoms can be divided into storage symptoms of frequency, urgency, nocturia and urgency incontinence, and voiding symptoms such as hesitancy, straining to void, weak stream, incomplete emptying, and any prior history of urinary retention. It is important to have an assessment of patient's baseline symptoms, if any, before the development of PD and their progression over time as the disease progresses. Many elderly male patients can also have similar urinary symptoms secondary to bladder outlet obstruction owing to prostatic hypertrophy and idiopathic overactive bladder (OAB). The provider should also ask about other comorbid conditions that can contribute to LUTS, such as cerebrovascular accident, multiple sclerosis, spinal cord injury, diabetes, constipation, chronic pelvic pain, prior pelvic operations, or pelvic malignancy.[16]

Taking a history regarding other symptoms from primary disease symptoms, such as tremor, bradykinesia, or postural instability, is important in developing an individualized approach. Often, patients do not understand the relationship between the movement disorder and autonomic symptoms.

Current use of any medication should be taken into consideration. Patients frequently use other medication that may alter bladder function and aggravate existing symptoms. For example, diuretics, beta-blockers, and parasympathomimetics can enhance detrusor activity, whereas tricyclic antidepressants abate detrusor activity but increase sphincter activity, possibly resulting in urinary retention. Alpha-blockers have a relaxing action on bladder outlet.

A validated questionnaire may be also useful in addressing primary bothersome urinary symptom and help in documenting the response to therapy. Commonly used questionnaires include the International Prostate Symptom Score and the Lower Urinary Tract Symptom Score.[17] In addition to an interview, a bladder diary is an important adjunct in assessment and directing treatment.

Physical Examination

Clinical examination should include an assessment of the stage of the disease, functional status, urologic examination, and a basic neurologic examination. Blood pressure should be routinely measured because some of these patients have postural hypotension, which can be exacerbated with the use of certain medications, like alpha blockers, that are used in men with PD. The abdomen should be inspected for any scar or a palpable urinary bladder. The local urogenital area should be screened for any skin excoriation from urine and, if possible, an account of the pad soakage and odor of urine should be elicited.

The clinician should assess for sphincteric bradykinesia in addition to the standard urologic examination, such as assessment of prostate size in men and presence of prolapse in women, as well as determination of the stage of PD. Asking the patient to contract their sphincter during the digital rectal examination can crudely do this. The inability to contract the sphincter quickly can have a substantial impact on the ability to prevent urgency incontinence. Urgency in patients with significant sphincteric bradykinesia, neurogenic OAB and mobility issues can result in urgency incontinence or functional incontinence; these conditions have substantial morbidity and a negative impact quality of life. The degree of sphincteric bradykinesia in patients with PD can profoundly affect the ability of patients to delay micturition. Many patients are unable to contract their sphincter quickly enough to delay the urge and

suffer from urge incontinence and decreased quality of life. In addition to affecting quality of life, the presence of sphincteric bradykinesia can also impact the efficacy of treatment, particularly behavioral modification.[16]

Rectal examination should also asses for resting tone, prior anal sphincter tears, fecal impaction, and other rectal pathology, including rectovaginal fistula, tumor, hemorrhoids, or fissure. If fecal impaction if uncovered, it should be treated aggressively because there is often an improvement in urinary symptoms and urinary incontinence as a result.

The neurologic assessment should include cognitive function, motor ability, and a focused neurologic examination to test for the integrity of sacral spinal cord segments. The anal wink and bulbocavernosus reflexes are useful in assessment of sacral arc integrity.[16]

ADDITIONAL DIAGNOSTIC TESTS
Bladder Diary and 24-Hour Pad Test

Bladder diaries provide useful information about a patient's fluid intake, voiding frequency, and voided volumes, as well as urine leakage episodes, pad usage, and so on. This can help in the diagnosis and treatment of urinary incontinence. A patient records the information about intake and voids, and leakage over a set period of time. Various time intervals have been used (24 hours, 2 days, 3 days, 1 week, etc). The 3-day diary seems to be a good balance between obtaining sufficient information and minimizing the burden of data collection for patients. Bladder diaries also are helpful in documenting symptoms, which can be useful in initiating behavioral changes and thus improving patient compliance. The diary should include the volume and time of each void, as well as the severity of the urge that prompted urination—the urge perception score.[18]

Another tool is a 24-hour pad test. This can help to quantify the degree of urine loss better than a standard 24-hour pad count. Patients are asked to bring in all the pads that they used in a 24-hour period and also to bring in a dry pad so the urine weight can be calculated. It must be noted that a pad count is a poor measure of urinary incontinence severity.[19] This procedure can be cumbersome, and may not alter therapy in this population.

Uroflowmetry, Postvoid Residual, and Transabdominal Ultrasonography

The Uroflow is a noninvasive measure of urinary velocity. The volume voided, average flow rate, and maximum flow rate should be reported. Additionally, the pattern of the flow can be commented on. The Uroflow, along with the postvoid residual, is a wonderful screening tool for voiding phase abnormalities. The postvoid residual alone is also a critical measure in treating patients with neurogenic conditions and those with urinary symptoms. Ultrasound imaging can assess for anatomic abnormalities that may have led to the presenting complaints and allows screening of the upper tracts. In men, determination of prostate volume can be helpful.

Urodynamics and Cystoscopy

Urodynamics is a minimally invasive procedure that can give the most accurate assessment of the underlying pathophysiology of lower urinary tract dysfunction in patients with PD. The pressure flow portion can give useful information about bladder sensation, compliance, contractility, the presence of overactivity, and in some cases the presence or absence of obstruction (ie, bladder outlet obstruction index, and bladder contractility index).[20] The addition of fluoroscopic images (videourodynamics) allows determination of the level of obstruction if present (bladder neck, prostate, sphincter, or other) and can add information about sphincter relaxation when electromyography is suboptimal or inconclusive.

The American Urological Association/Society of Urodynamics and Female Urology guidelines statement[21] recommend to consider periodic postvoid residual assessment as a standard (evidence strength grade B) in patients with neurogenic bladder dysfunction (PD and MSA) to monitor for progression regardless of symptoms. Urodynamics is recommended (evidence strength grade C) in these patients, especially in cases not showing symptomatic improvement with initial medical management or in which there is a progressive impairment in bladder emptying as a result of disease process or treatment for bladder dysfunction. However, the role of follow-up urodynamics and its association with the preservation of renal function is less clear, considering that upper urinary tract deterioration is less common in these patients.

Cystoscopy is useful to rule out other bladder pathology and assess bladder and bladder outlet anatomy. Cystoscopy and urodynamics carry a small risk of urinary tract infection, dysuria, hematuria, and postprocedural urinary retention. Postprocedural urinary retention is more common in men with PD. The patient should be informed of this potential risk.

DIFFERENTIAL DIAGNOSIS

The high prevalence of LUTS in the elderly population often precludes adequate diagnosis and treatment in many Parkinson's patients. Often, urinary complaints are accepted to be owing to the primary disease without considering the possibility of another etiology. It is important to have an understanding of all possible factors contributing to the urinary symptoms so as to provide adequate treatment to these patients. Some of the common differential diagnoses can include the following.

- Other causes for urinary incontinence in women. One of the most frequent causes of leakage of urine in elderly women is stress urinary incontinence, a condition that should not be caused by this neurodegenerative disease. Further, OAB secondary to subclinical ischemic brain insult is commonly seen in elderly females.
- Other causes of incomplete emptying in men include benign prostatic hyperplasia (BPH), a very prevalent condition in males. Symptoms may overlap with PD-related urinary symptoms. These patients, besides having frequency and urgency, present primarily with a weak stream and additional residual urine after voiding. Clinically, an enlarged prostate and a diligent history can lead to a correct diagnosis. In cases were there is doubt, additional testing with videourodynamics can be of help.

Differentiation Between Parkinson's Disease and Multiple System Atrophy

MSA is a neurodegenerative condition that presents with symptoms of Parkinsonism along with features of cerebellar ataxia and autonomic failure. As many as 50% of MSA patients are commonly misdiagnosed as having PD. It is important to distinguish these 2 similar clinical entities because their urologic management is different.[22] In MSA, urinary dysfunction may precede motor dysfunction and, therefore, these patients are more likely to be evaluated by an urologist first. At this point, the neurologic symptoms may be subtle. There is diffuse involvement of several neural systems in MSA. Suprapontine involvement is the cause for detrusor overactivity and atrophy of the efferent parasympathetic tracts may result in incomplete bladder emptying. Involvement of Onuf's nucleus is a distinct feature peculiar to MSA not seen in patients with PD. This is the reason for a weak outlet (bladder neck) and increased incidence of urinary incontinence in these patients (60%–100%). Some authors have used external sphincter electromyographic parameters to distinguish between the 2 conditions. Another distinct finding is an elevated postvoid residual seen in 66% versus 16% cases of PD and MSA, respectively (Table 2).[23]

Table 2
Urodynamic abnormalities may aid differentiation between MSA and PD

Urodynamic Parameter	PD	MSA
Detrusor overactivity	At small fill more profound	At larger fill less profound
Sensation	More sensate	Delayed
DESD	Rare	Common
Straining voiding/weak stream	Rare	Common
Voiding efficiency	Preserved	Impaired
PVR	Insignificant	High
Bladder neck on videourodynamics	Closed	Open

Abbreviations: DESD, detrusor–external sphincter dyssynergia; MSA, multisystem atrophy; PD, Parkinson's disease; PVR, postvoid residual.

Data from Sakakibara R, Hattori T, Uchiyama T, et al. Videourodynamic and sphincter motor unit potential analyses in Parkinson's disease and multiple system atrophy. J Neurol Neurosurg Psychiatr 2001;71:600–6; and Kirchhof K, Apostolidis AN, Mathias CJ, et al. Erectile and urinary dysfunction may be the presenting features in patients with multiple system atrophy: a retrospective study. Int J Impot Res 2003;15:293–8.

Sakakibara and colleagues[13,24] reported that 45% of patients with MSA to have detrusor external sphincter dyssynergia on urodynamic assessment. This may account for the higher incidence of incomplete bladder emptying and incontinence in these patients. Additionally, an open bladder neck at rest on voiding cystourethrogram is commonly seen in patients with MSA, although it is not seen in patients with PD, except in those who underwent prostatectomy.

Urinary frequency (33%–45%) and urgency (63%–67%) are also more common in MSA than PD. MSA patients carry a worse prognosis and poor response to surgery. These patients when treated with transurethral resection of the prostate (TURP) for BPH have a high rate of postoperative urinary incontinence (≤100%).

Medical management in the form of anticholinergics for detrusor overactivity, intermittent self-catheterization for high postvoid residual, and desmopressin for nocturnal frequency is the main line of therapy for patients with MSA. TURP and alpha-blockers should be avoided in MSA because they can result in incontinence and postural hypotension, respectively.

MANAGEMENT

Treatment of LUTS in PD should focus on improving quality of life by improving urinary symptoms and at the same time minimizing the morbidity and maximizing the outcomes of treatment options. The morbidity from bradykinesia and immobility and depression/cognitive impairment in these patients makes it extremely difficult to design effective treatment, even with dedicated caregivers. Patient motivation is essential to maximize treatment efficacy. Given the profound cognitive, psychological, and motor limitations, an honest discussion with the patient regarding likely outcomes needs to be accomplished at the onset of treatment (**Table 3**).

Conservative Management

Successful conservative management with behavioral modification can profoundly improve quality of life in patients with PD and LUTS. Behavioral modification includes a multipronged strategy involving patient education, bladder training, fluid and diet management, pelvic floor education, and biofeedback training. Consideration should be given to the patient's living facility, mobility, and dexterity. Patient education can include teaching activities like fluid consumption habits; a bedside commode or urinal when there is difficulty in making to the bathroom, given the motor limitations, is also helpful. Analysis of the bladder diary can give an idea about the patient's bladder capacity (through the maximum voided volume), the presence of polyuria, and the relationship of

Table 3
Detrusor overactivity treatment recommendations in Parkinson's disease

Therapy	Level of Evidence
Bladder training	1
Anticholinergics	2[25]
Botulinum toxin	2[26]
Surgical intervention	2[27]

Data from Sakakibara R, Panicker J, Finazzi-Agro E, et al. A guideline for the management of bladder dysfunction in Parkinson's disease and other gait disorders. Neurourol Urodyn 2016;35:551–63.

voided volume with incontinence, the correlation with grades of urgency (the urge perception score) and voided volume.[18] The patient is asked to start voiding at a shorter interval than her usual and once this is managed without any leakage, the intervals between the voids are gradually increased in a step ladder pattern taking into consideration their limited mobility. Patients with urgency incontinence without significant sphincteric bradykinesia can be given a trial of biofeedback to teach for contraction of their sphincter for preventing incontinence.[16]

Medical Management

Medical therapy should be started if lifestyle modifications prove ineffective. Consideration should be given to patient-specific bladder dysfunction, cognitive function, primary disease stage, and other factors, such as dexterity and constipation. Side effects of many drugs can exaggerate the primary disease and can make the situation worse.

The main drugs used for the treatment of motor symptoms are levodopa (L-dopa), dopamine agonists, and monoamine oxidase type B inhibitors.[28] Treatment for motor dysfunction have a mixed effect (either ameliorate or worsen) on bladder function in PD.

Levodopa

L-Dopa is a precursor of dopamine and has been the standard therapy for motor dysfunction in PD patients. It is generally prescribed in combination with a peripheral dopa-decarboxylase inhibitor (ie, carbidopa or benserazide). The effect of L-dopa on LUTS in PD patients is unclear. Studies have shown that acute D2 receptor activation worsens bladder function and tonic activation of D1 receptors inhibits bladder voiding. Dopamine's affinity for D1 receptors is lower when compared with D2 receptors.

L-Dopa and dopamine agonists both have been shown to have a mixed effect on bladder symptoms. Although L-dopa initially may exacerbate urinary symptoms, longer usage has been shown to improve bladder symptoms. Brusa and colleagues[29] evaluated 26 L-dopa–naive PD patients with urodynamic session in the off treatment condition and 1 hour after acute challenge with carbidopa/L-dopa 50/200 mg and then after 2 months of L-dopa therapy. They found that the first acute L-dopa challenge significantly worsened detrusor overactivity (32% worsening) and bladder capacity (22% worsening); in contrast, an L-dopa challenge during chronic administration ameliorated the first sensation of bladder filling (120% improvement), detrusor overactivity (93% improvement), and bladder capacity (33% improvement) versus the

values obtained with acute administration. Chronic L-dopa administration, possibly owing to the combined stimulation of both D1 and D2 receptors, may improve bladder capacity and the volume at which micturition reflex is activated.

It is likely that the D2-mediated effect prevails over the D1-mediated effect after acute L-dopa administration in naive patients, which might suppress the nigral cells and facilitate the micturition reflex. A long-term L-dopa treatment produces a higher synaptic concentration of the drug optimal for D1 and D2 activation, which can inhibit bladder voiding and improve bladder function. It can also cause a downregulation of dopamine receptors that correlates with the development of motor fluctuations.[17,28]

Dopamine agonists

Dopamine receptor agonists works by binding directly with the postsynaptic dopamine receptors. They are classified as ergolinine (bromocriptine, pergolide, cabergoline, lisuride) or nonergolinine (pramipexole, ropinirole, and apomorphine) drugs. Some studies have shown them to improve storage function in PD. One of the questionnaire-based studies reported voiding symptoms (intermittency and sensation of residual urine) to be greater in patients taking L-dopa and bromocriptine (D2-selective agonist) than in those taking L-dopa alone.

This was in contrast to where bromocriptine was changed to pergolide (D1 < D2 agonist), in which the incidence of nocturia lessened.[30] Apomorphine use has been shown to improve bladder capacity.[31] No randomized, controlled trials have been reported in literature with effects of L-dopa or dopamine agonists for the treatment of bladder dysfunction.

Monoamine oxidase type B inhibitors

Monoamine oxidase type B inhibitors (selegiline and rasagiline) work by blocking the metabolism of dopamine, thereby increasing its level. Recently rasagiline, was found to improve urodynamic findings in early mild PD patients. Rasagiline administration significantly ameliorated bladder volume measurements in comparison with baseline. A post hoc analysis showed a significant ($P<.001$) increase in bladder capacity and in first desire to void while significantly decreasing residual volume. However, further research is needed to substantiate their benefit in bladder dysfunction.[32]

Drugs for Overactive Bladder in Parkinson's Disease

Anticholinergics (muscarinic acetylcholine receptor antagonists) are used as a second-line of therapy for OAB (behavioral modification is considered a first-line therapy). However, side effects such as dry mouth, constipation, and cognitive dysfunction not only decrease adherence with these drugs, but can also exacerbate the symptoms of the Parkinson's, thereby limiting their use. It is important to balance the therapeutic benefits with the potential adverse effects.

Studies have shown the centrally acting anticholinergic, trihexyphenidyl (used in PD), to exacerbate cognitive function in humans.[33] Factors determining cognitive effects of these medications include (i) central muscarinic receptor affinity (high M1-receptor selectivity) and (ii) penetration of the blood–brain barrier and lipid solubility. Most of the anticholinergics for OAB are nonselective muscarinic blockers.[34]

Regarding blood–brain barrier penetration, oxybutynin, owing to its high lipophilicity and neutrality, can readily penetrate the central nervous system in comparison with other anticholinergic agents. This concern was first described by Donnellan and colleagues,[35] who reported 4 cases of acute confusional states in elderly patients with a preexisting cognitive impairment treated with oxybutynin. This cognitive dysfunction reversed after discontinuation of oxybutynin. There are numerous commercially available antimuscarinic agents. Listed below are those with some efficacy data in treating OAB in PD.

Oxybutynin

Bennett and colleagues[36] evaluated the efficacy and tolerability of higher doses of oxybutynin chloride in 7 PD patients. Extended release oxybutinin at a 5 mg weekly increment to a maximum dose of 30 mg/d was prescribed, guided by patient perception of efficacy versus side effects. At the end of the study, there were statistically significant decreases in the number of voids over 24 hours, episodes of nocturia, and incontinence episodes. Residual urine remained unchanged. No patient experienced serious adverse events. Currently, there are not many well-designed studies of clinical use of oxybutynin in PD patients.

Trospium

Trospium is a quaternary ammonium derivative with mainly antimuscarinic actions. Being a quaternary amine, trospium has a high polarity that may limit blood–brain barrier penetration and cognitive adverse events. It has not been studied regarding efficacy or morbidity in patients with Parkinson's. The European Association of Urology guidelines recommend that trospium be given to cognitively impaired patients when compared with anticholinergics.[37]

Solifenacin

Solifenacin is competitive against the M3 receptor antagonist. Recently, Zesiewicz and colleagues[38] conducted a placebo-based, randomized, controlled trial studying the use of solifenacin succinate for OAB in PD. In the double-blind phase, the primary outcome measure (mean number of micturitions per 24-hour period) was not seen to improve significantly with the use of solifenacin succinate. However, there was an average decrease of 1.18 urinary incontinence episodes per 24-hour period in the solifenacin group. In the open-label phase of the study, there was a significant improvements mean daily number of urinary incontinence episodes (from a baseline of 1.33 ± 1.54 to 0.52 ± 1.01), the number of nocturia episodes (from 2.67 ± 1.08 to 1.64 ± 1.09; $P = .01$), the patient's perception of their bladder condition ($P = .01$). By the end of the open-label phase, 56% of participants (9/16) took 10 mg solifenacin succinate daily. Solifenacin succinate was generally well-tolerated. Treatment associated adverse events during the double-blind period included constipation (1/9 participants on active treatment, 0/12 on placebo), xerostomia (2/9 participants on active treatment, 0/12 on placebo), and urinary retention (1/9 participants on active treatment, 0/12 on placebo), which all resolved upon treatment discontinuation. The authors concluded that treatment with solifenacin succinate decreases the number of urinary incontinence episodes; however, the clinical effect on other bladder symptoms was not significant.

Mirabegron

Mirabegron, a selective beta-3 adrenergic receptor agonist, has been extensively used for OAB without any significant cognitive adverse events. Currently, no specific well-designed studies have assessed the clinical use of mirabegron in PD. It could be a useful alternative to anticholinergics in these patients considering the side effect profile. However, there was a report of mirabegron precipitating dyskinesia in a 72-year-old women with PD. The authors commented that mirabegron could precipitate dyskinesia in those already prone to the disorder, owing to the changes in striatal pathways that occur with chronic dopamine depletion and use of L-dopa.[39] Larger observational studies would be required to determine whether mirabegron could precipitate dyskinetic movements in patients with PD who have not yet developed L-dopa-induced dyskinesia.

In general, anticholinergics remain the mainstay for treating OAB symptoms in PD patients. Perez-Lloret and colleagues[40] compared use of different antimuscarinic agents in women with PD and urinary incontinence. Fesoterodine was found to be the most effective in this study and the order of efficacy, as assessed by percent of women with restored continence, was fesoterodine > oxybutynin > trospium > solifenacin > tolterodine.

In 2006, Winge and Fowler[41] in their review found that in PD patients with a postvoid residual of greater than 100 mL, the use of clean intermittent self-catheterization in addition to antimuscarinic therapy is beneficial in relieving storage symptoms.

Use of selective serotonin reuptake inhibitors and desmopressin

The 5-hydroxytryptamine (or serotonin) reuptake inhibitors have been shown to facilitate urine storage. In PD, neuronal cell loss in the raphe nucleus has been documented. Therefore, serotonergic drugs, such as duloxetine and milnaciplan, can be an off-label choice to treat OAB in PD.[42] These drugs should be used with caution, especially in patients on L-dopa therapy, because there is an increased risk of serotonin toxicity. In patients with PD, the imbalance between diurnal and nocturnal production of urine can be observed in the course of the disease. Treatment with desmopressin proved to be effective in reducing nocturia in PD, although this medication requires extreme caution of water intoxication.[43]

Drugs for Voiding Lower Urinary Tract Symptoms

Alpha blockers

Alpha-blockers have been reported to be useful for the treatment of neurogenic bladder by decreasing urethral resistance during voiding. Gomes and colleagues[44] studied the correlation between LUTS improvement with doxazosin and neurologic disease status in PD patients. They used the Unified Parkinson's Disease Rating Scale for disease

classification and the International Continence Society Male Short Form questionnaire for Urologic symptom assessment. At 12 weeks of treatment with 4 mg extended release doxazosin, there was a reduction in the International Continence Society Male Short Form questionnaire for Urologic symptom assessment score from 17.4 ± 7.5 to 11.1 ± 6.9 (P = .001) and change in maximum urinary flow rate from 9.3 ± 4.4 to 11.2 ± 4.6 mL/s (P = .025). Patients with a Unified Parkinson's Disease Rating Scale score of less than 70 had a 3.1-fold higher chance of clinical improvement with doxazosin treatment than those with a higher Unified Parkinson's Disease Rating Scale score. This was a single arm study without a control group and improvement in symptoms could have been secondary to a placebo effect. A larger randomized trial could give better insight into the use of alpha-blockers in PD. Practitioners should use caution when prescribing alpha-blockers in PD patients because they can result in postural hypotension, especially in patients with MSA.

MINIMALLY INVASIVE MANAGEMENT

Both PD and BPH can present with LUTS in late middle-aged men, thus necessitating their differentiation. LUTS starts insidiously in PD and there can be considerable diagnostic difficulty in its early stage. **Table 4** summarizes urodynamic differences between PD and BPH patients with LUTS.

Limited data suggest that men with concomitant BPH and PD can safely be offered TURP whenever necessary to maximize patients' quality of life. In a retrospective study, 23 men with PD and BPH underwent TURP. At a median postoperative follow-up of 3 years after TURP, the procedure was successful in 16 of the 23 patients (70%), with no further need for catheterization in 9, complete urinary continence in 3, and normalization of urinary

Table 4
Urodynamic findings between lower urinary tract symptoms in Parkinson's disease and benign prostatic hyperplasia

Urodynamic Parameter	Parkinson's Disease	Benign Prostatic Hyperplasia
Detrusor overactivity	Phasic at low volume and more profound	Mostly terminal
Detrusor overactivity incontinence	More common	Less common
Pressure flow	Nonobstructed voiding	Obstructed voiding
Sphincteric activity	Bradykinesia	Normal guarding reflex
Postvoid residual	Insignificant	Can be elevated

Data from Defreitas GA, Lemack GE, Zimmern PE, et al. Distinguishing neurogenic from non-neurogenic detrusor overactivity: A urodynamic assessment of lower urinary tract symptoms in patients with and without Parkinson's disease. Urology 2003;62:651–5.

frequency in 4. The risk of de novo urinary incontinence is minimal.[45] Although these data are limited, we believe that TURP is a viable option for men with PD and refractory BPH.

However, as mentioned, it is important to make a clear distinction between MSA and PD (see **Table 2**) because the incontinence of MSA rarely improves after prostate surgery.[13,46] If there is a clinical suspicion that a patient has MSA, nonsurgical management of bladder symptoms should be considered (level of evidence 2).[16]

INTRAVESICAL BOTULINUM TOXIN INJECTION FOR OVERACTIVITY IN PARKINSON'S DISEASE

Intravesical injection of onabotulinumtoxinA (BOTOX) is the newest approved treatment for urinary incontinence in adult neurologic patients with an inadequate response to (or reduced tolerance of) anticholinergic medications (US Food and Drug Administration approval in 2011).[47] Patients with PD presents with further complexity because of age and general neuromuscular disability. There are limited data specifically on the use of botulinum toxin for bladder treatment in the PD population. In 2009, Giannantoni and colleagues[26] studied the effect with 200 U of onabotulinumtoxin type A in 4 patients with PD and 2 patients with MSA. The authors were of the conclusion that onabotulinumtoxin A injections into the detrusor muscle are an effective and safe treatment for refractory OAB symptoms and detrusor overactivity related to PD. In 2010, Kulaksizoglu and colleagues[48,49] reported a series of 16 patients—10 female and 6 male PD patients receiving an alternative formulation of abobotulinumtoxin A (Dysport) at a dosage of 500 IU. An overall improvement in voiding frequency was seen in all these patients. However, 6 patients were almost completely incontinent and used diapers, and thus the daily urinary frequency assessment could be skewed. None of these patients required intermittent or indwelling catheterization after the procedure.

The largest study of onabotulinumtoxin therapy for PD patients was from 2014. Anderson and colleagues[50] conducted a study to asses for the safety and effectiveness of low-dose (100 U) onabotulinumtoxinA in 20 patients with PD and incontinence. Twelve men and 8 women were treated with mean age of 70.4 years, median bladder contraction volume of 115 mL, maximum bladder pressure of 62 cm, and postvoid volume of 9 mL. Moderate to marked symptom relief at 3 months and a 50% incontinence decrease over 6 months relative to pretreatment was reported in 59%

patients ($P \leq .02$); 5 patients failed to complete the 6-month endpoint. No urinary retention required catheterization. The authors concluded that office cystoscopy with a low-dose onabotulinumtoxinA injection treatment is a potential long-term management strategy for patients with PD and urinary incontinence who do not respond to oral antimuscarinic agents.

We believe that some non-PD botulinum toxin studies can be extrapolated to suggest efficacy in the PD groups. For example, a non-PD patient trial studied the safety and effectiveness of using 200 U onabotulinumtoxinA in an elderly population (mean age, 81.2 years) with refractory idiopathic OAB. Of study population, 76% reported a greater than 50% improvement with no treatment complications. We suggest that, given the high degree of disability in this group, data may be potentially applicable to extrapolate to the patients with PD group.[48]

Similar to TURP, it is important to differentiate MSA from PD before completing botulinum injections because the risk of urinary retention is higher in patients with MSA. Currently, no recommendation for dosages, risk factors for retention, or difficulty voiding or long-term effectiveness are available for MSA. Careful patient selection with regard to urinary bladder contractility on urodynamics, postvoid residual, and bladder outlet obstruction in males can improve patient outcomes and minimize potential complications with therapy.

NEUROMODULATION FOR DETRUSOR OVERACTIVITY IN PARKINSON'S DISEASE

Although electrical neuromodulation technology is available and occasionally useful, it is incompletely studied in neurogenic bladder overactivity in patients with PD and the neuromodulation technology is not specifically Food and Drug Administration cleared for this indication in PD.[51] Kabay and colleagues[52] evaluated the acute effects of posterior tibia nerve stimulation on the clinical and urodynamic findings in PD patients with detrusor overactivity. Forty-seven patients underwent 12 weekly posterior tibia nerve stimulation treatments. At the end of 12 weeks, there was a statistically significant improvement in the first involuntary detrusor contraction volume and maximum cystometric capacity. Mean parametric changes in daytime frequency decreased by 5.6 voids daily, urge incontinence decreased by 3.1 episodes daily, urgency episodes decreased by 6.3 episodes daily, nocturia decreased by 2.7 voids, and voided volume improved by a mean of 92.6 mL. The authors concluded that these findings are encouraging for further evaluation of the effective use of posterior tibia nerve stimulation in clinical practice for detrusor overactivity in PD patients. These data should be verified with a prospective multicenter study before this treatment is introduced in routine clinical practice.

Newer Modalities: Deep Brain Stimulation

The STN is the key area in the basal ganglia that regulates the indirect pathway, which is dominant in the parkinsonian state. Deep brain stimulation (DBS) of the STN has shown promising results for motor symptoms in PD patients.[53] Multiple small studies with STN DBS have been performed in humans with bladder symptoms and have shown mixed results regarding efficacy. In 2012, Winge and Nielsen[54] studied patients with advanced PD receiving oral medications treated using either DBS in the STN or with anapomorphine pump. Patients treated with DBS in the STN had a similar amount of LUTS as patients treated with either conventional oral medication therapy or anapomorphine pump; however, these patients exhibited significantly less nocturia ($P = .007$). In another study, Kessler and colleagues[27] compared for urodynamic parameters in the on and off state of thalamic DBS in patients with essential tremor on DBS for 15 to 85. They found a significant decrease in bladder volume at first desire to void, at strong desire to void, and at maximum cytometric capacity in the on state when compared with 30 minutes in an off state. The authors concluded that thalamic DBS resulted in an earlier desire to void and decreased bladder capacity, suggesting a regulatory role of the thalamus in lower urinary tract function. Therefore, the thalamus may be a promising target for the development of new therapies for lower urinary tract dysfunction. Seif and colleagues[55] demonstrated STN-DBS to have a normalization effect on urodynamic parameters in the storage phase with a delayed first desire to void and an increased bladder capacity. Although DBS may be a promising therapy for LUTS based on a small number of studies, a very low number of cases described any worsening of urologic disorders. Further research on this topic can improve on the treatment strategy for LUTS in PD.

SUMMARY

The topic of lower urinary tract dysfunction in patients with PD is one of great importance given its impact on quality of life and potentially debilitating sequelae. An important area of understanding is in distinguishing centrally mediated LUTS secondary to PD from LUTS that are merely coincidental. Urodynamics is a key investigative tool to determining the presence (and potential cause) of bladder outlet obstruction as well as bladder function abnormalities. It can also help in differentiating patients with MSA. It should be actively incorporated in assessment of these patients when there is a specific question to answer and the study may help to guide therapy. In men with concomitant symptoms from an enlarged prostate, BPH treatments can be considered. Prostate reduction surgery (ie, TURP) for comorbid BPH in PD is no longer recognized as contraindicated, assuming MSA is excluded. In cases of storage symptoms, behavioral modification and pelvic floor exercises should be encouraged. Clinicians should consider regarding patient's living facility, mobility, dexterity, goals, and overall health status. With regard to bladder management, dopaminergic drugs have been shown to both improve and worsen LUTS in PD. Therefore, add-on therapy with anticholinergics is often required for bothersome OAB symptoms. Although there are limited data in PD, beta-3 adrenergic agonist they may have a role given the lack of cholinergic burden centrally. Botulinum toxin can be used for intractable urinary incontinence in PD with a risk of impairing bladder emptying. Data on other third-line therapies in this population are limited. Newer interventions, such as DBS, are expected to improve bladder dysfunction in PD. The collaboration of urologists with neurologists is highly recommended to maximize patients' bladder quality of life.

REFERENCES

1. Gilman S, Wenning GK, Low PA, et al. Second consensus statement on the diagnosis of multiple system atrophy. Neurology 2008;71:670–6.
2. Hughes AJ, Daniel SE, Ben Shlomo Y, et al. The accuracy of diagnosis of parkinsonian syndromes in a specialist movement disorder service. Brain 2002; 125:861–70.
3. Winge K. Lower urinary tract dysfunction in patients with parkinsonism and other neurodegenerative disorders. Handb Clin Neurol 2015;130:335–56.
4. National Collaborating Centre for Chronic Conditions. Parkinson's disease: national clinical guideline for diagnosis and management in primary and secondary care. London: Royal College of Physicians; 2006. p. 121–4.
5. Braak H, Ghebremedhin E, Rub U, et al. Stages in the development of Parkinson's disease related pathology. Cell Tissue Res 2004;318:121–34.
6. Hattori T, Yasuda K, Kita K, et al. Voiding dysfunction in Parkinson's disease. Jpn J Psychiatry Neurol 1992;46:181–6.

7. Campos-Sousa RN, Quagliato E, da Silva BB, et al. Urinary symptoms in Parkinson's disease: prevalence and associated factors. Arq Neuropsiquiatr 2003;61:359–63.

8. Fowler CJ. Integrated control of lower urinary tract: clinical perspective. Br J Pharmacol 2006;147:14–24.

9. Yokoyama O, Yoshiyama M, Namiki M, et al. Changes in dopaminergic and glutamatergic excitatory mechanisms of micturition reflex after middle cerebral artery occlusion in conscious rats. Exp Neurol 2002;173:129–35.

10. Sakakibara R, Tateno F, Kishi M, et al. Pathophysiology of bladder dysfunction in Parkinson's disease. Neurobiol Dis 2012;46:565–71.

11. Bonnet AM, Pichon J, Vidailhet M, et al. Urinary disturbances in striatonigral degeneration and Parkinson's disease: clinical and urodynamic aspects. Mov Disord 1997;12:509–13.

12. Gray R, Stern G, Malone-Lee J. Lower urinary tract dysfunction in Parkinson's disease: changes related to age and not disease. Age Ageing 1995; 24:499–504.

13. Sakakibara R, Hattori T, Uchiyama T, et al. Videourodynamic and sphincter motor unit potential analyses in Parkinson's disease and multiple system atrophy. J Neurol Neurosurg Psychiatr 2001;71:600–6.

14. Araki I, Kitahara M, Oida T, et al. Voiding dysfunction and Parkinson's disease: urodynamic abnormalities and urinary symptoms. J Urol 2000;164:1640–3.

15. Yamamoto T, Sakakibara R, Uchiyama T, et al. Neurological diseases that cause detrusor hyperactivity with impaired contractile function. Neurourol Urodyn 2006;25:356–60.

16. Sakakibara R, Panicker J, Finazzi-Agro E, et al. A guideline for the management of bladder dysfunction in Parkinson's disease and other gait disorders. Neurourol Urodyn 2016;35:551–63.

17. Araki I, Kuno S. Assessment of voiding dysfunction in Parkinson's disease by the international prostate symptom score. J Neurol Neurosurg Psychiatr 2000;68:429–33.

18. Blaivas JG, Panagopolous G, Weiss JP, et al. The urgency perception score: validation and test-retest. J Urol 2007;177:199–202.

19. Tsui JF, Shah MB, Weinberger JM, et al. Pad count is a poor measure of the severity of urinary incontinence. J Urol 2013;190:1787–90.

20. Nitti VW. Pressure flow urodynamic studies: the gold standard for diagnosing bladder outlet obstruction. Rev Urol 2005;7:14–21.

21. Winters JC, Dmochowski RR, Goldman HB, et al. Urodynamic studies in adults: AUA/SUFU guideline. J Urol 2012;188:2464–72.

22. Quinn N. Parkinsonism–recognition and differential diagnosis. Br Med J 1995;310:447–52.

23. Kirchhof K, Apostolidis AN, Mathias CJ, et al. Erectile and urinary dysfunction may be the presenting features in patients with multiple system atrophy: a retrospective study. Int J Impot Res 2003;15:293–8.

24. Sakakibara R, Uchiyama T, Yamanishi T, et al. Genitourinary dysfunction in Parkinson's disease. Mov Disord 2010;25:2–12.

25. Katzenschlager R, Sampaio C, Costa J, et al. Anticholinergics for symptomatic management of Parkinson's disease. Cochrane Database Syst Rev 2003;(2):CD003735.

26. Giannantoni A, Rossi A, Mearini E, et al. Botulinum toxin A for overactive bladder and detrusor muscle overactivity in patients with Parkinson's disease and multiple system atrophy. J Urol 2009;182:1453–7.

27. Kessler TM, Burkhard FC, Z'Brun S, et al. Effect of thalamic deep brain stimulation on lower urinary tract function. Eur Urol 2008;53:607–12.

28. The National Collaborating Centre for Chronic Conditions, editor. Symptomatic pharmacological therapy in Parkinson's disease. Parkinson's Disease. London: Royal College of Physicians; 2006. p. 59–100.

29. Brusa L, Petta F, Pisani A, et al. Acute vs chronic effects of L-dopa on bladder function in patients with mild Parkinson disease. Neurology 2007;68:1455–9.

30. Kuno S, Mizuta E, Yamasaki S, et al. Effects of pergolide on nocturia in Parkinson's disease: three female cases selected from over 400 patients. Parkinsonism Relat Disord 2004;10:181–7.

31. Aranda B, Cramer P. Effect of apomorphine and l-dopa on the parkinsonian bladder. Neurourol Urodyn 1993;12:203–9.

32. Brusa L, Musco S, Bernardi G, et al. Rasagiline effect on bladder disturbances in early mild Parkinson's disease patients. Parkinsonism Relat Disord 2014;20:931–2.

33. Schrag A, Schelosky L, Scholz U, et al. Reduction of parkinsonian signs in patients with Parkinson's disease by dopaminergic versus anticholinergic single-dose challenges. Mov Disord 1999;14:252–5.

34. Sakakibara R, Uchiyama T, Yamanishi T, et al. Dementia and lower urinary dysfunction: with a reference to anticholinergic use in elderly population. Int J Urol 2008;15:778–88.

35. Donnellan C, Fook L, McDonald P, et al. Oxybutynin and cognitive dysfunction. BMJ 1997;315:1363–4.

36. Bennett N, O'Leary M, Patel AS, et al. Can higher doses of oxybutynin improve efficacy in neurogenic bladder. J Urol 2004;171:749–51.

37. Staskin D, Kay G, Tannenbaum C, et al. Trospium chloride has no effect on memory testing and is assay undetectable in the central nervous system of older patients with overactive bladder. Int J Clin Pract 2010;64:1294–300.

38. Zesiewicz TA, Evatt M, Vaughan CP, et al. Randomized, controlled pilot trial of solifenacin succinate for overactive bladder in Parkinson's disease. Parkinsonism Relat Disord 2015;21:514–20.

39. Murchison AG, Fletcher C, Cheeran B. Recurrence of dyskinesia as a side-effect of mirabegron in a patient with Parkinson's disease on DBS (GPi). Parkinsonism Relat Disord 2016;27:107–8.

40. Perez-Lloret S, Rey MV, Pavy-Le Traon A, et al. Emerging drugs for autonomic dysfunction in Parkinson's disease. Expert Opin Emerg Drugs 2013;18:39–53.

41. Winge K, Fowler CJ. Bladder dysfunction in Parkinsonism: mechanisms, prevalence, symptoms and management. Mov Disord 2006;21:737–45.

42. Sakakibara R, Ito T, Uchiyama T, et al. Effects of milnacipran and paroxetine on overactive bladder due to neurologic diseases: a urodynamic assessment. Urol Int 2008;81:335–9.

43. Suchowersky O, Furtado S, Rohs G. Beneficial effect of intranasal desmopressin for nocturnal polyuria in Parkinson's disease. Mov Disord 1995;10:337–40.

44. Gomes CM, Sammour ZM, Bessa Junior JD, et al. Neurological status predicts response to alpha-blockers in men with voiding dysfunction and Parkinson's disease. Clinics (Sao Paulo) 2014;69:817–22.

45. Roth B, Studer UE, Fowler CJ, et al. Benign prostatic obstruction and Parkinson's disease should transurethral resection of the prostate be avoided. J Urol 2009;181:2209–13.

46. Sakakibara R, Shinotoh H, Uchiyama T, et al. Questionnaire-based assessment of pelvic organ dysfunction in Parkinson's disease. Auton Neurosci 2001;92:76–85.

47. Abrams P, Cardozo L, Khoury S, et al. Incontinence. International Consultation on Urological Diseases ICUD–EAU. 5th edition; 2013.

48. Kulaksizoglu H, Parman Y. Use of botulinum toxin-A for the treatment of overactive bladder symptoms in patients with Parkinson's disease. Parkinsonism Relat Disord 2010;16:531–4.

49. White WM, Pickens RB, Doggweiler R. Short-term efficacy of botulinum toxin A for refractory overactive bladder in the elderly population. J Urol 2008;180:2522–6.

50. Anderson RU, Orenberg EK, Glowe P. Onabotulinumtoxin A office treatment for neurogenic bladder incontinence in Parkinson's disease. Urology 2014;83:22–7.

51. Campeau L, Soler R, Ander E, et al. Bladder dysfunction and Parkinsonism: current pathophysiological understanding and management strategies. Curr Urol Rep 2011;12:396–403.

52. Kabay S, Canbaz KS, Cetiner M. The clinical and urodynamic results of percutaneous posterior tibial nerve stimulation on neurogenic detrusor overactivity in patients with Parkinson's disease. Urology 2016;87:76–81.

53. Krack P, Batir A, Van Blercom N, et al. Five-year follow-up of bilateral stimulation of the subthalamic nucleus in advanced Parkinson's disease. N Engl J Med 2003;349:1925–34.

54. Winge K, Nielsen KK. Bladder dysfunction in advanced Parkinson's disease. Neurourol Urodyn 2012;31:1279–83.

55. Seif C, Herzog J, van der Horst C. Effect of subthalamic deep brain stimulation on the function of the urinary bladder. Ann Neurol 2004;55:118–20.

Chronic Urinary Retention in Multiple Sclerosis Patients

Physiology, Systematic Review of Urodynamic Data, and Recommendations for Care

John T. Stoffel, MD

KEYWORDS

• Multiple sclerosis • Urinary retention • Neurogenic bladder • Urodynamics

KEY POINTS

• Urinary retention is common in patients with multiple sclerosis (MS). Cross-sectional self-reported survey data show that 1 in 4 MS patients performs intermittent catheterization.

• Urinary retention in patients with MS can be caused by neurogenic underactive bladder and/or bladder outlet obstruction from detrusor sphincter dyssynergia (DSD). Pooled urodynamic data (1997–2017) show that 53% of patients with MS have detrusor overactivity, 43% have DSD, and 12% have atonic bladder.

• It is recommended that urinary retention in patients with MS be defined as post–void residual volume greater than 300 mL. Prospective studies are needed to validate this threshold value.

• Relationship between elevated post–void residual and risk of urinary tract infection or upper tract pathophysiology has not been well defined.

• Treatment algorithm for management of MS-related urinary retention is proposed based on stratifying patients by risk of morbidity from chronic urinary retention and then bothersome symptoms. Low-risk, asymptomatic patients with MS with chronic urinary retention should not be followed conservatively and not treated until they become symptomatic.

INTRODUCTION

Multiple sclerosis (MS) is an inflammatory autoimmune disease that affects approximately 100 per 100,000 people.[1] The disease more commonly affects younger women and can be characterized into relapsing versus progressive disease types. Urinary symptoms are highly prevalent among patients with MS. The 2005 North American Research Committee on Multiple Sclerosis (NARCOMS) survey collated responses from almost 10,000 patients with MS and reported that 65% of the responders experienced at least one moderate to severe urinary symptom.[2] Over time, MS urinary symptoms tend to increase in severity. Tepavcevic and colleagues[3] recently studied 93 patients with MS over a 6-year timeframe, and demonstrated symptoms of bladder dysfunction were reported by approximately 50% of men and women with MS on presentation

Department of Urology, University of Michigan Hospital, University of Michigan, 3875 Taubman Center, 1500 East Medical Center Drive, Ann Arbor, MI 48109, USA
E-mail address: jstoffel@med.umich.edu

Urol Clin N Am 44 (2017) 429–439
http://dx.doi.org/10.1016/j.ucl.2017.04.009
0094-0143/17/© 2017 Elsevier Inc. All rights reserved.

and by 75% of men and women after 6 subsequent years with the disease.

Over the past 10 years, there have been significant improvements in diagnosing and treating MS. The McDonald criteria for diagnosing MS were revised in 2010 and now provide a greater degree of standardization for identifying patients with MS through clinical symptoms, MRI findings, and cerebral spinal fluid evaluations.[4] These revised criteria have resulted in earlier diagnosis of MS.[5] New treatment methodologies have also expanded care and support options for patients with MS. Compared with past treatments, contemporary treatment algorithms now include escalating disease-modifying therapies[6] and shared decision making in a team-based care environment.

Urologic care for the MS patient has also improved. Urologic symptom-specific treatment algorithms have been developed in the British, French, and Italian Health Systems.[7–9] Advances have occurred in understanding the efficacy of anticholinergic medications[10] and botulinum toxin[11] in treating MS-related overactive bladder. Similarly, studies have demonstrated significant improvement of MS-related nocturia for the patient taking desmopressin.[12] Published outcomes on surgical interventions for patients with MS with refractory neurogenic bladder symptoms are likewise becoming more common in the literature.[13,14]

However, despite these advances, there is uncertainty regarding the optimal strategy for managing MS-related urinary retention. The prevalence and impact of urinary retention among patients with MS are significant; Mahajan and colleagues[15] reanalyzed responses from the NARCOMS survey and found that approximately 1 in 4 MS patients performs some type of catheterization. Furthermore, the patients catheterized reported consistently lower quality of life across multiple domains. The purpose of this review is to describe the physiology, presentation, diagnosis, and treatment of MS-related urinary retention. A systematic review of MS-related urodynamic data was also performed.

PHYSIOLOGY OF URINARY RETENTION

The bladder detrusor consists of 3 layers of overlapping smooth muscle, which have no insertion or origin points. An extracellular matrix surrounds the detrusor muscle and acts a scaffold of support. It is a constantly remodeled matrix and consists of collagen (type 1 and 3), elastic fibers, adhesive proteins, glycans, and glycoproteins.[16] Bladder storage requires sympathetic nervous system stimulation of alpha- and beta-adrenergic receptors to close the bladder outlet and relax the detrusor muscle. There are 3 subtypes of $\alpha 1$ receptors ($\alpha 1a$, $\alpha 1b$, and $\alpha 1d$), but the $\alpha 1a$ subtype in the prostate and urethra is primarily responsible for contraction of the bladder outlet.[17] There are 3 subtypes of beta-receptors, and stimulation of $\beta 2$- and $\beta 3$-receptors facilitates detrusor smooth muscle relaxation and bladder storage.[18] Bladder contraction and emptying is facilitated by parasympathetic stimulation of the muscarinic cholinergic receptors. Although there are 5 known subtypes of muscarinic receptors (M1 to M5), the human detrusor has a preponderance of M2 (70%), M3 (20%), and M1 (10%) receptors.[19] M3 receptors are principally responsible for detrusor contraction, but inactivation of M3 in knockout mice models shows that M2 receptors can also stimulate detrusor activity. M2/M3 receptors may also trigger some afferent reflex activity based on a neurogenic bladder rat model, which may result in uninhibited contraction of the detrusor muscle.[20] It is unclear how muscarinic receptors function in an acontractile bladder, but mice models suggest that M3 receptors become dysregulated and not coupled to detrusor stimulator.[21]

When the bladder fills, afferent sensory nerves are stimulated. The bladder neck and proximal urethra have the greatest concentration of afferent nerve bundles, and the bladder dome has the lowest concentration.[22] In a rat model, 2 types of afferent nerves, myelinated A-delta and unmyelinated C fibers, carry sensory information from the bladder to the spinal cord through the pelvic and pudendal nerves. Delta fibers are located mostly in the detrusor muscle and are activated with bladder stretching. C fibers are located closer to the urothelium and respond to stimulus such as pain and temperature stimuli. C fibers are thought to have a higher threshold of activation.[23] It is postulated that some urinary retention may be related to detrusor muscle decompensation and/or poor afferent signaling.[24]

Afferent sensory nerves enter the dorsal spinal cord through the S2-S4 nerve roots. Sensory information is carried cephalad by the spinothalamic tract in the spinal cord to the periaqueductal gray (PAG) region in the midbrain region. In some cases, overstimulation of urethral afferent nerves may inhibit bladder afferent nerves and thus cause urinary retention through a loss of communication to the central nervous system.[25] When the bladder fills, the PAG activates and inhibits the pontine micturition complex (PMC) in the brainstem. The PMC is held in a state of inhibition by the PAG throughout bladder filling.[26] During storage, sympathetic efferent nerves exiting the spinal cord at T10-L2 and traveling through the hypogastric nerve in the pelvis stimulate B3 receptors in the detrusor and alpha 1 receptors in the bladder neck. Stimulation of the sympathetic nervous system causes the bladder to relax and the outlet to close. As the bladder fills, the medial prefrontal cortex and the hypothalamus modulate PAG activity and generate consciousness about bladder fullness.[26]

During bladder emptying, the PMC is no longer inhibited, and the parasympathetic nervous system is activated. Preganglionic parasympathetic efferent nerves exiting from the sacral spinal cord at the S2-4 then stimulate the parasympathetic nervous system through the pelvic nerve. When the parasympathetic system is active, interneurons in the spinal cord inhibit sympathetic stimulation and the bladder outlet relaxes.[27] The pelvic plexus ganglia then stimulate the detrusor muscarinic receptors and voiding commences. **Fig. 1** summarizes these pathways.

Patients with MS can develop urinary retention because of an underactive detrusor and/or and obstructed outlet. Basic and imaging research suggests that disruptions of neurologic signaling are most likely responsible for either of these causes, rather than primary detrusor failure. Altuntas and colleagues[28] demonstrated this in an experimental autoimmune encephalomyelitis (EAE) mouse model in which mice with urinary retention had notable inflammation found in the spinal cord after development of EAE, but minimal initial inflammation in the bladder. MRI findings also suggest MS-related urinary retention may be linked with lesions location in the central nervous system. Araki and colleagues[29] reviewed MRI and urodynamic studies from 32 patients with MS and found a strong correlation between pons lesions and detrusor underactivity. Similarly, Weissbart and colleagues[30] examined quality-of-life questionnaires of patients with MS with pontine lesions and noted that larger lesions were associated with weaker stream. Araki and colleagues[29] also showed a strong relationship between patients with cervical spinal cord lesions and detrusor sphincter dyssynergia (DSD) findings on urodynamics. Khavari and colleagues[31] studied 23 ambulatory women with MS and demonstrated that DSD findings were associated greater activation of the right caudate nucleus and brainstem. It is postulated that disruption of the signaling tracts between the PMC and the sacral spinal cord, particularly in the cervical spinal cord region, can cause high urethral closure pressures during a

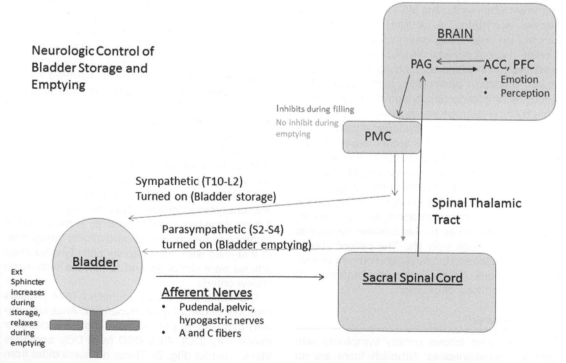

Fig. 1. Neurophysiology of urinary tract. PFC, prefrontal cortex. ACC, anterior cingulate cortex; PAG, periaqueductal grey; PFC, prefrontal cortex; PMC, pontine micturition center.

detrusor contraction and result in DSD for both men and women.[32]

DIAGNOSIS OF URINARY RETENTION IN PATIENTS WITH MULTIPLE SCLEROSIS
Definition

There is no universally accepted post–void residual (PVR) value that defines urinary retention in the MS population. In the United Kingdom, the consensus statement on management of MS-related urinary symptoms defined retention as greater than 100 mL. Amarenco and colleagues[8] recommended that French patients with MS with greater than 300 mL PVR should be referred for specialty assessment because this PVR adds to complexity of management. A consensus definition is needed for patients with MS. Without a standardized definition, it is challenging to compare risk among patients and treatment efficacy. The author recommends that greater than 300 mL, measured at least twice in 2 months, be used as a defacto threshold value for chronic urinary definition because this value has been proposed by the American Urological Association Chronic Urinary Retention Workgroup to define nonneurogenic urinary retention.[33]

History

A patient's urinary-specific history is critically important when evaluating MS-related neurogenic bladder symptoms. A detailed history follows focused on onset/progression of MS symptoms, current musculoskeletal impact, and additional systemic manifestations, such as cognitive and bowel function, particularly constipation. The author recommends classifying MS urinary symptoms by type (storage vs emptying), frequency of occurrence, severity, and systemic impact to the person. If incontinent, the author assesses not only for inability to delay urination and leakage with physical activity but also for functional incontinence (ie, limited mobility preventing timely micturition). When taking a history, voiding diaries should be reviewed for functional bladder capacity and to gain insight as to how bladder symptoms ultimately influence daily life. The patient should also be questioned about past and current urinary tract infections (UTIs), including frequency of infections and type of organism.

Questionnaires

The author also follows urinary symptoms with validated questionnaires. Although there are no specific questionnaires that focus exclusively on urinary retention, there are several effective questionnaires that can be used for following urinary symptoms in the MS population, including the American Urologic Associated Symptom Index,[34] urogenital distress index,[35] and Michigan incontinence severity index.[36] These questionnaires are not specific to the neurogenic bladder population but can be useful in characterizing general urinary symptoms. Additional neurogenic bladder-centric questionnaires continue to be developed. Welk and colleagues[37] have recently published a patient-reported neurogenic bladder symptom score that focuses on domains of incontinence, storage/voiding symptoms, and consequences. Regarding MS-specific urinary-specific questionnaires, the Actionable Bladder Symptom and Screening Tool was developed to identify and follow patients with MS with symptomatic neurogenic detrusor overactivity (NDO).[38] The cumulative information from both the history and validated questionnaire such as these will ultimately help the treating provider identify a current symptom baseline and the impact of symptoms. Any subsequent treatments should be compared against this clinical baseline to determine efficacy when addressing patient quality of life.

Urodynamics

There are no clear best recommendations as to when to use urodynamics for assessing urinary symptoms in the patient with MS. Dillon and Lemack[39] have pointed out that urinary symptoms do not always predict urodynamic findings in patients with MS. At the author's institution, thye perform urodynamics in patients with MS to differentiate whether a symptomatic elevated PVR is from bladder outlet obstruction or from underactive bladder. Both of these findings are prevalent among patients with MS with urinary symptoms.

The author examined the contemporary MS urodynamic literature and performed a systematic review of patients with MS undergoing screening urodynamics between January 1997 and January 2017. Literature search was performed for MS and urodynamic articles. Studies were excluded if there were less than 50 patients in the cohort, if incomplete description of urodynamic categories, or if studies were after intervention. Two hundred articles were identified, and 12 met the systematic review criteria.

The systematic review identified 1524 patients with MS undergoing urodynamics. Analysis showed that 53% of patients demonstrated detrusor overactivity (DO), 43% DSD (with DO), and 12% atonic bladder (**Fig. 2**). These numbers differ from a previous systematic review performed in 1999.[40] The author suggests that advances in MS

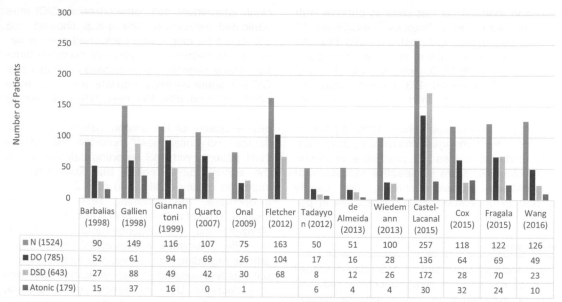

Fig. 2. System review of patients with MS studied with urodynamics 1997–2016. (*Data from* Refs.[41,44,62–68])

	Barbalias (1998)	Gallien (1998)	Giannan toni (1999)	Quarto (2007)	Onal (2009)	Fletcher (2012)	Tadayyo n (2012)	de Almeida (2013)	Wiedem ann (2013)	Castel-Lacanal (2015)	Cox (2015)	Fragala (2015)	Wang (2016)
■ N (1524)	90	149	116	107	75	163	50	51	100	257	118	122	126
■ DO (785)	52	61	94	69	26	104	17	16	28	136	64	69	49
■ DSD (643)	27	88	49	42	30	68	8	12	26	172	28	70	23
■ Atonic (179)	15	37	16	0	1		6	4	4	30	32	24	10

OAB treatments could have skewed referral patterns to urology such that urologists may be performing urodynamics on a different cohort of patients with MS compared with the past 20 years. It is possible that overactive bladder may be now treated more commonly by the patient's primary care team and thus may explain the marked increase in DSD findings (43% vs 25%) and reduction in DO.

MANAGING CHRONIC URINARY RETENTION IN PATIENTS WITH MULTIPLE SCLEROSIS
Identification of Risk Related to Chronic Urinary Retention

It is the author's practice to screen all patients with MS with a PVR at the first visit. Patients with a PVR greater than 300 mL are subsequently assessed as to whether the residual volume is associated with risk to the patient (chronic UTIs, hydronephrosis on imaging, fall risk from incontinence). There are some data suggesting that elevated PVR may increase risk of pyelonephritis and UTIs among patients with MS. Gallien and colleagues[41] retrospectively studied 179 patients with MS referred for urodynamics over a 5-year period and found that the patients with a history of pyelonephritis had a mean PVR of greater than 30% of the functional capacity on urodynamics. Kornhuber and Schutz[42] published a study in which 350 patients with MS were followed for urinary retention. They found that patients with PVR greater than 50 mL had more dementia and bactiuria.[42] There are few other data that draw associations between PVR, urinary symptom severity, and upper tract risk. **Box 1**

summaries some potential signs and symptoms of risk potentially associated with urinary retention in the MS population (extrapolated from American Urological Association nonneurogenic chronic urinary retention white paper).[33]

Patients with MS with DSD, with or without retention, may also be at risk for subsequent systemic morbidity. In other neurologic conditions, such as spinal cord injury and spina bifida, patients with DSD may develop low bladder compliance and subsequent risk renal failure over time.[32] However, the relationship between

---

Box 1
Indications of "high-risk" chronic urinary retention

Radiologic findings

- Hydronephrosis
- Hydroureter

Laboratory findings

- Stage 3 chronic kidney disease (estimated glomerular filtration rate 30–59 mL/min/1.73 m^2)
- Recurrent, symptomatic, culture-proven UTI
- Culture-proven systemic urosepsis

Signs and symptoms

- Urinary incontinence associated with perineal skin changes
- Urinary incontinence associated with sacral decubitus ulcers

DSD and morbidity is less clear in patients with MS. de Seze and colleagues[43] examined 11 studies comprising 1200 patients with MS and noted an increased risk of upper tract changes among those with DSD. However, Fletcher and colleagues[44] screened 173 patients with MS with renal ultrasound and found upper tract changes in only 6%. Over a median 61-month follow-up of a censured cohort, 12% of patients had upper tract changes. Urodynamic diagnosis, particularly DSD, was not predictive of developing changes. More prospective studies, with standardized inclusion criteria, are clearly needed to understand DSD-related risk in patients with MS.

Medications

Pharmacologic treatment of MS-related urinary retention has had not great success in reducing PVR or symptoms. In theory, pro–contractility medications such as bethanechol could help improve bladder emptying for patients with MS with underactive bladder. However, there are no randomized trials or large cohort studies that have examined the efficacy of bethanechol in the MS population. Anecdotally, the author has not seen much improvement in PVR when bethanechol is attempted as treatment in MS-related urinary retention. Similarly, there are little data examining the efficacy of alpha-blocker for reducing PVR or symptoms in patients with MS, either with or without DSD. Stankovich and colleagues[45] administered tamsulosin 0.4 mg to 28 patients with MS with DSD for 60 days and demonstrated a reduction in PVR and a 58% improvement in quality-of-life indexes. O'Riordan and colleagues[46] studied the effects of indoramin in 18 men over 4 weeks and found a 26% reduction of PVR compared with a 24% reduction in the placebo group. Based on the low quality of evidence currently available, the National Clinical Guideline Center in the United Kingdom recommended in 2012 that caregivers not give alpha-blockers for any bladder-emptying problem caused by a neurologic disease.

Catheterization

Intermittent and indwelling catheters have long been mainstay therapy for MS-related urinary retention. Intermittent catheterization is preferred for patients with good hand function and who are still able to void. Patients learning intermittent catheterization benefit from a rigorous instructional program, such as described by Wyndaele.[47] Vahter and colleagues[48] also demonstrated that 87% (20/23) of patients with MS could perform clean intermittent self-catheterization (CIC) after dedicated instruction. The group showed that CIC could be taught and performed even in patients with decreased physical or cognitive function. Many patients with MS have concerns that CIC will negatively impact quality of life and cause additional morbidity. However, NARCOM survey data suggest that catheterization generally improves quality of life among patients with MS. James and colleagues[49] reported that of the 1201 patients with MS reporting catheter use in the survey, 52% replied that catheterization improved quality of life, and only 25% reported a decrease. The remaining 19% reported no change. Type of catheter used in intermittent catheterization may also influence morbidity and quality of life. Shamout and colleagues[50] reviewed 31 articles regarding CIC among neurogenic bladder patients and concluded that hydrophilic catheters may decrease UTI's incidence, reduce urethral trauma, and improve satisfaction among neurogenic bladder patients.

If a patient with MS cannot perform CIC, an indwelling catheter may be beneficial. An indwelling urethral catheter can be temporarily placed until neurologic symptoms return to baseline in relapsing-remitting patients or used as long-term drainage as a suprapubic tube for advanced primary or secondary progressive patients. The UK MS treatment guidelines recommend long-term drainage with a suprapubic tube rather than a urethral catheter to limit catheter-related complications.[7] Kidd and colleagues[51] performed a systemic review of catheterization outcomes for hospitalized adults (neurogenic and nonneurogenic) and found that suprapubic tubes were associated with less asymptomatic bacteriuria, recatheterization, and pain. There are several case series reporting severe complications from selected patients with long-term indwelling urethral catheters.[52] More studies are needed to determine risk and quality of life related to catheterization in patients with MS.

Neuromodulation

Neuromodulation is an approved treatment for nonneurogenic, nonobstructive urinary retention. Although neuromodulation is increasingly being studied to treat neurogenic detrusor overactivity, little data exist that evaluate the efficacy of this modality for neurogenic, or MS specifically, urinary retention. However, some small case series show encouraging results. Engeler and colleagues[53] published an 18-patient series that examined staged neuromodulation outcomes for

MS-related urinary symptoms, including both detrusor overactivity and DSD. Sixteen of the 18 patients progressed to second-stage implantation. At 3 years' follow-up, the investigators reported that both the median voided volume increased (125 mL preimplantation to 265 mL post, $P = .001$) and the median PVR decreased (170 mL to 25 mL, $P = .01$). However, most patients underwent frequent reprogramming to maintain treatment benefit and 31% needed a formal revision. Marinkovic and Gillen[54] reported outcomes of sacral neuromodulation for 14 patients with MS with urinary retention and using intermittent catheterization. Twelve of the patients progressed to second-stage implantation and over a mean follow-up of 4 years decreased their PVR to a mean 50 mL.[54] Minardi and Muzzonigro[55] presented a case series of 5 patients with MS for 10 to 44 years treated with neuromodulation and commented that 4/5 patients had lower PVRs or decreased frequency of intermittent catheterization. Although the numbers in these series are small, many of the patients who responded to neuromodulation had a longstanding diagnosis of MS.

These data may argue for attempts to be focused in patients with MS with longstanding, rather than acute, urinary retention.

Posterior tibia nerve stimulation (PTNS) offers a different type of less invasive neuromodulation. PTNS could be a particularly important to patients with MS because an implantable, non MRI compatible, sacral neuromodulator will limit the patient's ability to have body MRI evaluations. There are some data showing improved bladder emptying after PTNS. Gobbi and colleagues[56] reported outcomes for PTNS treatment of 21 patients with MS (mean duration of disease 10 years) and found the PVR decreased from 98 to 43 mL ($P = .02$) over a 12-week treatment period. Kabay and colleagues[57] similarly published that PVR decreased from 83 mL to 48 mL ($P = .006$) after PTNS. However, none these patients had a primary diagnosis of urinary retention, so it is difficult to extrapolate efficacy. Similar to sacral neuromodulation, there are a few large prospective studies examining PTNS in the MS population,[58,59] and the cohorts that exist have few patients with chronic urinary retention.

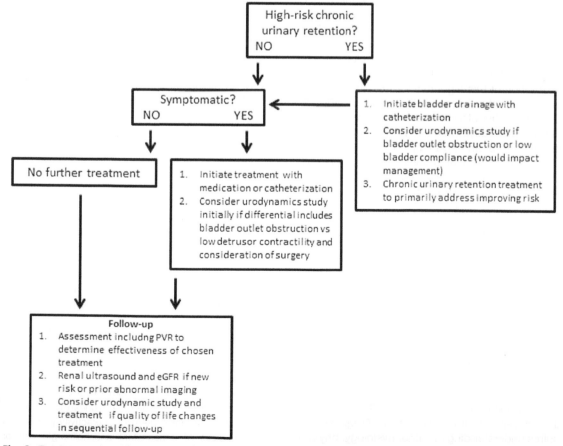

Fig. 3. Treatment algorithm proposed. eGFR, estimated glomerular filtration rate.

40. Litwiller SE, Frohman EM, Zimmern PE. Multiple sclerosis and the urologist. J Urol 1999;161(3): 743–57.

41. Gallien P, Robineau S, Nicolas B, et al. Vesicoure- thral dysfunction and urodynamic findings in multi- ple sclerosis: a study of 149 cases. Arch Phys Med Rehabil 1998;79(3):255–7.

42. Kornhuber HH, Schutz A. Efficient treatment of neurogenic bladder disorders in multiple sclerosis with initial intermittent catheterization and ultrasound-controlled training. Eur Neurol 1990; 30(5):260–7.

43. de Seze M, Ruffion A, Denys P, et al. The neurogenic bladder in multiple sclerosis: review of the literature and proposal of management guidelines. Mult Scler 2007;13(7):915–28.

44. Fletcher SG, Dillon BE, Gilchrist AS, et al. Renal deterioration in multiple sclerosis patients with neu- rovesical dysfunction. Mult Scler 2013;19(9): 1169–74.

45. Stankovich E, Borisov VV, Demina TL. Tamsulosin in the treatment of detrusor-sphincter dyssynergia of the urinary bladder in patients with multiple scle- rosis. Urologiia 2004;(4):48–51 [in Russian].

46. O'Riordan JI, Doherty C, Javed M, et al. Do alpha- blockers have a role in lower urinary tract dysfunc- tion in multiple sclerosis? J Urol 1995;153(4): 1114–6.

47. Wyndaele JJ. Self-intermittent catheterization in mul- tiple sclerosis. Ann Phys Rehabil Med 2014;57(5): 315–20.

48. Vahter L, Zopp I, Kreegipuu M, et al. Clean intermit- tent self-catheterization in persons with multiple sclerosis: the influence of cognitive dysfunction. Mult Scler 2009;15(3):379–84.

49. James R, Frasure HE, Mahajan ST. Urinary catheter- ization may not adversely impact quality of life in multiple sclerosis patients. ISRN Neurol 2014;2014: 167030.

50. Shamout S, Biardeau X, Corcos J, et al. Out- come comparison of different approaches to self- intermittent catheterization in neurogenic patients: a systematic review. Spinal Cord 2017. [Epub ahead of print].

51. Kidd EA, Stewart F, Kassis NC, et al. Urethral (indwelling or intermittent) or suprapubic routes for short-term catheterisation in hospitalised adults. Cochrane Database Syst Rev 2015;(12):CD004203.

52. Stoffel JT, McGuire EJ. Outcome of urethral closure in patients with neurologic impairment and complete urethral destruction. Neurourol Urodyn 2006;25(1): 19–22.

53. Engeler DS, Meyer D, Abt D, et al. Sacral neuromo- dulation for the treatment of neurogenic lower uri- nary tract dysfunction caused by multiple sclerosis: a single-centre prospective series. BMC Urol 2015;15:105.

54. Marinkovic SP, Gillen LM. Sacral neuromodulation for multiple sclerosis patients with urinary retention and clean intermittent catheterization. Int Urogyne- col J 2010;21(2):223–8.

55. Minardi D, Muzzonigro G. Sacral neuromodulation in patients with multiple sclerosis. World J Urol 2012; 30(1):123–8.

56. Gobbi C, Digesu GA, Khullar V, et al. Percutaneous posterior tibial nerve stimulation as an effective treat- ment of refractory lower urinary tract symptoms in patients with multiple sclerosis: preliminary data from a multicentre, prospective, open label trial. Mult Scler 2011;17(12):1514–9.

57. Kabay S, Kabay SC, Yucel M, et al. The clinical and urodynamic results of a 3-month percutaneous posterior tibial nerve stimulation treatment in pa- tients with multiple sclerosis-related neurogenic bladder dysfunction. Neurourol Urodyn 2009; 28(8):964–8.

58. de Seze M, Raibaut P, Gallien P, et al. Transcuta- neous posterior tibial nerve stimulation for treat- ment of the overactive bladder syndrome in multiple sclerosis: results of a multicenter pro- spective study. Neurourol Urodyn 2011;30(3): 306–11.

59. Zecca C, Panicari L, Disanto G, et al. Posterior tibial nerve stimulation in the management of lower urinary tract symptoms in patients with multiple sclerosis. Int Urogynecol J 2016;27(4):521–7.

60. Gallien P, Reymann JM, Amarenco G, et al. Pla- cebo controlled, randomised, double blind study of the effects of botulinum A toxin on detrusor sphincter dyssynergia in multiple sclerosis pa- tients. J Neurol Neurosurg Psychiatry 2005; 76(12):1670–6.

61. Utomo E, Groen J, Blok BF. Surgical management of functional bladder outlet obstruction in adults with neurogenic bladder dysfunction. Cochrane Data- base Syst Rev 2014;(5):CD004927.

62. Barbalias GA, Nikiforidis G, Liatsikos EN. Vesicoure- thral dysfunction associated with multiple sclerosis: clinical and urodynamic perspectives. J Urol 1998; 160(1):106–11.

63. Cox LCA, Wittman D, Papin JE, et al. Analysis of uri- nary symptoms and urodynamic findings in multiple sclerosis patients by gender and disease subtype. J Neurol Neurobiol 2015;1(2):1–5.

64. Wang T, Huang W, Zhang Y. Clinical characteristics and urodynamic analysis of urinary dysfunction in multiple sclerosis. Chin Med J (Engl) 2016;129(6): 645–50.

65. de Almeida CR, Carneiro K, Fiorelli R, et al. Urinary dysfunction in women with multiple sclerosis: anal- ysis of 61 patients from rio de janeiro, Brazil. Neurol Int 2013;5(4):e23.

66. Fragala E, Russo GI, Di Rosa A, et al. Association between the neurogenic bladder symptom score

and urodynamic examination in multiple sclerosis patients with lower urinary tract dysfunction. Int Neurourol J 2015;19(4):272–7.

67. Wiedemann A, Kaeder M, Greulich W, et al. Which clinical risk factors determine a pathological urodynamic evaluation in patients with multiple sclerosis? An analysis of 100 prospective cases. World J Urol 2013;31(1):229–33.

68. Giannantoni A, Scivoletto G, Di Stasi SM, et al. Lower urinary tract dysfunction and disability status in patients with multiple sclerosis. Arch Phys Med Rehabil 1999;80(4):437–41.

Identifying Patients with High-Risk Neurogenic Bladder
Beyond Detrusor Leak Point Pressure

Elizabeth V. Dray, MD, Anne P. Cameron, MD, FRCSC, FPMRS*

KEYWORDS

- Neurogenic bladder • Spinal cord injury • Urodynamics

KEY POINTS

- The standard workup of neurogenic bladder dysfunction should include patient-based assessments, such as validated questionnaires and 2- to 3-day voiding diaries, a thorough history and physical examination, and baseline urodynamics for patients with spinal cord injury (SCI) and spina bifida. Urodynamic studies (UDS) should be repeated every 1 to 2 years in patients with recent SCI and at regular intervals for children with spina bifida. In adult patients with spina bifida whose linear growth is complete and for patients with chronic SCI whose urinary symptoms have stabilized, UDS should be repeated if urologic symptoms change. In individuals with multiple sclerosis, a history of cerebral vascular accidents, movement disorders, and diabetes, urodynamics may be used more judiciously to help define bladder function if conservative measures fail.
- Nephrolithiasis and bladder stones are more common in patients with SCI and spina bifida than in the general population. Renal and bladder ultrasound every 1 to 2 years should be used both to screen for upper tract changes and evaluate for stone formation.
- Patients with neurogenic bladder should not be treated with antibiotics for bacteriuria alone. Intervention should be prompted by leukocyturia and bacteriuria combined with symptoms of urinary infection, systemic infection, or significant changes in urologic symptoms only.
- Patients managed with indwelling Foley catheters are at increased risk for multiple urologic complications, and alternative bladder management strategies should be pursued.

INTRODUCTION

More than 12,000 spinal cord injuries (SCI) occur annually in the United States, and more than 80% of these individuals will experience urinary tract dysfunction.[1] When combined with the population of patients who have neurogenic bladder as a result of cerebrovascular accidents (CVA), spina bifida, Parkinson disease (PD), multiple sclerosis (MS), and diabetic cystopathy, the number of people with neurologic illness who require urologic care is significant. Despite the clinical demand, there is a paucity of guidelines for the care of these patients. Although most urologists are familiar with dangerous urodynamic parameters and the benefits of clean intermittent catheterization (CIC), these patients face a myriad of risks that may go unrecognized. In this article, the authors briefly discuss the impact of specific neurologic diseases on the urinary tract; examine the risks inherent to

The authors have no pertinent commercial or financial conflicts of interest to disclose, and no funding was used for the creation of this article.
Urology, University of Michigan, 1500 East, Medical Center Drive, Ann Arbor, MI 48109, USA
* Corresponding author.
E-mail address: annepell@med.umich.edu

Urol Clin N Am 44 (2017) 441–452
http://dx.doi.org/10.1016/j.ucl.2017.04.010
0094-0143/17/© 2017 Elsevier Inc. All rights reserved.

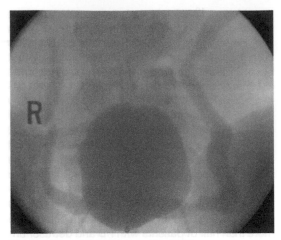

Fig. 2. Upper tract changes and VUR.

1980s, when Ghoniem and colleagues[26] noted that poor compliance on UDS predicted poor renal outcomes in children with myelodysplasia. In the same year, analysis of the adult SCI population showed similar trends. In a study by Hackler and colleagues[27] of 254 patients with SCI, 64% of patients with low compliance had hydronephrosis and 46% had VUR compared with 21% hydronephrosis and 6% VUR in the normal-compliance group (defined by compliance of >20 mL/cm H_2O at 100-mL volume). The cumulative findings of this era suggested an interplay between elevated outlet pressures, either via the fixed sphincter activity produced by sacral lesions and many myelomeningoceles or the DSD common to suprasacral injuries, and progressive loss of detrusor compliance and increased bladder pressure. In turn, increased bladder pressure leads to impaired delivery of urine from the kidneys as well as increased risk of VUR and pyelonephritis and ultimately renal impairment. The validity of this connection was bolstered by several studies that demonstrated stabilization or improvement in upper tract deterioration when outlet pressures were pharmacologically or surgically lessened.[28,29] Unfortunately, reduced outlet pressures may exacerbate underlying incontinence and are, therefore, a treatment option only in a very select group of patients, such as patients with DSD who manage their bladder with sphincterotomy and condom catheters.

The contemporary approach to avoiding unsafe bladder pressures and subsequent upper tract deterioration in patients with neurogenic voiding dysfunction typically focuses on pharmacologic interventions for decreasing bladder pressures, typically anticholinergic medication, β-3 agonists, or intravesical botulinum toxin, plus or minus the addition of alpha-blockers to lower outlet resistance and improve compliance, in conjunction with regular

CIC.[29–31] If this conservative approach fails, bladder augmentation with or without a continent channel that can be catheterized may be offered. With this strategy, most patients will have preserved renal function, with cystectomy and urinary diversion being a last resort in the most severe cases.[32]

Of course, a problem must be identified before it can be addressed. The most important tool in identifying neurogenic patients at risk of renal failure remains properly performed urodynamics and upper tract imaging. Compliance must be assessed over the entire range of volumes typically seen by the bladder, which can be determined by either self-reported voiding diaries or CIC volumes. Meaning, if patients routinely have bladder volumes more than 700 mL, then the study should continue filling until it reaches that volume. Although the definition of reduced compliance remains controversial, generally accepted normal values are less than 12.5 to 15.0 mL/cm H_2O in the absence of a detrusor contraction.[33] Once an intervention to reduce bladder pressures has been undertaken for patients with reduced compliance, UDS should be repeated after a few months to ensure that the treatment has been successful. Although renal ultrasonography is very sensitive in detecting upper tract abnormalities, hydronephrosis is likely a late manifestation of impaired compliance and should not be relied on for early diagnosis of unsafe bladder storage pressures. Serum creatinine is also a poor indicator of renal function in this group. Although 24-hour creatinine clearance is more accurate, appropriate correction factors must be used to address the low creatinine production of spinal cord patients versus age-matched controls because of their low muscle mass.[34]

Disease-specific risk factors for impaired compliance exist. Multiple studies have shown a reduction in compliance with sacral injuries when compared with suprasacral injuries.[27,33] Upper tract changes are less frequently seen in patients with MS, even in the setting of DSD.[14] Patients whose bladders are primarily managed with indwelling catheters, either SPT or urethral Foley, are also at increased risk of loss of compliance over time when compared with those managed with CIC or voiding.[33] Alternative methods of bladder drainage should be pursued when possible, and increased frequency of UDS should be performed if long-term catheter drainage is necessary.

UROLITHIASIS

Before 1980, approximately 40% of patients with SCI developed urolithiasis.[35] Contemporary studies have shown the overall risk to be closer to 7% over a 10-year follow-up, with the greatest risk occurring in the first several months following injury due to bone resorption from immobilization.[36] Among children with myelomeningocele, the risk of urinary calculi is 4.0%, compared with 0.2% in normal controls.[37] Urinary stasis; foreign bodies, such as debris or indwelling catheters; and metabolic changes from immobilization likely all contribute to the risk of stone formation. Recurrent urinary tract infections (UTIs) and chronic bacteriuria are other probable drivers. Older analyses of upper urinary tract stones removed from patients with SCI actually demonstrated a marked predominance of infection stones, such as struvite and apatite.[38] However, newer studies, although still demonstrating higher than baseline levels of infection stones, particularly apatite, have noted increased incidence of metabolic stones in SCI and spina bifida populations.[39,40] Other risk factors for upper tract stones include VUR, indwelling catheters (although data on this are conflicting), and prior stone disease.[36,41,42] Risk factors for bladder stones in this population include indwelling Foley catheter and older age.[43] Environmental and behavioral risk factors are consistent with those found in the general population.[44]

Kidney stone disease may contribute to renal insufficiency and seed recurrent UTIs, increasing patients' risk of potentially life-threatening sepsis. It is, therefore, imperative to diagnose urolithiasis in this population. Unfortunately, renal colic may present atypically in patients with SCI and preexisting incontinence may obscure symptoms of bladder stones. Annual screening with renal ultrasonography is, therefore, advisable for patients with SCI.[34] The high prevalence of fecal loading and risk for radiolucent stones reduces the sensitivity of abdominal radiographs and makes them less useful as a screening tools for stone disease in patients with SCI than in the general population.[45] Although the risk of urolithiasis in other neurogenic populations is less well defined, recurrent UTIs in patients with impaired emptying should prompt imaging to evaluate for an underlying stone burden.

Treatment of stone disease in patients with SCI, spina bifida, or advanced MS poses several unique challenges. Recurrent UTIs are common in this population, and frequent antibiotic use may increase the risk of multidrug-resistant organisms. It is, therefore, imperative that a urine culture is sent preoperatively and culture-specific antibiotics started before surgical intervention.[46] Intraoperative or stone cultures should be considered to aid in accurately treating postoperative infection. Operative positioning in the setting of contractures or severe spinal curvature can be difficult, and lithotomy position for retrograde interventions may not be feasible. Extracorporeal shockwave lithotripsy offers easier positioning; however, stone clearance rates are poorer than in the general population (in limited case series); fragments may take longer to pass, an unfortunate outcome in the setting of infected stones. Stone clearance rates for percutaneous nephrolithotomy (PCNL) fare better. A retrospective study by Rubenstein and colleagues[47] reporting on outcomes for 23 patients with neurogenic bladder secondary to a variety of causes showed a 96% stone-free rate following PCNL. There was an increased risk of postoperative complications in the cohort, a finding which has been demonstrated in prior studies.[48] PCNL can also be used for patients with urinary tract diversions. Bladder stones may be treated retrograde, via a percutaneous approach or with cystolithotomy.

Stone recurrence is common in this population, with bladder stones recurring in 30% of patients within 1 year and upper tract stones recurring in 34% over a 5-year period (vs 20% in the general population).[49–51] Strategies for prevention include increased hydration and standard dietary interventions. Specific to the neurogenic bladder population, avoidance of indwelling catheters decreases the risk of both upper and lower urinary tract stones as does the maintenance of safe bladder pressures.[52] Urease-splitting organisms should be aggressively treated to discourage formation of struvite stones. Finally, regular bladder irrigation in patients prone to urinary debris or mucous production (such as those with augmented bladders) may be helpful in preventing recurrence of bladder stones.[53]

URINARY TRACT INFECTION

Despite modern improvement over historical rates of UTI and sepsis in the neurogenic bladder population, infection remains one of the most common and morbid complications of neurogenic bladder. Manack and colleagues[54] recently analyzed 46,000 patients with neurogenic bladder and found that between 29.2% and 36.4% of patients with neurogenic bladder (NGB) were diagnosed with lower UTI annually. In another recent study, 81% of patients with SCI and NGB were diagnosed with a UTI over a 5-year period, 35% percent of which met criteria for recurrent UTI.[55] Although urosepsis has been supplanted by pulmonary complications as the leading cause of death in this population, sepsis from a urinary source still accounts for 10% of mortality in patients with NGB.[56]

The high prevalence of recurrent UTIs in this populations is likely multifactorial. Changes to the vaginal and urethral flora in women, alterations in the glycosaminoglycan (GAG) layer of the bladder, and impaired mucosal immunity have all been implicated as potential risk factors in the neurogenic population.[57–61] Bladder ischemia from overdistension, poor bladder compliance, and impaired bacterial washout from incomplete emptying are other likely contributors.[60,62–65] The use of indwelling catheters independently elevates the risk of UTI by negating the protective effect of urethral length on prevention of UTI, producing chronic inflammation, which may contribute to alterations in defense mechanisms, such as the GAG layer, and encouraging the formation of biofilms.[60] Although CIC has been shown in multiple studies to decrease the risk of UTI when compared with indwelling catheters, bacteriuria is still present in most patients by the third week of bladder management.[66,67] Low frequency of CIC (<4 times daily) and high mean catheterization volumes are thought to increase the risk of UTI, but little evidence supports this common-sense claim.[68] Single versus multiuse catheters and hydrophilic coating have not been shown to substantially decrease the frequency of UTI.[69,70]

Demographic and modifiable risk factors for recurrent UTIs in this population are poorly understood. No definitive findings exist regarding correlation between UTIs and hygiene or level of SCI; there is conflicting evidence regarding gender, and no studies have examined a link between domicile and infection risk.[66] Studies indicate that UTIs are more common and severe in patients with SCI than patients with other forms of neurogenic bladder.[54] In neurogenic patients who void, elevated postvoid residual (PVR) is a risk factor for development of UTI. In stroke patients, a PVR of 150 mL has been defined as the threshold for elevated infection risk.[71] Epididymo-orchitis and prostatitis are also common complications of CIC, indwelling catheter use and reflex voiding.[52,68]

The diagnosis of UTI in neurogenic bladder patients can also prove challenging, due to the high rate of baseline voiding symptoms and chronic bacteriuria in this population. The National Institute on Disability and Rehabilitation Research defines significant bacteriuria as greater than 10^2 colony-forming units (CFU) per milliliter for patients performing CIC, greater than 10^4 CFU/mL for patients using a condom catheter, and any amount of bacteria from an indwelling catheter.[72] However, this definition is rarely used and many laboratories do not routinely report low colony counts. Pyuria on urinalysis is a vital part of the diagnostic workup, and bacteriuria should only be considered to indicate UTI in the setting of leukocyturia.[73]

Symptoms of UTI may differ in this group: in addition to *new or worsened* urinary frequency, urgency, dysuria, or suprapubic pain, symptoms may include sweating, fatigue, restlessness, and increased spasticity.[74] In order to avoid overtreatment of asymptomatic bacteriuria, urine cultures should not be sent in the absence of relevant urinary symptoms. Prophylactic antibiotics and antimicrobial agents to prevent bacteriuria or symptomatic UTI in this population have been met with variable success and should be used on a patient-to-patient basis. In the setting of neurogenic bladder and recurrent UTIs, the authors advocate renal and bladder imaging to rule out stone disease, as well as UDS, as worsening bladder physiology may predispose patients to infections and mimic UTI symptoms.

MALIGNANCY

In the general population, bladder cancer is a relatively rare disease, with an incidence of 20.1 and mortality of 4.4 individuals per 100,000 in the United States.[75] Historically, the incidence of bladder cancer in the SCI population has been thought to be significantly increased. This relationship was first reported in the 1960s by Melzak[76] and was reinforced by multiple small studies over the subsequent 4 decades.[76–78] Recent studies have called this conventional wisdom into question. A 2016 meta-analysis examining SCI and bladder cancer risk found a pooled lifetime incidence of 6% in patients with SCI overall, whereas the most recent large cohort studies have shown an incidence of 0.1% to 2.4%, which is comparable with controls.[79,80] When compared with neurologically intact individuals, however, bladder cancer does seem to be more deadly in this group. In the largest study to date, Nahm and colleagues[81] analyzed the risk of bladder cancer mortality in 45,486 patients with SCI and found it to be 6.7 times that of controls. This mortality ratio has been reported to be as high as 71:1 in earlier literature.[82] In fact, the 1-year overall survival in patients with SCI diagnosed with bladder cancer is a mere 62.1% versus a 5-year overall survival of 77.5% in non-SCI individuals.[75,79] Additionally, bladder cancer was found to occur at a younger age in the SCI cohort (50 vs 73 years). This demographic shift has been reported in multiple studies.[80,81] Up to 24% of patients with bladder cancer in the setting of SCI will be diagnosed before 40 years of age.[80] The incidence of malignancy increases with duration of neurogenic bladder; few studies show a statistically significant difference in risk before 10 years postinjury.[79,81,83,84] Other independent risk factors include complete motor injuries, bladder stones, and long-term indwelling catheter use (>8 years).[79,81,85] In patients with spina bifida, the risk of bladder cancer is also elevated.[86] Like the SCI population, they tend to present at a younger age and with more advanced disease. Prior bladder augmentation is also implicated in development of malignancy.[87] MS, even in the setting of disease-modifying agents, does not seem to increase incidence of bladder cancer, although concomitant risk factors, such as long-term indwelling catheters, should be considered.[88]

Bladder cancer subtypes differ in this population as well. Although urothelial cell cancer comprises 90% of bladder cancer overall in the general population, in SCI populations 36.8% of cancers are of squamous cell histology.[79,89] It is notable that earlier reports cited squamous cell carcinoma as being the most common histology, but more recent studies reveal a shift to a slight preponderance of urothelial cell cancers in this group.[90] This variant histology is generally thought to be related to chronic irritation from indwelling catheter use, although this is being called into question. Although a correlation is found between indwelling catheter use and cancer in many studies, higher-than-baseline rates of bladder cancer still occur in patients with neurogenic bladder whose bladders are managed by CIC or volitional voiding.[91]

The role of bladder cancer surveillance for patients with neurogenic bladder is controversial. In an oft-cited article, Navon and colleagues[84] concluded that screening patients with SCI and recurrent UTI with cystoscopy resulted in early stage diagnosis of bladder cancer and likely conferred a survival advantage but was not a study on screening cystoscopy. Although other studies have advocated surveillance cystoscopy, objective measures of benefit have been lacking.[91,92] Studies by Hamid and colleagues[92] and Yang and Clowers[93] did not reveal a single bladder cancer diagnosis in screening arms. A retrospective study by Groah and colleagues[94] actually showed that patients with successful 5-year bladder cancer survival had fewer numbers of screening cystoscopies overall versus those who died of their disease. In their analysis, the sensitivity of cystoscopy in detecting bladder cancer in SCI was only 64%; similarly, low sensitivities have been reported in multiple studies.[79,94] The low reported sensitivity of cystoscopy in this population may be related to the high rates of benign bladder abnormalities found in patients with neurogenic bladder. In a study by Delnay and colleagues,[90] 23% of cystoscopies performed on patients with SCI had biopsy-proven nonmalignant urothelial changes, most commonly keratinizing squamous metaplasia, a purported precursor to squamous

cell carcinoma, and cystitis glandularis. Chronic inflammation from indwelling catheters and cystitis are other possible confounders. Urine cytology generally has decreased sensitivity in detecting squamous cell carcinoma, and interpretation may be difficult in the setting of infection. Although some studies have advocated the use of cytology for screening in this population, a meta-analysis of these results have shown a sensitivity of only 46.2%, far too low for a screening tool.[34,95] Similarly, no improvement in diagnostic accuracy has been seen with voided tumor markers.[96,97]

No guidelines currently encourage routine annual cystoscopy in asymptomatic patients with neurogenic bladder. However, new onset of hematuria, worsening lower urinary tract symptoms, and new-onset leakage around an indwelling catheter should prompt a workup, as bladder malignancies are common and deadly in this population. Given the morbidity and cost of screening cystoscopy and the absence of proven benefit to patients, at this time routine screening cannot be recommended.

SOFT TISSUE COMPLICATIONS OF NEUROGENIC BLADDER

Chronic indwelling catheters pose a distinct risk of soft tissue erosion. Traumatic hypospadias, resulting from pressure of an indwelling catheter on the glans penis, has been reported in up to 21% of male patients with NGB managed with a urethral catheter (**Fig. 3**).[98] Urethral erosion may also occur in women following prolonged catheterization (**Fig. 4**). Because of the short female urethra and proximity of the bladder neck, this often results

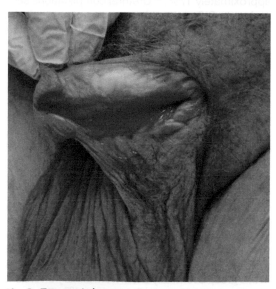

Fig. 3. Traumatic hypospadias.

35. DeVivo MJ, Fine PR, Cutter GR, et al. The risk of bladder calculi in patients with spinal cord injuries. Arch Intern Med 1985;145(3):428–30.

36. Chen Y, DeVivo MJ, Roseman JM. Current trend and risk factors for kidney stones in persons with spinal cord injury: a longitudinal study. Spinal Cord 2000;38(6):346–53.

37. Ramachandra P, Palazzi KL, Holmes NM, et al. Children with spinal abnormalities have an increased health burden from upper tract urolithiasis. Urology 2014;83(6):1378–82.

38. Burr RG. Urinary calculi composition in patients with spinal cord lesions. Arch Phys Med Rehabil 1978;59(2):84–8.

39. Matlaga BR, Kim SC, Watkins SL, et al. Changing composition of renal calculi in patients with neurogenic bladder. J Urol 2006;175(5):1716–9 [discussion: 1719].

40. Gnessin E, Mandeville JA, Handa SE, et al. Changing composition of renal calculi in patients with musculoskeletal anomalies. J Endourol 2011; 25(9):1519–23.

41. Cameron AP, Wallner LP, Forchheimer MB, et al. Medical and psychosocial complications associated with method of bladder management after traumatic spinal cord injury. Arch Phys Med Rehabil 2011;92(3):449–56.

42. DeVivo MJ, Fine PR. Predicting renal calculus occurrence in spinal cord injury patients. Arch Phys Med Rehabil 1986;67(10):722–5.

43. Favazza T, Midha M, Martin J, et al. Factors influencing bladder stone formation in patients with spinal cord injury. J Spinal Cord Med 2004;27(3):252–4.

44. Chen YY, Roseman JM, Devivo MJ, et al. Geographic variation and environmental risk factors for the incidence of initial kidney stones in patients with spinal cord injury. J Urol 2000;164(1):21–6.

45. Linsenmeyer MA, Linsenmeyer TA. Accuracy of bladder stone detection using abdominal x-ray after spinal cord injury. J Spinal Cord Med 2004; 27(5):438–42.

46. Ost MC, Lee BR. Urolithiasis in patients with spinal cord injuries: risk factors, management, and outcomes. Curr Opin Urol 2006;16(2):93–9.

47. Rubenstein JN, Gonzalez CM, Blunt LW, et al. Safety and efficacy of percutaneous nephrolithotomy in patients with neurogenic bladder dysfunction. Urology 2004;63(4):636–40.

48. Culkin DJ, Wheeler JS, Nemchausky BA, et al. Percutaneous nephrolithotomy: spinal cord injury vs. ambulatory patients. J Am Paraplegia Soc 1990;13(2):4–6.

49. Khan AA, Mathur S, Feneley R, et al. Developing a strategy to reduce the high morbidity of patients with long-term urinary catheters: the BioMed catheter research clinic. BJU Int 2007;100(6): 1298–301.

50. Chen Y, DeVivo MJ, Stover SL, et al. Recurrent kidney stone: a 25-year follow-up study in persons with spinal cord injury. Urology 2002;60(2): 228–32.

51. Rule AD, Lieske JC, Li X, et al. The ROKS nomogram for predicting a second symptomatic stone episode. J Am Soc Nephrol 2014;25(12):2878–86.

52. Gormley EA. Urologic complications of the neurogenic bladder. Urol Clin North Am 2010;37(4): 601–7.

53. Kronner KM, Casale AJ, Cain MP, et al. Bladder calculi in the pediatric augmented bladder. J Urol 1998;160(3 Pt 2):1096–8 [discussion: 1103].

54. Manack A, Motsko SP, Haag-Molkenteller C, et al. Epidemiology and healthcare utilization of neurogenic bladder patients in a US claims database. Neurourol Urodyn 2011;30(3):395–401.

55. Biering-Sørensen F, Nielans HM, Dørflinger T, et al. Urological situation five years after spinal cord injury. Scand J Urol Nephrol 1999;33(3): 157–61.

56. García Leoni ME, De Ruz AE. Management of urinary tract infection in patients with spinal cord injuries. Clin Microbiol Infect 2003;9(8): 780–5.

57. Taylor TA, Waites KB. A quantitative study of genital skin flora in male spinal cord-injured outpatients. Am J Phys Med Rehabil 1993;72(3):117–21.

58. Perlow DL, Gikas PW, Horowitz EM. Effect of vesical overdistention on bladder mucin. Urology 1981;18(4):380–3.

59. Vaidyanathan S, McDicken IW, Soni BM, et al. Secretory immunoglobulin A in the vesical urothelium of patients with neuropathic bladder–an immunohistochemical study. Spinal Cord 2000;38(6): 378–81.

60. Vasudeva P, Madersbacher H. Factors implicated in pathogenesis of urinary tract infections in neurogenic bladders: some revered, few forgotten, others ignored. Neurourol Urodyn 2014;33(1):95–100.

61. Schlager TA, Grady R, Mills SE, et al. Bladder epithelium is abnormal in patients with neurogenic bladder due to myelomeningocele. Spinal Cord 2004;42(3):163–8.

62. Cox CE, Hinman F. Experiments with induced bacteriuria, vesical emptying and bacterial growth on the mechanism of bladder defense to infection. J Urol 1961;86:739–48.

63. Merritt JL. Residual urine volume: correlate of urinary tract infection in patients with spinal cord injury. Arch Phys Med Rehabil 1981;62(11): 558–61.

64. Bakke A, Digranes A, Høisaeter PA. Physical predictors of infection in patients treated with clean intermittent catheterization: a prospective 7-year study. Br J Urol 1997;79(1):85–90.

65. Peters KM, Kandagatla P, Killinger KA, et al. Clinical outcomes of sacral neuromodulation in patients with neurologic conditions. Urology 2013; 81(4):738–43.

66. Shekelle PG, Morton SC, Clark KA, et al. Systematic review of risk factors for urinary tract infection in adults with spinal cord dysfunction. J Spinal Cord Med 1999;22(4):258–72.

67. Wyndaele JJ, Brauner A, Geerlings SE, et al. Clean intermittent catheterization and urinary tract infection: review and guide for future research. BJU Int 2012;110(11 Pt C):E910–7.

68. Wyndaele JJ. Complications of intermittent catheterization: their prevention and treatment. Spinal Cord 2002;40(10):536–41.

69. Bakke A, Vollset SE. Risk factors for bacteriuria and clinical urinary tract infection in patients treated with clean intermittent catheterization. J Urol 1993;149(3):527–31.

70. Prieto JA, Murphy C, Moore KN, et al. Intermittent catheterisation for long-term bladder management (abridged Cochrane review). Neurourol Urodyn 2015;34(7):648–53.

71. Dromerick AW, Edwards DF. Relation of postvoid residual to urinary tract infection during stroke rehabilitation. Arch Phys Med Rehabil 2003;84(9): 1369–72.

72. The prevention and management of urinary tract infections among people with spinal cord injuries. National Institute on Disability and Rehabilitation Research consensus statement. January 27-29, 1992. SCI Nurs 1993; 10(2):49–61.

73. Averch TD, Stoffel J, Goldman HB, et al. AUA white paper on catheter associated urinary tract infections: definitions and significance in the urological patient. Urol Pract 2015;2(6):321–8.

74. Sauerwein D. Urinary tract infection in patients with neurogenic bladder dysfunction. Int J Antimicrob Agents 2002;19(6):592–7.

75. Fact Sheet- Bladder Cancer. National Cancer Institute: surveillance epidemiology and end results program. 2016. Available at: https://seer.cancer.gov/statfacts/html/urinb.html. Accessed January 1, 2016.

76. Melzak J. The incidence of bladder cancer in paraplegia. Paraplegia 1966;4(2):85–96.

77. Esrig D, McEvoy K, Bennett CJ. Bladder cancer in the spinal cord-injured patient with long-term catheterization: a casual relationship? Semin Urol 1992; 10(2):102–8.

78. Kaufman JM, Fam B, Jacobs SC, et al. Bladder cancer and squamous metaplasia in spinal cord injury patients. J Urol 1977;118(6):967–71.

79. Gui-Zhong L, Li-Bo M. Bladder cancer in individuals with spinal cord injuries: a meta-analysis. Spinal Cord 2016;51(7):516–21.

80. Welk B, McIntyre A, Teasell R, et al. Bladder cancer in individuals with spinal cord injuries. Spinal Cord 2013;51(7):516–21.

81. Nahm LS, Chen Y, DeVivo MJ, et al. Bladder cancer mortality after spinal cord injury over 4 decades. J Urol 2015;193(6):1923–8.

82. Groah SL, Weitzenkamp DA, Lammertse DP, et al. Excess risk of bladder cancer in spinal cord injury: evidence for an association between indwelling catheter use and bladder cancer. Arch Phys Med Rehabil 2002;83(3):346–51.

83. Lee WY, Sun LM, Lin CL, et al. Risk of prostate and bladder cancers in patients with spinal cord injury: a population-based cohort study. Urol Oncol 2014; 32(1):51.e1-7.

84. Navon JD, Soliman H, Khonsari F, et al. Screening cystoscopy and survival of spinal cord injured patients with squamous cell cancer of the bladder. J Urol 1997;157(6):2109–11.

85. Stonehill WH, Dmochowski RR, Patterson LA, et al. Risk factors for bladder tumors in spinal cord injury patients. J Urol 1996;155(4):1248–50.

86. Austin JC, Elliott S, Cooper CS. Patients with spina bifida and bladder cancer: atypical presentation, advanced stage and poor survival. J Urol 2007; 178(3):798–801.

87. Gurung PMS, Attar KH, Abdul-Rahman A, et al. Long-term outcomes of augmentation ileocystoplasty in patients with spinal cord injury: a minimum 10-year follow-up. BJU Int 2012;109(8):1236–42.

88. Lebrun C, Debouverie M, Vermersch P, et al. Cancer risk and impact of disease-modifying treatments in patients with multiple sclerosis. Mult Scler 2008;14(3):399–405.

89. Silverman DT, Hartge P, Morrison AS, et al. Epidemiology of bladder cancer. Hematol Oncol Clin North Am 1992;6(1):1–30.

90. Delnay KM, Stonehill WH, Goldman H, et al. Bladder histological changes associated with chronic indwelling urinary catheter. J Urol 1999; 161(4):1106–8.

91. Kalisvaart JF, Katsumi HK, Ronningen LD, et al. Bladder cancer in spinal cord injury patients. Spinal Cord 2010;48(3):257–61.

92. Hamid R, Bycroft J, Arya M, et al. Screening cystoscopy and biopsy in patients with neuropathic bladder and chronic suprapubic indwelling catheters: is it valid? J Urol 2003; 170(2):425–7.

93. Yang CC, Clowers DE. Screening cystoscopy in chronically catheterized spinal cord injury patients. Spinal Cord 1999;37(3):204–7.

94. Groah SL, Lammertse DP. Factors associated with survival after bladder cancer in spinal cord injury. J Spinal Cord Med 2003;26(4):339–44.

95. Stonehill WH, Goldman HB, Dmochowski RR. The use of urine cytology for diagnosing bladder

cancer in spinal cord injured patients. J Urol 1997; 157(6):2112–4.

96. Davies B, Chen JJ, McMurry T, et al. Efficacy of BTA stat, cytology, and survivin in bladder cancer surveillance over 5 years in patients with spinal cord injury. Urology 2005;66(4):908–11.

97. Konety BR, Nguyen TS, Brenes G, et al. Clinical usefulness of the novel marker BLCA-4 for the detection of bladder cancer. J Urol 2000; 164(3 Pt 1):634–9.

98. Larsen LD, Chamberlin DA, Khonsari F, et al. Retrospective analysis of urologic complications in male patients with spinal cord injury managed with and without indwelling urinary catheters. Urology 1997;50(3):418–22.

99. Meeks JJ, Erickson BA, Helfand BT, et al. Reconstruction of urethral erosion in men with a neurogenic bladder. BJU Int 2009;103(3):378–81.

100. Stoffel JT, McGuire EJ. Outcome of urethral closure in patients with neurologic impairment and complete urethral destruction. Neurourol Urodyn 2006;25(1): 19–22.

101. Lindehall B, Abrahamsson K, Jodal U, et al. Complications of clean intermittent catheterization in young females with myelomeningocele: 10 to 19 years of follow-up. J Urol 2007;178(3 Pt 1): 1053–5.

102. Raup VT, Eswara JR, Weese JR, et al. Urinary-cutaneous fistulae in patients with neurogenic bladder. Urology 2015;86(6):1222–6.

103. Fowler CJ, Panicker JN, Drake M, et al. A UK consensus on the management of the bladder in multiple sclerosis. Postgrad Med J 2009;85(1008):552–9.

104. de Sèze M, Ruffion A, Denys P, et al. The neurogenic bladder in multiple sclerosis: review of the literature and proposal of management guidelines. Mult Scler 2007;13(7):915–28.

Peripheral and Sacral Neuromodulation in the Treatment of Neurogenic Lower Urinary Tract Dysfunction

CrossMark

Paholo G. Barboglio Romo, MBBS, MPH[a], Priyanka Gupta, MD[b],*

KEYWORDS

- Neurogenic bladder • Neuromodulation • Sacral • Posterior tibial • Multiple sclerosis
- Spinal cord injury • Overactive bladder

KEY POINTS

- Sacral and peripheral neuromodulation are not approved for treating urinary symptoms related to neurogenic bladder; however, small case studies show that this the treatment has promise for treating lower urinary tract symptoms.
- Neuromodulation may be effective in patients with spinal cord injury and multiple sclerosis in reducing neurogenic detrusor overactivity and symptomatic urinary retention requiring of intermittent catheterization.
- Small studies of patients with spinal cord injuries have shown improvement in fecal incontinence with neuromodulation.

INTRODUCTION

Neuromodulation is a widely accepted tertiary treatment option for patients with refractory non-neurogenic overactive bladder symptoms and urinary retention. Recently, there has been interest in the utilization of this therapy for other groups of patients with overactive bladder, urinary retention, and pain, including patients with neurologic disease.

Neurogenic patients encompass a wide spectrum of disease processes that can alter bladder and bowel function depending on the location of the neurologic lesion. Neurologic disorders affect both storage and voiding functions. Management of neurogenic lower urinary tract dysfunction (NLUTD) can involve a combination of several treatment modalities, including behavioral modification, intermittent catheterization, indwelling catheterization, medical therapy, botulinum toxin injection, bladder augmentation, urinary diversion, and neuromodulation.

In this review, the authors explore the mechanism of action of peripheral and sacral neuromodulation (SNM), the operative technique, and its use in the neurogenic population.

PATIENT SCENARIO

A 42-year-old woman is diagnosed with relapsing-remitting multiple sclerosis (MS) and is referred to urology to address overactive bladder symptoms refractory to oral drug therapy. The patient complains of mild visual disturbances and severe urinary urgency with urge incontinence episodes that occur 3 to 4 times per week. She reports no

Disclosure: The authors have nothing to disclose.
[a] Female Pelvic Medicine and Reconstructive Surgery, Department of Urology, University of Michigan, 1500 East Medical Center Drive, 3875 Taubman Center, Ann Arbor, MI 48109-5330, USA; [b] Department of Urology, University of Michigan, 1500 East Medical Center Drive, 3875 Taubman Center, Ann Arbor, MI 48109-5330, USA
* Corresponding author.
E-mail address: guptapr@med.umich.edu

Urol Clin N Am 44 (2017) 453–461
http://dx.doi.org/10.1016/j.ucl.2017.04.011
0094-0143/17/© 2017 Elsevier Inc. All rights reserved.

difficulty emptying, and her postvoid residual volume is 100 mL. Her physical examination is otherwise unremarkable. Her urinary symptoms have not improved after behavioral modification, pelvic floor physical therapy, and a 1-month trial of an anticholinergic medication. She is fairly active, works full time, and is negatively impacted by her urinary symptoms. She has no recent history of urinary tract infections. She is very apprehensive of having to use catheters to drain her bladder at this early stage of her MS. Because of her stable disease she will not require any MRI studies in the near future.

HISTORY AND MECHANISM OF NEUROMODULATION

Significant advances in the understanding of neuromodulation and the neurophysiology of the urinary tract were made by Tanagho and colleagues[1] at the University of California, San Francisco in the 1970s. They determined that the S3 nerve was responsible for innervation to the bladder, pelvic floor muscles, and external urethral sphincter[2,3] and that external sacral nerve root stimulation would lead to bladder contraction. In the frequently cited study by Tanagho and colleagues[1] from 1989, they performed a dorsal rhizotomy and selective ventral neurotomy in dog models. They then performed sacral nerve stimulation using an electrical implant and demonstrated that this autonomic efferent activation restored normal bladder emptying.[1]

Medtronic, Inc (Minneapolis, MN) developed an implantable neuroprosthesis that was first tested in the 1990s during a multicenter phase II trial in patients with non-neurogenic overactive bladder (OAB). The first device was the Pisces Quad foramen electrode, which required a paraspinous incision with splitting of the lumbodorsal fascia and paraspinous musculature to place the needle into the S3 foramen. The electrode was then sutured to the posterior sacral periosteum and tunneled to the generator. The generator was then implanted into the abdominal wall and fixed above the fascia. The results from the US study showed complete symptom improvement in 6 of 12 patients who had permanent implantation. The European results showed greater than 50% symptom improvement in 19 of 23 patients. The results led to the Food and Drug Administration (FDA) approval of the device for urge incontinence in 1997.[4]

Neuromodulation can be performed via the sacral nerve or peripherally via the posterior tibial nerve. The authors review the operative technique for both approaches, the outcomes, and adverse events associated with each technique.

SACRAL NEUROMODULATION

SNM is a technique in which the S3 nerve is percutaneously targeted via a tined electrode that is placed through the S3 foramen. Currently, there is one device on the market that has been approved by the FDA for the treatment of nonobstructive urinary retention and overactive bladder in 1997 and fecal incontinence in 2011 (InterStim, Medtronic Inc, Minneapolis, MN).

Operative Technique

This procedure is performed via a 2-stage process. The first stage can be performed as an office-based procedure called a percutaneous nerve evaluation or in the operating room as a first-stage lead placement. Both methods allow patients to test the clinical effectiveness of the stimulation before having the full device and battery implanted. A quadripolar lead is placed in S3 foramina as illustrated in **Figs. 1–3**, while confirming motor and sensory appropriate responses, and then the lead is plugged to an external generator to test for 1 or 2 weeks.[5,6]

Outcomes

In the late nineties, researchers soon began investigating the efficacy of SNM treatments for treating neurogenic urinary tract symptoms. However, the data supporting the use of SNM for neurogenic bladder were limited by small sample sizes. This population is particularly difficult to study as NLUTD encompasses a wide variety of neurologic causes with differing symptom profiles. The literature includes largely retrospective data that assesses heterogeneous populations and different outcomes.

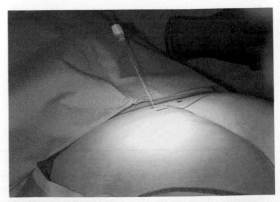

Fig. 1. Needle placement for SNM. The needle is passed at a 60° angle into the entrance point to access the foramen and advanced to the edge of the inferior sacral bone plate.

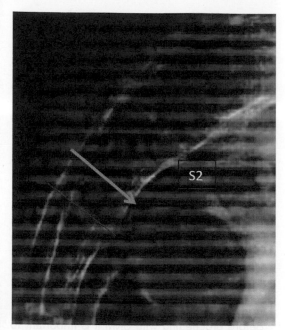

Fig. 2. Determining ideal lateral location. Needle should be placed above the S3 hillock, which is marked with the red dotted line. The arrow indicates the ideal entry point for the lead into the S3 foramen above the hillock. (Reprinted with the permission of Medtronic, Inc. ©.)

A meta-analysis published in 2010 was able to combine the available data from 26 trials with a mean follow-up of 26 months. Only 6 of the included trials were prospective studies, and the sample size in half of all the included trials was less than 10 patients. Success was defined as improvement of greater than 50% in bladder diary

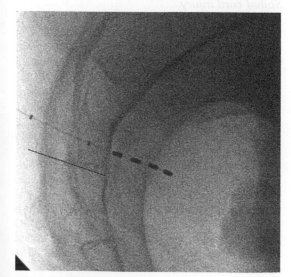

Fig. 3. Ideal lateral radiograph. The red dotted line shows the S3 hillock with the lead entering above.

variables (number of leakages, pad use, number of voids, number of catheterizations).[7] This study reported a pooled success rate of 68% in 256 patients and 92% in 224 patients with neurologic lower urinary tract disease during the test and implantation phases, respectively, with a mean follow-up of 26 months. Results are shown in **Table 1** for specific urinary outcomes.

Analysis of outcomes during both testing and permanent phases suggested a stable and improved success with SNM therapy over time. One significant limitation of the study is the patient drop-off over time during the testing period compared with permanent implantation.

Peters and colleagues[8] reported outcomes for 340 patients who had a sacral lead placed from 2004 to 2012. Of the 71 patients with neurogenic bladder, 63 (89%) underwent permanent implantation. Outcomes were compared with a cohort of non-neurogenic patients. Stroke, MS, and Parkinson disease represented the most common causes. Objective outcomes were measured using 3-day voiding diaries and showed a statistically and clinically significant improvement in patients with neurogenic bladder in regard to urinary frequency and urgency at 3, 6, 12, and 24 months. However, although urinary incontinence episodes improved during the first 12 months, the improvement was not sustained at 24 months in the neurogenic group. Subjective data from the questionnaires showed a clear improvement in the non-neurogenic patients and mixed results in the neurogenic group.[8]

The Peters and colleagues'[8] study suggests that SNM did not sustain long-term improvement in urinary incontinence for neurogenic bladder, which could be explained by the small sample size of patients with neurogenic bladder when compared with non-neurogenic bladder (frequency n = 215 vs 53; urgency n = 155 vs 35; incontinence n = 118 vs 33, non-neurogenic vs neurogenic, respectively) at baseline. Given the heterogeneity of this population and the small sample size, the

Table 1 Urinary outcomes from sacral neuromodulation in neurogenic bladder		
Success Rates for Specific Urinary Outcomes[7]		
	Testing Phase	**Last Follow-up**
Urinary retention	56% (67 of 119)	73% (65 of 89)
Urgency incontinence	60% (46 of 77)	74% (62 of 84)
Urinary frequency	75% (6 of 8)	86% (12 of 14)

study results are limited and further investigation is needed to prospectively assess outcomes. It is possible that the lack of a durable response to SNM was due to lack of sustained efficacy or the outcomes reflect disease progression of a specific neurologic ailment.[8]

A 2011 study assessed neurogenic bladder outcomes in 62 patients with neurogenic detrusor overactivity (34) and urinary retention (28) secondary to a variety of neurologic diseases. They reported a significant improvement in urinary urgency, frequency, and incontinence episodes via 3-day voiding diary data (mean test duration 17 ±10 days). The testing phase was successful in 41 (66%); 37 underwent an implant, of which 28 of 37 (76%) reported a persistent improvement after 4 years. A subgroup analysis suggested that patients with peripheral neuropathy responded better than those with Parkinson disease. The investigators commented that half of the patients with a loss of efficacy had MS and recommended that SNM only be considered in patients with MS with relapsing-remitting disease who have not had a relapse for 2 years.[9]

One of the few prospective studies was by Spinelli[10] and Chartier-Kastler's[11] groups who found improvement in both incomplete emptying (up to 66% not doing clean intermittent catheterization [CIC] at 6 months) and overactive urinary symptoms in patients with NLUTD (more than 50% improvement in all patients and 5 of 9 were dry). Other clinical studies with small sample sizes have followed; however, in the last 30 years, there has not been a large sample trial that has been able to provide level-one data for the efficacy of SNM in neurogenic patients.

The authors now examine studies that have reported individually on specific outcomes and neurologic causes. **Table 2** displays the most representative contemporary studies addressing urinary symptom outcomes with a minimum follow-up of 3 months in this neurogenic population.

Multiple sclerosis

MS is a unique disease in that it can manifest a variety of urologic symptoms depending on the timeline of the disease, stage of neurologic impairment, and the location of the neurologic lesions. Urinary symptoms can oscillate from overactive bladder, dry or wet symptoms, to incomplete emptying.

Early research on SNM was undertaken to address neurogenic bladder symptoms in the setting of MS. Ruud Bosch and Groen[18] were some of the pioneers in this field investigating patients with stable/slowly progressive MS. In 1996, they reported more than 50% improvement in

urinary incontinence episodes in 4 of 5 patients with SNM.[12] Marinkovic and Gillen[14] retrospectively studied a group of 14 patients with MS. Results showed an 86% success rate for reducing urinary retention in 12 of 14 patients after a mean follow-up of 9 years. All patients were doing CIC before SNM; 12 no longer required CIC at their last follow-up, 9 years after surgery. The mean postoperative postvoid residual was well less than 100 mL. The investigators commented these 12 patients were ambulatory compared with the 2 patients who were wheelchair bound at baseline. Interestingly, only 40% underwent battery replacement despite the long follow-up period of this study.[14] A study by Minardi and Muzzonigro[15] on 25 patients with MS suggested that patients with urinary retention who were diagnosed with a weak detrusor on urodynamics (UDS) testing did not have favorable outcomes. However, these findings have not been reproduced, and the data supporting this finding are limited.[15]

Before proceeding with SNM it is important to discuss with patients with MS and the neurologist the need for future MRI scans, which may make patients ineligible for SNM. In addition, disease progression can be associated with worsening urinary symptoms, incomplete emptying, and upper extremity impairment, which can lead to difficulty with intermittent catheterization. The role of SNM is yet to be defined to address refractory neurogenic bladder symptoms in this population. Further studies are needed to better understand when this treatment may be most effective and impactful in the spectrum of MS disease and improving patients' quality of life.

Spinal cord injury

Urinary symptoms from spinal cord injury (SCI) depend on the level of the lesion and whether it is complete or incomplete. The available data regarding SNM and SCI are conflicting with a wide range of success ranging from 29% to 40% in the testing phase and 58% to 80% in the permanent phase.[7]

Lombardi and Del Popolo[16] performed a retrospective review of 24 patients with incomplete SCI, including 13 with urinary retention and 11 with urinary incontinence. Outcomes were evaluated with voiding diaries and urodynamics, and the median follow-up was 61 months. After implantation, patients with urinary retention had a more than 50% decrease in mean number of CIC episodes per day from 3.7 ±1.0 to 0.6 ±0.7 at first postoperative check and 0.7 ±0.8 at last follow-up. There was a significant decrease in catheterized volume, an increase in mean voided volume, and a decrease in mean urinary frequency of

Table 2
Urinary symptoms outcomes for sacral neuromodulation in patients with neurogenic bladder

Author	Cause	Success Test (Phase I)	Follow-up	Urinary Retention (CIC), Mean Baseline, Postop, Improvement (%)	Urinary Frequency, Mean Baseline, Postop, Improvement (50%)	Urinary Incontinence, Mean Baseline, Postop, Improvement (50%)
Wallace,[12] 2007	Various	N = 28 of 33 (85%)	12	3.8–1.6 ± 1.9 ($P<.02$) N = 8 of 16 (50%)	10.5–6.0 ± 1.4 ($P<.0001$)	4.0–1.3 ± 2.4 ($P<.0001$)
Daniels,[13] 2010	DM	N = 26 of 32 (81%)	29	N = 6 of 9 (66.7%)	N = 12 of 14 (85.7%)	N = 18 of 26 (69.2%)
Marinkovic,[14] 2010	MS	N = 12 of 14 (86%)	52	N = 12 of 14 (86%)	—	—
Chabaane,[9] 2011	Various	N = 41 of 62 (66%)	52	N = 28 of 37 (76%)	—	—
Minardi,[15] 2011	MS	N = 15 of 25 (60%)	49	3.3 ± 1.3–1.2 ± 0.7 (N = 9)	17.7 ± 3.5–9 ± 0 (N = 6)	13 ± 2.6–3.3 ± 31 (N = 6)
Peters et al,[8] 2013	Various	N = 63 of 71 (88.7%)	24	—	11.6 ± 4.1–10.2 ± 3.9 ($P = .02$)	6.7 ± 5.3–5.5 ± 4.8 ($P = .06$)
Lombardi,[16] 2013	SCI (incomp)	N = 36 of 85 (42%)	61	N = 13 of 13 (100%)	13.5 ± 2.1–7.4 ± 0.9 ($P<.05$)	2.5 ± 0.19–0.7 ± 0.8 ($P<.05$)
Wollner,[17] 2015	Various	N = 35 of 50 (70%)	16	—	9.9 ± 4.2–5.7 ± 1.5 ($P<.05$)	—

Abbreviations: DM, diabetes mellitus; incomp, incomplete; postop, postoperative; SCI, spinal cord injury.

micturition.[16] Patients with overactive bladder symptoms also had more than 50% improvement and registered a decrease in mean urinary frequency, urinary incontinence, pads used, and nocturia as well as an increase in mean voided volume.

About 30% of the cohort (4 of 14) required a second lead placement during the first year, which was not associated with lead or battery complications or neurologic disease progression. These patients had a second lead deployed on the contralateral side and regained more than 50% improvement. The investigators reported 22 adverse events, which all resulted in at least one additional visit.[16]

Interestingly, the same group reported their updated results in 2014 showing a moderate success rate of 42% after testing 85 high-functioning patients (73% traumatic, 25% myelitis, 3% vascular). Patients who had bladder sensation during filling on UDS were more likely to have a positive testing response (P<.05). In the 11 of 34 (32%) patients who had inconsistent improvement after implantation, a contralateral lead was subsequently implanted. Additionally, the investigators placed a lead in the S4 foramen on 2 patients who failed prior contralateral placement.[19]

Recent studies have reported promising results in patients with complete SCI. Sievert and colleagues were able to prevent the development of neurogenic detrusor overactivity and reported a low-pressure acontractile bladder with no evidence of incontinence with the use of early SNM. Subjects had an American Spinal Injury Association T2-11 injury and underwent bilateral 2-electrode lead placement within 4.5 months of the initial injury. They were compared with a similar control group. Subjects with SCI had compliance greater than 30, no incontinence, no neurogenic detrusor overactivity (DO), decreased incidence of urinary tract infections and improved bowel and erectile function and quality of life when compared with controls.[20]

Diabetic patients

Daniels and colleagues[13] studied 32 patients with neurogenic lower urinary tract symptoms from diabetes mellitus (DM) and compared them with 211 non-neurogenic and nondiabetic patients. They reported good long-term success in the neurogenic patients that was comparable with the controls. There was no difference in the explant rate 38% (9 of 24) in diabetic versus 26% (36 of 141) in non-DM (P = .224) patients. However, when examining the reason for explantation, infectious cause was higher in diabetic patients (16.7%) compared with nondiabetic patients (4.3%; P = .018).[13]

Adverse events

Adverse events after SNM are infrequent but include lead migration, infection, and need for revision of the implanted pulse generator (**Table 3**). Meta-analysis showed a pooled complication rate of zero and 24% for the test and the implantation phases, which corresponded to 69 patients who reported at least one adverse event. Lead migration (15 of 224), pain at the site of the implanted permanent generator (12 of 224) and infection at the site of implantation (11 of 224) were the most common complications. Explantation of both the

---

Table 3
Adverse events associated with sacral neuromodulation implantation in patients with neurogenic bladder

	N	Follow-up	Revision Surgery	Battery Replacement	Infection	Explant
Wallace,[12] 2007	28 of 33	12	NR	NR	NR	(3 of 28) 11%
Daniels,[13] 2010	24 of 32	29	NR	(1 of 24) 4%	(4 of 24) 17%	(9 of 24) 37.5%
Marinkovic,[14] 2010	12 of 14	52	NR	(5 of 12) 40%	NR	NR
Chabaane,[9] 2011	28 of 37	52	(8 of 37) 22%	(2 of 37) 5%	(2 of 37) 5%	NR
Minardi,[15] 2011	5 of 25	49	0	NR	NR	NR
Lombardi,[16] 2013	24 of 24	61	(5 of 24) 21%	(4 of 24) 17%	(1 of 24) 4%	NR
Peters et al,[8] 2013	63	24	(5 of 63) 8%	NR	(1 of 63) 1.6%	(6 of 63) 9.5%
Wollner,[17] 2015	35 of 50	16	(6 of 35) 17%	NR	(2 of 35) 5.7%	(2 of 35) 5.7%

Abbreviation: NR, None reported.

lead and permanent device was performed in 25 of 224 and the lead only in 8 of 224.[7] Peters and colleagues[8] reported similar adverse event rates for neurogenic and non-neurogenic patients in his trial of 11%, lead revision in 8%, and explantation in 10%.[8] In the presence of DM, the infection and explant rate can increase up to 38%[13]

Neurogenic Bowel Outcomes

Neuromodulation was also introduced for the treatment of idiopathic fecal incontinence in 1995.[21] The operative technique is the same as for urinary symptoms with electrode placement through the S3 sacral foramina. A 50% improvement in fecal incontinence episodes is accepted as a successful outcome. Stimulation parameters are adopted from urinary treatment data (pulse width of 210 μs, a frequency of 15 Hz, and the amplitude set individually usually in the range between 0.1 V and 10.0 V).[22] This topic is another area of interest in neurogenic patients.

Small sample studies have shown an improvement in fecal incontinence ranging from 59% to 92% in patients with incomplete SCI.[22] The effects of SNM on anorectal physiology in patients with neurogenic bladder are still controversial, and it is not clear who are ideal candidates for this therapy. **Table 4** displays the success outcomes after SNM in the neurogenic setting.

Holzer and colleagues[26] performed a retrospective review of 36 patients with neurogenic bladder, of which 29 (81%) underwent a permanent implant with a median follow-up of 35 (range 3–71) months. Causes of neurogenic bladder were complications after surgical intervention to address spinal stenosis, spinal protrusion, or spinal trauma. Significant fecal continence improvement was seen in 28 of 29 patients. Incontinence to solid or liquid stool decreased from a median of 7 (range 4–15) to 2 (range 0–5) episodes in 21 days (P = .002). Saline retention time increased from a median of 2 (range 0–5) to 7 (range 2–15) minutes (P = .002). Maximum resting and squeeze anal canal pressures

increased compared with preoperative values. Significant improvement in quality of life was noted among all patients with a permanent implant that remained at 2 years of follow-up.[26]

Neuromodulation can also be potentially effective for treating fecal symptoms in patients with myelomeningocele. Lansen-Koch and colleagues[28] reported outcomes on 10 myelomeningocele patients who underwent SNM, and 3 of 10 reported more than 50% improvement during a 3-week testing period and went onto permanent implantation. The investigators commented that peripheral stimulation of the nerve was not possible in 2 candidates during testing (phase I) and in one patient during permanent placement (phase II).[28] Overall, this therapy is promising for an issue for which there are relatively few effective treatment options.

Posterior Tibial Nerve Stimulation

The procedure has been previously described[29] and consists of placing a 34-gauge needle inserted 3 fingerbreadths above the medial malleolus and advanced approximately 3 cm (**Fig. 4**) depending on the depth of the subcutaneous tissue. The needle is tested with the electrical generator, and the depth of the needle may be adjusted based on patients' response.[29]

Literature supporting posterior tibial nerve stimulation (PTNS) efficacy in patients with neurogenic bladder is similarly limited by few numbers of studies, small sample size, retrospective type, heterogeneous neurologic causes, and different outcome measures. A meta-analysis was performed to assess the outcomes of PTNS for urinary symptoms. Although only 3 of the 32 studies evaluated neurogenic bladder, they were prospective trials. Outcomes ranged from 40% to 100% improvement of urinary symptoms and varied among different neurologic diseases.[30]

Kabay's group has published outcomes regarding PTNS therapy in patients with MS and Parkinson disease with refractory urinary

---

Table 4
Bowel symptoms outcomes for sacral neuromodulation in patients with neurogenic bowel

	Mean Age (y)	Follow-up	Cause	Fecal Incontinence Improvement	Constipation
Ganio,[23] 2001	10	19	Various	N = 6 of 10 (60%)	—
Rosen,[24] 2001	15	15	Various	N = 11 of 15 (73%)	—
Jarret,[25] 2005	13	12	Various	N = 12 of 13 (92%)	—
Holzer,[26] 2007	25	12	Various	N = 18 of 25 (72%)	—
Gstaltner,[27] 2008	11	12	Cauda equina	N = 8 of 11 (73%)	—
Lombardi,[19] 2009	23	38	SCI	N = 11 of 11 (100%)	N = 12 of 12 (100%)

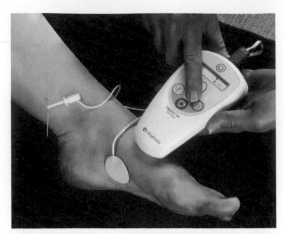

Fig. 4. PTNS. (*Courtesy of* Kenneth Peters, MD, Beaumont Hospital, Royal Oak, MI; Cogentix Medical, Minnetonka, MN)

symptoms. They assessed urinary outcomes with UDS after 12 weeks of PTNS and reported improvement in neurogenic DO (124.0 ±38 mL to 217.5 ±66 mL; P<.001) and increasing cystometric capacity (200 ±29 mL to 267 ±37 mL; P<.0001) in patients with MS.[31] These results were similar in 32 patients with Parkinson disease after 12 weeks of PTNS with UDS.[32] PTNS can potentially provide successful clinical outcomes when addressing urinary symptoms in the ambulatory setting after completing the initial 12 weeks of therapy. A study of 70 patients with MS with refractory urinary symptoms showed improvement in urinary urgency (83%), and half of the patients had complete resolution of urgency. There were 62% of patients who reported significant improvement in incontinence, and 45% had complete resolution of incontinence.[33]

There are also data examining the efficacy of PTNS on urinary symptoms after an ischemic cerebrovascular event. Twenty-four subjects without prior urinary symptoms were randomized to PTNS twice weekly for 6 weeks or general advice (control group). PTNS showed improvement in urinary symptoms, reducing urinary urgency and frequency, and reported subjective improvement after treatment when compared with baseline. When compared with the control group, only urinary frequency was superior after 12 months of follow-up.[34] A longer follow-up period may have unmasked a placebo effect, therefore, making the outcomes between the groups mostly equivalent.

Another randomized control trial study evaluated the effect of PTNS in patients with SCI. One hundred patients with complete SCI were randomized to PTNS or solifenacin. Improvement in all bladder diary parameters was statistically significant within each group after 2 and 4 weeks after

treatment compared with baseline (P<.05). However, there was no difference between the two groups when comparing efficacy of treatment head-to-head. The investigators commented that PTNS was not associated with any adverse events, whereas 5% of patients complained of side effects in the solifenacin group. These side effects led to 2 subjects withdrawing from the trial.[35]

PTNS therapy is well tolerated with minimal side effects. The main disadvantage is the time associated with weekly ambulatory sessions. It has shown to be promising in neurogenic patients, but more research is needed to better understand its efficacy for various neurologic disorders.

SUMMARY

Sacral and peripheral neuromodulation are promising therapies for the neurogenic population. Literature in this area remains sparse and difficult to interpret given the small sample sizes, heterogeneous population, and different outcomes measured. Further prospective studies are needed to see the impact of neuromodulation on urinary and bowel symptoms and should be further stratified according to disease type and presentation.

REFERENCES

1. Tanagho EA, Schmidt RA, Orvis BR. Neural stimulation for control of voiding dysfunction: a preliminary report in 22 patients with serious neuropathic voiding disorders. J Urol 1989;142:340–5.
2. Bross S, Braun P, Weiß J, et al. The role of the carbachol test and concomitant diseases in patients with nonobstructive urinary retention undergoing sacral neuromodulation. World J Urol 2003;346–9. http://dx.doi.org/10.1007/s00345-002-0305-0.
3. Fisch M, Wammack R, Hohenfellner R. The sigma rectum pouch (Mainz pouch II). World J Urol 1996; 14:68–72.
4. Dijkema HE, Weil EH, Mijs PT, Janknegt RA. Neuromodulation of sacral nerves for incontinence and voiding dysfunctions. Clinical results and complications. Eur Urol 1993;24:72–6.
5. Bartley JM, Killinger KA, Boura JA, et al. The impact of prior back surgery on neuromodulation outcomes: a review of over 500 patients. Neurourol Urodyn 2016;1–8. http://dx.doi.org/10.1002/nau.23140.
6. Appell RA, Dmochowski RR, Blaivas JM, et al. Guideline for the surgical management of female stress urinary incontinence: 2009 update. AUA Guidel 799. 2009.
7. Kessler TM, La Framboise D, Trelle S, et al. Sacral neuromodulation for neurogenic lower urinary tract dysfunction: Systematic review and meta-analysis. Eur Urol 2010;58:865–74.

8. Peters KM, Kandagatla P, Killinger KA, et al. Clinical outcomes of sacral neuromodulation in patients with neurologic conditions. Urology 2013;81:738–43.

9. Chaabane W, Guillotreau J, Castel-Lacanal E, et al. Sacral neuromodulation for treating neurogenic bladder dysfunction: clinical and urodynamic study. Neurourol Urodyn 2011;30:547–50.

10. Spinelli M, Bertapelle P, Cappellano F, et al. Chronic sacral neuromodulation in patients with lower urinary tract symptoms: results from a national register. J Urol 2001;166:541–5.

11. Chartier-Kastler EJ, Ruud Bosch JL, Perrigot M, et al. Long-term results of sacral nerve stimulation (S3) for the treatment of neurogenic refractory urge incontinence related to detrusor hyperreflexia. J Urol 2000;164:1476–80.

12. Wallace PA, Lane FL, Noblett KL. Sacral nerve neuromodulation in patients with underlying neurologic disease. Am J Obstet Gynecol 2007;197:96.e1-5.

13. Daniels DH, Powell CR, Braasch MR, Kreder KJ. Sacral neuromodulation in diabetic patients: success and complications in the treatment of voiding dysfunction. Neurourol Urodyn 2010;581:578–81.

14. Marinkovic SP, Gillen LM. Sacral neuromodulation for multiple sclerosis patients with urinary retention and clean intermittent catheterization. Int Urogynecol J 2010;223–8. http://dx.doi.org/10.1007/s00192-009-1023-6.

15. Minardi D, Muzzonigro G. Sacral neuromodulation in patients with multiple sclerosis. World J Urol 2012;30:123–8.

16. Lombardi G, Musco S, Celso M, et al. Sacral neuromodulation for neurogenic non-obstructive urinary retention in incomplete spinal cord patients: a ten-year follow-up single-centre experience. Spinal Cord 2014;52:1–5.

17. Wöllner J, Krebs J, Pannek J. Sacral neuromodulation in patients with neurogenic lower urinary tract dysfunction. Spinal Cord 2016;54:137–40.

18. Bosch JLHR, Groen J. Treatment of refractory urge urinary incontinence with sacral spinal nerve stimulation in multiple sclerosis patients. Lancet 1996;348:717–9.

19. Lombardi G, Del Popolo G. Clinical outcome of sacral neuromodulation in incomplete spinal cord injured patients suffering from neurogenic lower urinary tract symptoms. Spinal Cord 2009;47:486–91.

20. Sievert K-D, Amend B, Gakis G, et al. Early sacral neuromodulation prevents urinary incontinence after complete spinal cord injury. Ann Neurol 2010;67:74–84.

21. Matzel KE, Stadelmaier U, Hohenfellner M, Gall FP. Electrical stimulation of sacral spinal nerves for treatment of faecal incontinence. Lancet 1995;346:1124–7.

22. Worsøe J, Rasmussen M, Christensen P, Krogh K. Neurostimulation for neurogenic bowel dysfunction. Gastroenterol Res Pract 2013. http://dx.doi.org/10.1155/2013/563294.

23. Ganio E, Luc AR, Clerico G, Trompetto M. Sacral nerve stimulation for treatment of fecal incontinence - a novel approach for intractable fecal incontinence. Dis Colon Rectum 2001;44:619–29.

24. Rosen HR, Urbarz C, Holzer B, et al. Sacral nerve stimulation as a treatment for fecal incontinence. Gastroenterology 2001;121:536–41.

25. Jarrett MED, Matzel KE, Christiansen J, et al. Sacral nerve stimulation for faecal incontinence in patients with previous partial spinal injury including disc prolapse. Br J Surg 2005;92:734–9.

26. Holzer B, Rosen HR, Novi G, et al. Sacral nerve stimulation for neurogenic faecal incontinence. Br J Surg 2007;94:749–53.

27. Gstaltner K, Rosen H, Hufgard J, et al. Sacral nerve stimulation as an option for the treatment of faecal incontinence in patients suffering from cauda equina syndrome. Spinal Cord 2008;46:644–7.

28. Lansen-Koch SMP, Govaert B, Oerlemans D, et al. Sacral nerve modulation for defaecation and micturition disorders in patients with spina bifida. Colorectal Dis 2012;14:508–14.

29. Gupta P, Ehlert MJ, Sirls LT, et al. Percutaneous tibial nerve stimulation and sacral neuromodulation: an update. Curr Urol Rep 2015;16:4.

30. Gaziev G, Topazio L, Iacovelli V, et al. Percutaneous Tibial Nerve Stimulation (PTNS) efficacy in the treatment of lower urinary tract dysfunctions: a systematic review. BMC Urol 2013;13:61.

31. Kabay S, Kabay SC, Yucel M, et al. The clinical and urodynamic results of a 3-month percutaneous posterior tibial nerve stimulation treatment in patients with multiple sclerosis-related neurogenic bladder dysfunction. Neurourol Urodyn 2009;28:964–8.

32. Kabay SC, Kabay S, Yucel M, Ozden H. Acute urodynamic effects of percutaneous posterior tibial nerve stimulation on neurogenic detrusor overactivity in patients with Parkinson's disease. Neurourol Urodyn 2009;28:62–7.

33. de Sèze M, Raibaut P, Gallien P, et al. Transcutaneous posterior tibial nerve stimulation for treatment of the overactive bladder syndrome in multiple sclerosis: results of a multicenter prospective study. Neurourol Urodyn 2011;30:306–11.

34. Monteiro ÉS, De Carvalho LBC, Fukujima MM, et al. Electrical stimulation of the posterior tibialis nerve improves symptoms of poststroke neurogenic overactive bladder in men: a randomized controlled trial. Urology 2014;84:509–14.

35. Chen G, Liao L, Li Y. The possible role of percutaneous tibial nerve stimulation using adhesive skin surface electrodes in patients with neurogenic detrusor overactivity secondary to spinal cord injury. Int Urol Nephrol 2015;47:451–5.

Disease-Specific Outcomes of Botulinum Toxin Injections for Neurogenic Detrusor Overactivity

Aaron Kaviani, MD, Rose Khavari, MD*

KEYWORDS

- Botulinum toxin • Overactive bladder • Neurogenic • Detrusor overactivity • Urinary incontinence
- Parkinson's disease • Myelomeningocele • Multiple sclerosis

KEY POINTS

- Intradetrusor injection of onabotulinumtoxinA for refractory neurogenic detrusor overactivity is effective in patients with multiple sclerosis (MS) and spinal cord injury (SCI) (level I evidence).
- Botulinum toxin A might be effective in patients with cerebrovascular accidents and Parkinson's disease, but results are not be as favorable as MS and SCI.
- Botulinum toxin A seems to be effective in children with myelomeningocele (low level of evidence). Data in adults is missing.
- Cost and morbid adverse events associated with Botulinum toxin A such as de novo clean intermittent catheterization, urinary tract infections, and the failure to adhere to therapy need to be considered during shared decision making in this setting.

INTRODUCTION

Neurogenic detrusor overactivity (NDO) is a bladder dysfunction caused by a neurologic disease such as multiple sclerosis (MS), spinal cord injury (SCI), Parkinson's disease (PD), cerebrovascular accident (CVA), or myelomeningocele (MMC). NDO might be associated with urinary frequency, nocturia, urgency, and urinary incontinence (UI). A systematic review of 189 articles by Ruffion and colleagues[1] showed that the prevalence of UI was 50.9%, 52.3%, 33.1%, and 23.6% in patients with MS, SCI, PD, and CVA, respectively. NDO leads to a negative impact on a patient's quality of life (QOL)[2] and may contribute to deterioration of the upper urinary tract.[3]

Accordingly, urodynamic study (UDS) findings including impaired detrusor compliance with a high detrusor leak point pressure, detrusor sphincter dyssynergia, and vesicoureteral reflux require special attention in patients with neurogenic bladder.[3]

Even though anticholinergic or beta agonist drugs have limited effectiveness and moderate adverse side effect profiles, they are the first-line pharmacotherapy for patients with NDO.[4] However, long-term treatment with these medications may be suboptimal, and many patients discontinue their medications because of lack of efficacy, and/or significant bothersome side effects, especially patients with neurogenic bladders in whom higher doses of medications are needed. In

Disclosure: R. Khavari is a scholar supported in part by NIH grant K12 DK0083014, the multidisciplinary K12 urologic research (KURe) career development program grant awarded to Dolores J Lamb by the national institute of diabetes and digestive and kidney diseases (NIDDK) (12 DK083014-09), national institutes of health (NIH). Department of Urology, Houston Methodist Hospital, 6560 Fannin Street, Suite 2100, Houston, TX 77030, USA
* Corresponding author.
E-mail address: rkhavari@houstonmethodist.org

addition, recent studies highlight the possibility of cortical atrophy, cognitive decline, and an increased risk of dementia with chronic use of strong anticholinergics such as oxybutynin.[5,6] These data are of significant concern for urologists, who would otherwise prescribe high doses of anticholinergics for the management of NDO in patients with preexisting neurologic compromise and cognitive decline, such as patients with MS, PD, MMC, or CVA. Until recently, augmentation cystoplasty was the next step in the management of refractory neurogenic bladder. However, augmentation cystoplasty is a major reconstructive surgery with significant immediate and long-term morbidity.[7,8]

Botulinum toxin A (BTX-A) blocks the release of acetylcholine at the neuromuscular junction and leads to a temporary chemodenervation of the bladder. Motor effects of BTX-A on the bladder have been studied extensively,[9] which has led to its approval by the US Food and Drug Administration in August of 2011 for the treatment of refractory NDO in patients with MS and SCI.

In this review, we appraised the disease-specific outcome of BTX-A injection in patients with NDO. Neurogenic bladder encompasses a broad spectrum of patients because of the heterogeneity of neurologic diseases. Our review focuses on the more common patient populations, including patients with MS, SCI, CVA, PD, and MMC. We performed a search in PubMed for all abstracts that contained the terms "bladder" and "botulinum." To not restrict our PubMed search to MEDLINE we did not use MeSH terms. Other searches of PubMed were also carried out to obtain additional related information. A total of 301 abstracts were identified and reviewed. The articles most relevant to the purpose of this article were then selected.

EFFICACY OF INTRADETRUSOR INJECTION OF BOTULINUM TOXIN A

Two forms of BTX-A—onabotulinumtoxinA (OnabotA, Botox) and abobotulinumtoxinA (AbobotA, Dysport)—have been evaluated for the treatment of refractory NDO[10] with comparable outcomes. In this review, the abbreviation BTX-A is used when we refer to botulinum toxin A in general (both available forms).

The first phase II randomized, double-blind, placebo-controlled clinical trial using BTX-A to treat NDO was reported by Schurch and colleagues[11] in 2005. They randomized a total of 59 patients (53 with SCI and 6 with MS) to receive a single dose of onabotulinumtoxinA (200 or 300 U) or placebo and concluded that intradetrusor injection of

onabotulinumtoxinA was associated with a clinically significant improvement in UI caused by NDO. Another randomized, double-blind, placebo-controlled trial was reported by Herschorn and colleagues[12] in 2011. Patients had experienced a reduction in their UI by 50% at week 6 after onabotulinumtoxinA injection. In a systematic review by Duthie[13] in 2011 of a heterogeneous population of NDO and idiopathic overactive bladder patients, BTX-A results were superior to those with a placebo in all 19 included studies. OnabotulinumtoxinA and abobotulinumtoxinA were used in 17 and 2 studies, respectively. Patients receiving repeated doses did not become refractory to BTX-A. Other systematic reviews by Zhou and colleagues[14] (2015), Cui and colleagues[15] (2015), and Lopez and colleagues[16] (2016) also concluded that intravesical injections of BTX-A significantly improve NDO symptoms. Zhou and colleagues[14] identified 4 randomized, double-blind, placebo-controlled trials combining a total of 807 patients, and reported that onabotulinumtoxinA effectively improved clinical outcomes and UDS findings in patients with NDO. Moreover, BTX-A injection seems to be cost effective in the management of UI related to NDO compared with costs of supportive care, which consists of incontinence pads and possible use of anticholinergics and clean intermittent catheterization (CIC).[17]

Pivotal Clinical Trials

The data offering strongest support for the use of onabotulinumtoxinA in NDO comes from 2 double-blind, placebo-controlled, phase III studies that were carried out after several phase II studies.[18] These 2 pivotal clinical trials constitute the 2 trials of the DIGNITY clinical research program (Double-Blind Investigation of Purified Neurotoxin Complex in Neurogenic Detrusor Overactivity). DIGNITY compared response to onabotulinumtoxinA with response to placebo in patients with NDO owing to SCI or MS.[19] MS or SCI patients with NDO who had 14 or more incidents of UI per week were randomized to receive 200 or 300 U of onabotulinumtoxinA or placebo, and the outcomes were assessed at week 6 after injection.[20] In 2011, Cruz and colleagues[21] published the results of the first trial of DIGNITY, which was conducted in 63 centers in Europe, North America, South America, South Africa, and the Asia Pacific. They enrolled and randomized a total of 275 patients (**Table 1**).[22] In 2012, Ginsberg and colleagues[23] reported the results of the second trial of DIGNITY from 85 centers and 416 patients randomized to intradetrusor injections of placebo or onabotulinumtoxinA

Table 1
Outcomes of intradetrusor injection of OnabotA in patients with NDO, 6 weeks after injection

		Patients (n)	UI (n)	Dry (%)	No IDC (%)	MCC (Mean, mL)	PdetmaxIDC (Mean, cmH$_2$O)	UR (%)
Cruz et al,[21] 2011	Saline	92	−13.2	7.6	17.4	6.5	+6.4	12.0
	200 U	92	−21.8	38.0	64.4	+157.0	−28.5	30.0
	300 U	91	−19.5	39.6	59.5	+157.2	−26.9	42.0
Ginsberg et al,[23] 2012	Saline	149	−8.8	0.0	19.0	+16.0	−2.4	10.0
	200 U	135	−21.0	36.0	64.0	+151.0	−35.1	35.0
	300 U	132	−22.0	41.0	69.0	+168	−33.3	42.0
DIGNITY[a]	Saline	241	−10.5	9.1	18.4	+11.9	+1.1	7.1
	200 U	227	−21.3	37.0	64.1	+153.6	−32.4	30.8
	300 U	223	−21.3	40.4	65.1	+163.1	−30.1	44.0

Abbreviations: IDC, involuntary detrusor contractions; MCC, maximum cystometric capacity; OnabotA, onabotulinumtoxinA; PdetmaxIDC, maximum detrusor pressure during involuntary detrusor contraction; UI, urinary urge incontinence episodes per week; UR, urinary retention.
[a] DIGNITY pooled data.

200 U or onabotulinumtoxinA 300 U (see **Table 1**). In addition, a follow-up study that pooled the data from these 2 trials of 691 patients is summarized in **Table 1**.[24] To evaluate the long-term efficacy of onabotulinumtoxinA injection for NDO in MS and SCI patients, Kennelly and colleagues[25] performed a prospective, multicenter extension trial on the patients in the initial DIGNITY study. The number of UI incidents/week at week 6 was significantly decreased after repeated onabotulinumtoxinA injections. The reductions from baseline were −22.7, −23.3, −23.1, −25.3, and −31.9 in the 200 U dose group and −23.8, −25.0, −23.6, −24.1, and −29.5 in the 300 U dose group in treatment rounds 1 to 5, respectively.[25] Final analysis of patients who completed 4 years of treatment showed that the decrease in UI episodes, which was 4.3 UI episodes per day at the baseline, consistently ranged from −3.4 to −3.9 episodes per day.[26]

Recommended dose and injection template

Phase III trials reported by Cruz, Ginsberg, Kennelly, and their colleagues found no statistically significant differences in efficacy between 200 and 300 U of onabotulinumtoxinA.[18] Other trials have shown 200 U to be more effective than 50 and 100 U in NDO.[18,27] The US Food and Drug Administration approved intradetrusor injection of 200 U of onabotulinumtoxinA (OnabotA, BOTOX) for NDO in 2011. There is no standard method of injection onabotulinumtoxinA; however, the phase III studies we analyzed used a trigone-sparing template. Two randomized clinical trials administered BTX-A to include versus exclude the trigone in SCI patients and both favored trigone-including template with improvements in

efficacy, as measured by detrusor pressure, higher volume to void, and episodes of incontinence without any difference in complications.[28,29] At our institution and in the clinic setting, we would use a rigid or flexible cystoscope with a intradetrusor/suburethral combination technique to deliver 200 U of onabotulinumtoxinA in 20 mL at 20 to 30 sites including the trigone, base, lateral, and dome of the bladder.

SHORTCOMINGS OF BOTULINUM TOXIN A
Adverse Event and Precautions

The adverse events associated with intradetrusor injection of BTX-A are not negligible. The most common adverse events reported are urinary tract infections (UTI) and increased postvoid residual, especially in patients with MS or diabetes mellitus with the incidence of UTI reported to be between 51.8% and 56%.[24] In addition, BTX-A should be avoided in settings where concomitant neuromuscular disorder may exacerbate clinical effects of treatment, such as myasthenia gravis or Lambert-Eaton syndrome. Caution must be taken when BTX-A is used in specific patient population with neurogenic bladder, such as patients under age 18 years of age and in geriatric patients. BTX-A is specified as pregnancy category C, where there are no adequate and well-controlled studies in humans, and it should only be used if the potential benefits justify the potential risk to the fetus.

Adherence to Therapy

In the extension trial of 2 phase III trials of DIGNITY study, in which 388 patients were offered repeat injections for up to 5 cycles, only 241 and 113 received the fourth and fifth cycles, respectively.[25]

Authors report that discontinuation as a result of AEs and lack of efficacy was noted in only 12 (3.1%) and 8 (2.1%) of the 388 patients, respectively.[26]

DISEASE-SPECIFIC FINDINGS
Multiple Sclerosis

MS is a chronic multifocal demyelinating disease that can affect any part of the central nervous system. Up to 90% of patients with MS develop lower urinary tract dysfunction within the first 18 years of the disease.[30] Neurogenic lower urinary tract dysfunction symptoms experienced by patients with MS can include abnormalities in the storage phase, voiding phase, or both.[30] Because of the diffuse, multifocal involvement of central nervous system in patients with MS, symptom severity and impact on QOL may vary from patient to patient. Urinary frequency, urgency, and urgency incontinence are the most common symptoms, occurring in 37% to 99% of MS patients[31] in whom they negatively impact health-related QOL.[32]

Analysis of the pooled DIGNITY study, which included 381 patients with MS, demonstrated that onabotulinumtoxinA injections improved clinical outcomes and UDS findings in these patients (**Table 2**).[33] Patients were considered overall responders if one of their goals was reached. These goals were to "be dry," "reduce incontinence," "reduce other urinary symptoms," "reduce activity limitations," "improve bladder control," improve QOL, sleep, and emotions," "reduce number of oral medication therapies," and "other." Patients

with MS or SCI reported significantly greater overall goal accomplishment with onabotulinumtoxinA injection than with placebo (P< .001).[34] **Table 2** summarizes the urodynamic outcomes after onabotulinumtoxinA injections in MS patients.[33]

Despite overall improvements in UI, QOL, and cystometric bladder capacity in these patients, some effects were modest in MS patients. In the pooled DIGNITY data analysis, being dry, the highest reported goal at baseline, was reached in only 42.9% of MS patients at week 6 after treatment, whereas dryness occurred in 21.7% of MS patients who received only a placebo.[34] In addition, in contrast with SCI patients, of whom only 13.5% were voiding voluntarily at baseline, the majority of MS patients were voiding spontaneously and were not using CIC at the baseline (69.6%). In this group at week 2, the overall percentage of patients who required initiation of CIC because of urinary retention was 30.8% to 44.0%. Therefore, it is recommended that all MS patients who are planning to undergo BTX-A should be taught, or agree to learn to do, CIC because as many as up to 88% of patients may need to perform CIC.[35] Initiating CIC is a burden in general, and it is even more so to patients in whom lower extremity spasms, compromised hand dexterity, or visual disturbances may be present. The cost and side effects (hematuria, pain, trauma, strictures, and UTI) associated with CIC also need to be considered.[36] Clinicians should also be aware that UTIs worsen urinary symptoms in MS patients and significantly impact their QOL[37] and may trigger pathways that result in exacerbation of MS and its neurologic progression.[38,39]

Table 2
Outcomes of DIGNITY study in MS versus SCI patients

	MS			SCI		
	Placebo	**200 U**	**300 U**	**Placebo**	**200 U**	**300 U**
No of patients	131	130	120	110	97	103
Age (y)	50.2	49.7	49.9	41.5	40.7	40.6
Male (%)	23.7	20	10.8	77.3	69.1	67
Baseline CIC (%)	32.1	31.5	24.2	88.2	80.4	85.4
UI (n)	−14.0	−22.6	−24.0	−6.4	−19.6	−18.2
Dry (%)	10.7	41.5	44.2	7.3	30.9	35.9
No IDC (%)	18.5	68	79	18.2	58.7	57.6
MCC (mL)	6.8	149.3	165.1	18.6	159.5	160.6
PdetmaxIDC (cm H_2O)	10.7	−22.1	−24.1	−10.9	−42.7	−35.3
UTI	29.2	53.3	59	44.8	49.5	52.5
Urinary retention (%)	4.6	29.5	39.3	1.9	7.2	4

Abbreviations: CIC, clean intermittent catheterization; IDC, involuntary detrusor contractions; MCC, maximum cystometric capacity; MS, multiple sclerosis; PdetmaxIDC, maximum detrusor pressure during involuntary detrusor contraction; SCI, spinal cord injury; UI, urge urinary incontinence episodes per week; UTI, urinary tract infection.

Furthermore, in the longest follow-up study of the use of onabotulinumtoxinA (15 years), the overall discontinuation rate among all neurogenic patients (SCI, MS, MMC) was 40%, and only 14% of MS patients continued with the treatment.[40]

In summary, there is level I evidence that intradetrusor injection of onabotulinumtoxinA for the treatment of refractory NDO in patients with MS is associated with significant achievement of patients' goals and improvement in UDS performance. However, the authors believe that, despite these overall improvements in urinary symptoms, UDS parameters, and QOL after onabotulinumtoxinA injection, its efficacy in MS patients who do not perform CIC is modest compared with the burden of initiating CIC. The cost, adverse events associated with onabotulinumtoxinA, and the significantly low adherence to therapy in MS patients who do not perform CIC need to be considered during shared decision making regarding NDO management in this specific patient group.

Spinal Cord Injury

More than 50% of patients with SCI suffer from UI.[1] Some of these patients do not respond to or tolerate oral medications to control their NDO. In this group, intravesical injection of BTX-A has been shown to decrease UI, improve UDS parameters, and increase QOL.[41] A systematic review by Mehta and colleagues[42] in 2013 of 14 studies representing data from 734 patients with SCI demonstrated that the average proportion of patients that experienced incidents of UI was reduced from a mean of 23% to 1.31% per day after BTX-A treatment. The DIGNITY study, which included 310 patients with SCI, showed that onabotulinumtoxinA injections effectively improve clinical outcomes and UDS parameters (see **Table 2**).[33]

Another clinically important consideration of BTX-A use in patients with SCI is its potential effect on autonomic dysreflexia. Bladder-related events, including NDO, are an important cause of autonomic dysreflexia in SCI patients. Animal and human studies have shown that intradetrusor injections of BTX-A decrease the severity and frequency of bladder-related incidents of autonomic dysreflexia in this setting.[43,44] In summary, there is level I evidence that intradetrusor injection of onabotulinumtoxinA for the treatment of refractory NDO in patients with SCI is associated with significantly improved UDS performance and achievement of patients' goals.

Parkinson's Disease

Fifty percent of patients with PD suffer from UI. Some of these patients do not tolerate or do not respond to oral medications to control their NDO. In addition, the anticholinergic action of the medications may complicate their PD medications to ameliorate the cholinergic system neurologic deficits present with the disease. Intradetrusor injection of BTX-A has been used by a few groups in patients with PD and NDO with good outcomes (**Table 3**). However, currently the literature does not provide a high level of evidence for BTX-A efficacy or indicate dosage and risk factors for retention or difficulty voiding in PD patients.[45] International Continence Society guidelines for the management of bladder dysfunction in PD published in 2016 mention that BTX-A can be used for intractable UI in PD.[45]

Cerebrovascular Accident

Of patients with a history of CVA, 23.6% suffer from NDO.[1] Intravesical injection of onabotulinumtoxinA has been reported in just a few groups of such patients (see **Table 3**). These data indicate that onabotulinumtoxinA might be effective in these patients, but the results might not be as favorable as in other settings. In addition, the possibility of urinary retention and UTI must receive serious consideration in this chronically ill and fragile group of patients.

Myelomeningocele

For many years, bladder management in patients with MMC has been dependent on CIC and high doses of oral anticholinergics. However, some patients do not respond to anticholinergics or their neurogenic constipation can be worsened by their side effects. Intradetrusor injection of BTX-A has been used in various groups to delay or avoid the need for augmentation cystoplasty.[46] The most commonly used dose of onabotulinumtoxinA in these patients is 10 to 12 U/kg with a maximal dose of 360 U.[47] A systematic review was performed by Hascoet and colleagues[48] in 2016 and included 12 studies and 293 patients who were all younger than 18 years of age (**Table 4**). In this review, there was no randomized trial comparing BTX-A versus placebo and most studies had no control group. This review concluded that most studies demonstrated an improvement in both clinical symptoms and UDS parameters. Complete resolution of incontinence occurred in 32% to 100% of patients. Two studies suggested that BTX-A has lower efficacy in patients with low bladder compliance. Intradetrusor injections of BTX-A could be effective in children with MMC, but this possibility is not supported by a high level of evidence.[48] Currently, there are no published data available in BTX-A use in adult MMC patients.

Table 3
Outcomes of BTX-A in patients with Parkinson's disease and cerebrovascular accident

Author, Year	Diagnosis	Method (Level of Evidence)	No of Patients	Mean Age (y)	Toxin Type	Clinical Outcomes	UDC after Tx	MCC after Tx (mL)	UR (%)
Anderson et al,[49] 2014	PD	Prospective No control (4)	20	70.4	OnabotA (100 U)	50% ↓ in UI in 59% of patients	NR	NR	0
Knüpfer et al,[50] 2016	PD	Retrospective No control (4)	10	67.9	OnabotA (200 U)	Pad use/d = 1 ± 0.94 (2.8 ± 2.35)[a]	20% of patients (90%)[a]	332.6 (196.2)[a]	0
Jiang et al,[51] 2014	PD	Retrospective No control (4)	9	73.6	OnabotA (100 U)	UI/3 d = 9.6[c] (10.8)[a]	NR	283 (266)[a]	11.1
Kulaksizoglu et al,[52] 2010	PD	Prospective No control (4)	16	67.2	AbobotA (500 U)	No UI = 6 patients Other patients = 1[c] of UI/1–3 d	Mean pressure M 40[d] (68)[a] F 29[d] (41)[a]	319 (198.6)[a]	0
Giannantoni et al,[53] 2011	PD	Prospective No control (4)	8	66	OnabotA (100 U)	No UI = 3 patients	First vol[b] ↑ significantly	↑[b] significantly	0
Giannantoni et al,[54] 2009	PD	Prospective No control (4)	4	76.25	OnabotA (200 U)	No UI	First vol 385 (158)[a]	468.25 (241.5)[a]	0
Kuo et al,[55] 2006	CVA	Prospective No control (4)	12	72.4	OnabotA (200 U)	8.3% became dry UI improved in 41.7%	First vol 328.1 (188.2)[a]	343.2 (198.3)[a]	25
Jiang et al,[51] 2014	CVA	Retrospective No control (4)	23	73.6	OnabotA (100 U)	UI/3 d = 5.7[c] (13.5)[a]	NR	358 (198)[a]	17.4

Studies outlined have used different variables as their clinical and UDS outcomes. Data in this table were reproduced as is.

Abbreviations: ↓, decrease(d); ↑, increase(d); AbobotA, abobotulinumtoxin A; CVA, cerebrovascular accident; d, day; F, female; M, male; MCC, maximum cystometric capacity; mL, milliliter; No, number; NR, not recorded; OnabotA, onabotulinumtoxinA; PD, Parkinson's disease; Tx, treatment; UDC, uninhibited detrusor contractions; UI, urinary incontinence; UR, urinary retention; vol, volume.

[a] Values before treatment.
[b] Only graphs have been used in this article.
[c] Episode(s).
[d] cmH_2O.

Table 4
Outcomes of BTX-A in patients with myelomeningocele

Author, Year	Method (Level of Evidence)	Number of Patients	Mean Age (y)	Toxin Type	Dry After Tx (%)	DO After Tx	Pdetmax Before Tx (cmH$_2$O)	Pdetmax After Tx (cmH$_2$O)	MCC Before Tx (mL)	MCC After Tx (mL)
Tiryaki et al,[56] 2015	Retrospective No control (4)	16	9	OnabotA	55	No	NR	NR	NR	NR
Tarcan et al,[57] 2014	Prospective No control (4)	31	7.95	NR	96	No	64.6	30.1	53.9	233.3
Marte,[58] 2013	Retrospective No control (4)	47	10.7	OnabotA	100	No	NR	NR	NR	NR
Zeino et al,[59] 2012	Retrospective No control (4)	28	6.45	OnabotA	32	Yes	60.2	33.14	120	153
Horst et al,[60] 2011	Retrospective No control (4)	11	6.7	OnabotA	NR	NR	56	46	208	279
Safari et al,[61] 2010	Prospective With control[a] (2)	60	6.65	AbobotA	63	Yes	133	62.53	176.2	246.3
Neel,[62] 2010	Prospective No control	13	5.3	NR	87	NR	58	36	75	150

(continued on next page)

Table 4
(continued)

Author, Year	Method (Level of Evidence)	Number of Patients	Mean Age (y)	Toxin Type	Dry After Tx (%)	DO After Tx	Pdetmax Before Tx (cmH$_2$O)	Pdetmax After Tx (cmH$_2$O)	MCC Before Tx (mL)	MCC After Tx (mL)
Deshpande et al,[63] 2009	Prospective No control (4)	7	16	OnabotA	NR	NR	NR	NR	257	344
Kajbafzadeh et al,[64] 2006	Prospective No control (4)	26	6.9	OnabotA	73	Yes	139	83.2	102.8	270.2
Altaweel et al,[65] 2006	Prospective No control (4)	20	13	NR	65	NR	43 (40.1)[b]	21.6 (40.1)[b]	215.6 (146)[b]	338.3 (164)[b]
Riccabona et al,[66] 2004	Prospective No control (4)	15	5.8	NR	87	NR	78.8	42.76	136.3	297
Schulte-Baukloh et al,[67] 2002	Prospective No control (4)	17	10.8	OnabotA	NR	Yes	58.9	39.7	137.5	215

Abbreviations: AboboA, abobotulinumtoxin A; DO, detrusor overactivity; MCC, maximum cystometric capacity; NR, not recorded; OnabotA, onabotulinumtoxinA; Pdetmax, maximum detrusor pressure; Tx, treatment.

[a] Data of control group have not been shown.

[b] Data in and out of parenthesis refer to incontinent and continent patients, respectively.

However, recently, we investigated the outcomes of intravesical injection of onbotulinumtoxinA in adults with spinal dysraphism.

Billing codes were used to identify patients who underwent onabotulinumtoxinA injection between 2012 and 2016 at our institution and within our transitional urology clinic. A total of 18 patients (8 males and 10 females) with mean age of 20.8 years with a history of spinal dysraphism were identified, and all patients reported refractory UI from native urethra or continent catheterizable channel. Fourteen patients had MMC, 2 sacral agenesis, 1 tethered cord, and 1 occult spina bifida. All patients completed UDS before onabotulinumtoxinA injection. UI improved by onabotulinumtoxinA injection in 81.25% of patients and 63.66% of them became dry ($P = .023$). The degree of hydronephrosis improved in 3 of 4 patients (75%) who had follow-up imaging. Repeat UDS after injection was done in 11 patients who did not improve clinically or who had loss of bladder compliance on their baseline UDS (29.34 mL/cmH$_2$O vs 67.24 mL/cmH$_2$O). The mean maximum cystometric capacity before and after injection was 310.18 mL and 380.27 mL, respectively ($P = .045$). However, mean bladder compliance before and after treatment was 29.26 mL/cmH$_2$O and 28.76 mL/cmH$_2$O, respectively ($P = .48$). Therefore, we believe that intravesical onabotulinumtoxinA injection may improve refractory UI in a selected group of adults with spinal dysraphism. However, despite improvement in maximum cystometric capacity, bladder compliance does not seem to improve after therapy in patients who had loss of compliance at baseline. We propose that possibly earlier intervention might be more beneficial in this specific patient population, when significant bladder remodeling has not occurred. Future prospective and multicenter trials are needed to evaluate the effects of onabotulinumtoxinA in adults with spinal dysraphism.

Another possibly unique and interesting use of BTX-A in neuropathic patients could be in the setting of history of prior augmentation cystoplasty. Augmentation cystoplasty has been used in the treatment of refractory overactive or neurogenic bladder for decades. In a very small number of patients, symptoms persist or recur after the surgery and there is little guidance on the management of these patients. At our institution, we reviewed the efficacy of intradetrusor and intra-augment onabotulinumtoxinA injections in this setting. We identified 13 patients (9 females, 4 males) with the mean age of 31.61 years and a history of prior augmentation cystoplasty. The indications for onabotulinumtoxinA injections were UI and refractory storage (irritative) symptoms in 12 (92.3%) and 1 (7.6%) patients, respectively. All patients completed urodynamic studies before treatment. Intradetrusor and intraaugment injections were done in 10 patients and 3 patients just received intradetrusor injections. Ten patients (77%) reported improvement in all subjective parameters (frequency, urgency, incontinence). One patient with history of ileocystoplasty and Mitrofanoff appendicovesicostomy continued to have incontinence per urethra. Video urodynamic testing in this patient after onabotulinumtoxinA injection showed persistence detrusor overactivity, decreased compliance, and hourglass configuration, and the patient underwent a repeat augmentation cystoplasty. Therefore, we propose that intradetrusor and intraaugment injection of BTX-A may improve refractory storage symptoms and continence after augmentation cystoplasty in the carefully selected patients. However, prospective studies are needed to better evaluate the efficacy and ideal sites of injection of BTX-A in the setting of augmentation cystoplasty.

Follow-up after botulinum toxin A

Currently, there are no guidelines available for the management of neurogenic bladder patients or their follow-up after intravesical BTX-A therapy. Because neurourologic disorders are usually progressive, we recommend obtaining a videourodynamic and validated questionnaires at baseline. If patient is high risk based on his or her UDS findings, as measured by vesicoureteral reflux, elevated detrusor pressures, and decreased bladder compliance, worsening of upper urinary tracts (hydronephrosis or renal function), we would also recommend repeating UDS after BTX-A therapy despite its clinical outcome. However, in a setting of the low-risk patient where the baseline UDS demonstrates low detrusor storage pressures and appropriate compliance, and other clinical evaluations also suggest stable lower and upper urinary tracts in a nonprogressive neurologic disease where the patient clinically responds to BTX-A treatment, we may delay the repeat UDS after treatment.

SUMMARY

There is level I evidence that intradetrusor injection of onabotulinumtoxinA is beneficial for the treatment of refractory NDO in patients with MS and SCI, and provides significantly better results than a placebo. BTX-A use is also supported by pilot studies for patients with PD. Current data indicate that BTX-A might have a limited efficacy in patients with CVA. In addition, the morbidity of urinary retention and UTI must be given serious consideration in this chronically ill and fragile group of patients. Intradetrusor injections of BTX-A could be effective in children with MMC, but this possibility is not supported by a high level of evidence. Cost, adverse events associated with BTX-A, including the need for de novo CIC, and the failure to adhere to therapy by some patients, especially patients who do not already perform CIC, requires careful consideration during shared decision making regarding management of NDO.

REFERENCES

1. Ruffion A, Castro-Diaz D, Patel H, et al. Systematic review of the epidemiology of urinary incontinence and detrusor overactivity among patients with neurogenic overactive bladder. Neuroepidemiology 2013; 41(3–4):146–55.
2. Haab F. Chapter 1: The conditions of neurogenic detrusor overactivity and overactive bladder. Neurourol Urodyn 2014;33(S3):S2–5.
3. Drake MJ, Apostolidis A, Cocci A, et al. Neurogenic lower urinary tract dysfunction: clinical management recommendations of the Neurologic Incontinence committee of the fifth International Consultation on Incontinence 2013. Neurourol Urodyn 2016;35(6): 657–65.
4. Buser N, Ivic S, Kessler TM, et al. Efficacy and adverse events of antimuscarinics for treating overactive bladder: network meta-analyses. Eur Urol 2012;62(6):1040–60.
5. Gray SL, Anderson ML, Dublin S, et al. Cumulative use of strong anticholinergics and incident dementia: a prospective cohort study. JAMA Intern Med 2015;175(3):401–7.
6. Risacher SL, McDonald BC, Tallman EF, et al. Association between anticholinergic medication use and cognition, brain metabolism, and brain atrophy in cognitively normal older adults. JAMA Neurol 2016; 73(6):721–32.
7. Khavari R, Fletcher SG, Liu J, et al. A modification to augmentation cystoplasty with catheterizable stoma for neurogenic patients: technique and long-term results. Urology 2012;80(2):460–4.
8. Krebs J, Bartel P, Pannek J. Functional outcome of supratrigonal cystectomy and augmentation ileocystoplasty in adult patients with refractory neurogenic lower urinary tract dysfunction. Neurourol Urodyn 2016;35(2):260–6.
9. Cruz F. Targets for botulinum toxin in the lower urinary tract. Neurourol Urodyn 2014;33(1):31–8.
10. Behr-Roussel D, Oger S, Pignol B, et al. Minimal effective dose of dysport and botox in a rat model of neurogenic detrusor overactivity. Eur Urol 2012; 61(5):1054–61.

11. Schurch B, de Seze M, Denys P, et al. Botulinum toxin type a is a safe and effective treatment for neurogenic urinary incontinence: results of a single treatment, randomized, placebo controlled 6-month study. J Urol 2005;174(1):196–200.
12. Herschorn S, Gajewski J, Ethans K, et al. Efficacy of botulinum toxin A injection for neurogenic detrusor overactivity and urinary incontinence: a randomized, double-blind trial. J Urol 2011;185(6):2229–35.
13. Duthie JB. Botulinum toxin injections for adults with overactive bladder syndrome. Cochrane Database Syst Rev 2011;(12):CD005493.
14. Zhou X, Yan HL, Cui YS, et al. Efficacy and safety of onabotulinumtoxinA in treating neurogenic detrusor overactivity: a systematic review and meta-analysis. Chin Med J (Engl) 2015;128(7):963–8.
15. Cui Y, Zhou X, Zong H, et al. The efficacy and safety of onabotulinumtoxinA in treating idiopathic OAB: a systematic review and meta-analysis. Neurourol Urodyn 2015;34(5):413–9.
16. Lopez Ramos HE, Torres Castellanos L, Ponce Esparza I, et al. Management of overactive bladder with onabotulinumtoxinA: systematic review and meta-analysis. Urology 2017;100:53–8.
17. Carlson JJ, Hansen RN, Dmochowski RR, et al. Estimating the cost-effectiveness of onabotulinumtoxinA for neurogenic detrusor overactivity in the United States. Clin Ther 2013;35(4):414–24.
18. Moore DC, Cohn JA, Dmochowski RR. Use of botulinum toxin A in the treatment of lower urinary tract disorders: a review of the literature. Toxins (Basel) 2016;8(4):88.
19. Cruz F, Nitti V. Chapter 5: clinical data in neurogenic detrusor overactivity (NDO) and overactive bladder (OAB). Neurourol Urodyn 2014;33(Suppl 3):S26–31.
20. Santos-Silva A, da Silva CM, Cruz F. Botulinum toxin treatment for bladder dysfunction. Int J Urol 2013; 20(10):956–62.
21. Cruz F, Herschorn S, Aliotta P, et al. Efficacy and safety of onabotulinumtoxinA in patients with urinary incontinence due to neurogenic detrusor overactivity: a randomised, double-blind, placebo-controlled trial. Eur Urol 2011;60(4):742–50.
22. Schurch B, Carda S. OnabotulinumtoxinA and multiple sclerosis. Ann Phys Rehabil Med 2014;57(5): 302–14.
23. Ginsberg D, Gousse A, Keppenne V, et al. Phase 3 efficacy and tolerability study of onabotulinumtoxinA for urinary incontinence from neurogenic detrusor overactivity. J Urol 2012;187(6):2131–9.
24. Rovner E, Dmochowski R, Chapple C, et al. OnabotulinumtoxinA improves urodynamic outcomes in patients with neurogenic detrusor overactivity. Neurourol Urodyn 2013;32(8):1109–15.
25. Kennelly M, Dmochowski R, Ethans K, et al. Long-term efficacy and safety of onabotulinumtoxinA in patients with urinary incontinence due to neurogenic

detrusor overactivity: an interim analysis. Urology 2013;81(3):491–7.

26. Rovner E, Kohan A, Chartier-Kastler E, et al. Long-term efficacy and safety of onabotulinumtoxinA in patients with neurogenic detrusor overactivity who completed 4 years of treatment. J Urol 2016; 196(3):801–8.

27. Apostolidis A, Thompson C, Yan X, et al. An exploratory, placebo-controlled, dose-response study of the efficacy and safety of onabotulinumtoxinA in spinal cord injury patients with urinary incontinence due to neurogenic detrusor overactivity. World J Urol 2013;31(6):1469–74.

28. Hui C, Keji X, Chonghe J, et al. Combined detrusor-trigone BTX-A injections for urinary incontinence secondary to neurogenic detrusor overactivity. Spinal Cord 2016;54(1):46–50.

29. Abdel-Meguid TA. Botulinum toxin-A injections into neurogenic overactive bladder–to include or exclude the trigone? A prospective, randomized, controlled trial. J Urol 2010;184(6):2423–8.

30. Phe V, Chartier-Kastler E, Panicker JN. Management of neurogenic bladder in patients with multiple sclerosis. Nat Rev Urol 2016;13(5):275–88.

31. Dillon BE, Lemack GE. Urodynamics in the evaluation of the patient with multiple sclerosis: when are they helpful and how do we use them? Urol Clin North Am 2014;41(3):439–44, ix.

32. Khalaf KM, Coyne KS, Globe DR, et al. The impact of lower urinary tract symptoms on health-related quality of life among patients with multiple sclerosis. Neurourol Urodyn 2016;35(1):48–54.

33. Ginsberg D, Cruz F, Herschorn S, et al. OnabotulinumtoxinA is effective in patients with urinary incontinence due to neurogenic detrusor overactivity [corrected] regardless of concomitant anticholinergic use or neurologic etiology. Adv Ther 2013; 30(9):819–33.

34. Chartier-Kastler E, Rovner E, Hepp Z, et al. Patient-reported goal achievement following onabotulinumtoxinA treatment in patients with neurogenic detrusor overactivity. Neurourol Urodyn 2016; 35(5):595–600.

35. Kalsi V, Gonzales G, Popat R, et al. Botulinum injections for the treatment of bladder symptoms of multiple sclerosis. Ann Neurol 2007;62(5):452–7.

36. Prieto J, Murphy CL, Moore KN, et al. Intermittent catheterisation for long-term bladder management. Cochrane Database Syst Rev 2014;(9):CD006008.

37. Phe V, Pakzad M, Curtis C, et al. Urinary tract infections in multiple sclerosis. Mult Scler 2016;22(7): 855–61.

38. Metz LM, McGuinness SD, Harris C. Urinary tract infections may trigger relapse in multiple sclerosis. Axone 1998;19(4):67–70.

39. Tauber SC, Nau R, Gerber J. Systemic infections in multiple sclerosis and experimental autoimmune encephalomyelitis. Arch Physiol Biochem 2007; 113(3):124–30.

40. Leitner L, Guggenbuhl-Roy S, Knupfer SC, et al. More than 15 years of experience with intradetrusor onabotulinumtoxinA injections for treating refractory neurogenic detrusor overactivity: lessons to be learned. Eur Urol 2016;70(3):522–8.

41. da Silva CM, Chancellor MB, Smith CP, et al. Use of botulinum toxin for genitourinary conditions: what is the evidence? Toxicon 2015;107(Pt A):141–7.

42. Mehta S, Hill D, McIntyre A, et al. Meta-analysis of botulinum toxin A detrusor injections in the treatment of neurogenic detrusor overactivity after spinal cord injury. Arch Phys Med Rehabil 2013; 94(8):1473–81.

43. Fougere RJ, Currie KD, Nigro MK, et al. Reduction in bladder-related autonomic dysreflexia after onabotulinumtoxinA treatment in spinal cord injury. J Neurotrauma 2016;33(18):1651–7.

44. Elkelini MS, Bagli DJ, Fehlings M, et al. Effects of intravesical onabotulinumtoxinA on bladder dysfunction and autonomic dysreflexia after spinal cord injury: role of nerve growth factor. BJU Int 2012; 109(3):402–7.

45. Sakakibara R, Panicker J, Finazzi-Agro E, et al. A guideline for the management of bladder dysfunction in Parkinson's disease and other gait disorders. Neurourol Urodyn 2016;35(5):551–63.

46. Hassouna T, Gleason JM, Lorenzo AJ. Botulinum toxin A's expanding role in the management of pediatric lower urinary tract dysfunction. Curr Urol Rep 2014;15(8):426.

47. Game X, Mouracade P, Chartier-Kastler E, et al. Botulinum toxin-A (Botox) intradetrusor injections in children with neurogenic detrusor overactivity/neurogenic overactive bladder: a systematic literature review. J Pediatr Urol 2009;5(3):156–64.

48. Hascoet J, Manunta A, Brochard C, et al. Outcomes of intra-detrusor injections of botulinum toxin in patients with spina bifida: a systematic review. Neurourol Urodyn 2017;36(3):557–64.

49. Anderson RU, Orenberg EK, Glowe P. OnabotulinumtoxinA office treatment for neurogenic bladder incontinence in Parkinson's disease. Urology 2014; 83(1):22–7.

50. Knupfer SC, Schneider SA, Averhoff MM, et al. Preserved micturition after intradetrusor onabotulinumtoxinA injection for treatment of neurogenic bladder dysfunction in Parkinson's disease. BMC Urol 2016;16(1):55.

51. Jiang YH, Liao CH, Tang DL, et al. Efficacy and safety of intravesical onabotulinumtoxinA injection on elderly patients with chronic central nervous system lesions and overactive bladder. PLoS One 2014; 9(8):e105989.

52. Kulaksizoglu H, Parman Y. Use of botulinim toxin-A for the treatment of overactive bladder symptoms

in patients with Parkinsons's disease. Parkinsonism Relat Disord 2010;16(8):531–4.

53. Giannantoni A, Conte A, Proietti S, et al. Botulinum toxin type A in patients with Parkinson's disease and refractory overactive bladder. J Urol 2011; 186(3):960–4.

54. Giannantoni A, Rossi A, Mearini E, et al. Botulinum toxin A for overactive bladder and detrusor muscle overactivity in patients with Parkinson's disease and multiple system atrophy. J Urol 2009;182(4):1453–7.

55. Kuo HC. Therapeutic effects of suburothelial injection of botulinum a toxin for neurogenic detrusor overactivity due to chronic cerebrovascular accident and spinal cord lesions. Urology 2006;67(2):232–6.

56. Tiryaki S, Yagmur I, Parlar Y, et al. Botulinum injection is useless on fibrotic neuropathic bladders. J Pediatr Urol 2015;11(1):27.e1-4.

57. Tarcan T, Akbal C, Şekerci ÇA, et al. Intradetrusor injections of onabotulinum toxin-A in children with urinary incontinence due to neurogenic detrusor overactivity refractory to antimuscarinic treatment. Korean J Urol 2014;55(4):281–7.

58. Marte A. Onabotulinumtoxin A for treating overactive/poor compliant bladders in children and adolescents with neurogenic bladder secondary to myelomeningocele. Toxins (Basel) 2013;5(1):16.

59. Zeino M, Becker T, Koen M, et al. Long-term follow-up after botulinum toxin A (BTX-A) injection into the detrusor for treatment of neurogenic detrusor hyperactivity in children. Cent European J Urol 2012; 65(3):156–61.

60. Horst M, Weber DM, Bodmer C, et al. Repeated botulinum-a toxin injection in the treatment of neuropathic bladder dysfunction and poor bladder compliance in children with myelomeningocele. Neurourol Urodyn 2011;30(8):1546–9.

61. Safari S, Jamali S, Habibollahi P, et al. Intravesical injections of botulinum toxin type A for management of neuropathic bladder: a comparison of two methods. Urology 2010;76(1):225–30.

62. Neel KF. Total endoscopic and anal irrigation management approach to noncompliant neuropathic bladder in children: a good alternative. J Urol 2010;184(1):315–8.

63. Deshpande AV, Sampang R, Smith GH. Study of botulinum toxin A in neurogenic bladder due to spina bifida in children. ANZ J Surg 2010;80(4):250–3.

64. Kajbafzadeh A-M, Moosavi S, Tajik P, et al. Intravesical injection of botulinum toxin type A: management of neuropathic bladder and bowel dysfunction in children with myelomeningocele. Urology 2006; 68(5):1091–6.

65. Altaweel W, Jednack R, Bilodeau C, et al. Repeated intradetrusor botulinum toxin type A in children with neurogenic bladder due to myelomeningocele. J Urol 2006;175(3):1102–5.

66. Riccabona M, Koen M, Schindler M, et al. Botulinum-A toxin injection into the detrusor: a safe alternative in the treatment of children with myelomeningocele with detrusor hyperreflexia. J Urol 2004; 171(2, Part 1):845–8.

67. Schulte-Baukloh H, Michael T, Schobert J, et al. Efficacy of botulinum-a toxin in children with detrusor hyperreflexia due to myelomeningocele: preliminary results. Urology 2002;59(3):325–7 [discussion: 327–8].

Surgical Management of Neurogenic Lower Urinary Tract Dysfunction

Ronak A. Gor, DO, Sean P. Elliott, MD, MS*

KEYWORDS

- Neurogenic bladder • Urinary diversion • Spina bifida • Urinary reconstruction • Transitional urology
- Congenital urology

KEY POINTS

- Surgery serves to augment, enhance, or obviate medical therapy for patients with neurogenic lower urinary tract dysfunction.
- Indications for surgery include failure of maximal medical therapy, inability to perform or aversion to clean intermittent catheterization, refractory incontinence, and complications from chronic, indwelling catheters.
- The catheterizable ileocecocystoplasty augments the bladder and creates a "custom fit" catheterizable channel while creating a single bowel anastomosis and obviating the need for a detrusor tunnel.
- Complications from surgery are high. Patients and their caregivers must provide adequate maintenance of their reconstruction to ensure longevity while mitigating complications.
- Surgeons must account for individual characteristics, including physical/cognitive function, financial/social support, access to care, motivation, comorbidities, and natural history of their underlying neurologic dysfunction when fashioning a plan.

INTRODUCTION AND NATURE OF THE PROBLEM

Neurogenic lower urinary tract dysfunction (nLUTD) can have a profound impact on the quality of life of patients with congenital or acquired neurologic disease.[1] Spina bifida/myelomeningocele (SB) is the most common cause of congenital nLUTD and comprises the largest group of adult congenital urologic patients in the United States.[2] Other causes of congenital nLUTD progressing into adulthood include cerebral palsy, epispadias/exstrophy complex, and Eagle-Barrett syndrome.

Improvements in perinatal, pediatric, and adolescent care have extended the life expectancy of patients with SB and other congenital conditions. Unfortunately, the transition of care from child to adulthood has proved challenging, with less than 50% of children successfully establishing adult care.[3] Adult urologists often lack appropriate training in the management of congenital urologic patients; as such, this population is at significant risk for upper and lower urinary tract deterioration stemming from nLUTD.

Acquired causes of nLUTD include spinal cord injury (SCI), stroke, multiple sclerosis, Parkinson's disease, and a variety of other central and peripheral nervous system disorders that may impact the lower urinary tract. An aging, growing population will certainly increase the prevalence of patients

Disclosure Statement: R.A. Gor: None; S.P. Elliott: Consultant for Boston Scientific/American Medical Systems.
Department of Urology, University of Minnesota, 420 Delaware Street Southeast, MMC 394, Minneapolis, MN 55455, USA
* Corresponding author.
E-mail address: selliott@umn.edu

Urol Clin N Am 44 (2017) 475–490
http://dx.doi.org/10.1016/j.ucl.2017.04.013
0094-0143/17/© 2017 Elsevier Inc. All rights reserved.

urologic.theclinics.com

with significant nLUTD from acquired conditions. As such, there is an increasing need for physicians dedicated to the care of patients with nLUTD. Herein, we broadly review the role of surgery in patients with nLUTD.

INDICATIONS FOR SURGERY

Optimal management for patients with nLUTD results in a lower urinary tract with (1) a low pressure, highly compliant bladder that protects the upper urinary tracts, (2) has predictable and controlled urine emptying, and (3) is dry. Surgery serves to add to, enhance, or obviate medical therapy to achieve these goals and preserve renal function. There are a variety of indications for surgical intervention (**Table 1**). For purposes of this article, surgical intervention excludes suprapubic catheter, intradetrusor botulinum injection, and sacral/peripheral nerve stimulation.

Individuals with congenital or acquired nLUTD require a nuanced approach to surgical management because their age, social and financial support, physical and cognitive faculties, and comorbidities contribute to both the decision to perform surgery and which surgery to perform.

Although indwelling urinary catheters carry the perception of improving the health and quality of life in patients with nLUTD by maintaining low bladder pressures and keeping patients dry, many untoward sequelae can result, including infections, obstruction, urethral atrophy, erosion,

necrosis, and fistula. Many of these complications are exacerbated by sequential catheter upsizing in reaction to pericatheter leakage.[4,5]

Surgery for Sphincteric Incontinence

Although congenital and acquired nLUTD often arise from disparate neuroanatomic origins, both can result in denervation of the sphincter, resulting in stress urinary incontinence (SUI) from intrinsic sphincter deficiency (ISD). Surgical options, in general, include bulking agents, pubovaginal/bladder neck slings, bulbar urethral sling, artificial urinary sphincter (AUS), bladder neck closure (BNC), and submucosal bulking.

BULKING AGENTS
Indications

First described in 1974 for nonneurogenic SUI in women, injectable bulking agents placed at the bladder neck or posterior urethra lead to submucosal expansion resulting in increased bladder outlet resistance.[6] The European Association of Urology Guidelines on nLUTD and the Neurologic Incontinence Committee of the International Consultation on Incontinence recommend bulking agent use for short-term improvement when there is a demand for a minimally invasive treatment.[7] Although many patients with nLUTD may experience SUI secondary to chronic catheter use, patients with sacral spina bifida or sacral/conus

---

Table 1
Surgical indications for patients with nLUTD

Indication	Sequelae if Untreated	Goals for Surgery	Surgical Intervention(s)
Failure of maximal medical therapy for elevated bladder pressure	↑ Detrusor pressure ↓ Renal function Recurrent infection	↓ Detrusor pressure	1. SPC 2. Augment ± CCC 3. Urinary diversion
Inability to perform or aversion to urethral CIC	Urinary retention ↑ Detrusor pressure ↓ Renal function	Facilitate CIC Maintain or ↓ detrusor pressure	1. SPC 2. CCC ± augment 3. Urinary diversion
Urinary incontinence	Personal/social embarrassment Skin maceration/breakdown	Achieve continence	1. SPC 2. Sling 3. AUS 4. BNR
Complications from chronic, indwelling catheters	Pubovesical fistula Urethral erosion Bladder perforation End-stage, contracted bladder	Repair and diversion	1. Urinary diversion 2. Cystectomy ± prostatectomy

Abbreviations: Augment, augmentation cystoplasty; AUS, artificial urinary sphincter; BNR, bladder neck reconstruction; CCC, continent catheterizable channel; CIC, clean intermittent catheterization; nLUTD, neurologic urinary tract dysfunction; SPC, suprapubic cystostomy.

medullaris lesions are populations that commonly experience ISD.

Contraindications

Patients who are otherwise appropriate candidates for sling or AUS and are interested in long-term treatment of ISD should not be offered bulking agents. Additionally, patients with urethral diverticulum, chronic urethritis, or fistula should not receive bulking agents.

Approach and Technique

Submucosal injection of bulking agents can be performed using standard cystoscopic equipment, with or without a working element. Contemporary material choices include dextranomer/hyaluronic acid (Deflux), polydimethylsiloxane (Macroplastique), pyrolytic carbon coated beads (Durasphere), and calcium hydroxylapatite beads (Coaptite). Injections are directed to the bladder neck in women and the bladder neck or posterior urethra in men. Direct visual feedback confirms appropriate needle position. Complete mucosal coaptation should be seen. Care must be taken to not pass the needle through the bladder neck, which will result in ineffective deposition of the agent into the bladder lumen.

Outcomes and Complications

Numerous pediatric series are available, with varying durations of efficacy depending on severity of incontinence and definition of success.[8–12] Typically, cure is the exception, and improvement duration spans months to less than 1 year, which is consistent with our clinical experience. Adult series are few and have inadequate follow-up to draw meaningful conclusions.[13,14] Although well-tolerated and efficacious as adjunctive treatment in the post midurethral sling setting in women with nonneurogenic SUI,[15,16] similar results have not been seen in patients with nLUTD.[9] Periurethral abscess, urethral prolapse, and bulking agent migration have been reported in several case reports, but major complications are rare.[17–22]

PUBOVAGINAL AND BLADDER NECK SLINGS
Indications

Slings are indicated in patients with ISD secondary to nLUTD. They improve continence by increasing bladder outlet resistance through direct suburethral or bladder neck compression. In women, they are placed as a pubovaginal sling (PVS) and in men as bladder neck slings. Although bulbar urethral slings are commonly used for men with ISD after radical prostatectomy, they are not approved for use in nLUTD and there are few data in nLUTD.

Contraindications

Many neurogenic patients are typically unable to generate sufficient abdominal pressure using Valsalva and Crede maneuvers to spontaneously void. As such, slings are contraindicated as the primary treatment in patients lacking the independent or dependent faculties to perform clean intermittent catheterization (CIC). Additionally, in patients with poor bladder compliance, a sling should not be used alone, for the risk of high-pressure transmission to the upper tracts is high.

Approach and Technique

Women with nLUTD may undergo PVS as an independent procedure, or concomitantly during augmentation cystoplasty (AC) with or without continent catheterizable channel (CCC) creation. In patients deemed high risk for these reconstructions, an SPC or ileovesicostomy are technically simpler alternative adjuncts to PVS. Chronic SPC presence carries similar risks of indwelling urethral catheters, and a poorly draining ileovesicostomy often necessitates surgical revision. Up to one-third of children who undergo bladder neck reconstruction/sling without AC require an AC within 10 years[23]; however, adults demonstrating low bladder pressures before PVS do not seem to develop high pressures postoperatively and may avoid an AC.[24] The surgical technique for autologous fascial PVS has remained largely unchanged since it was streamlined and popularized by McGuire and Lytton in 1978.[25]

Bladder neck sling placement in men is a significantly more invasive procedure, requiring an abdominal approach with sling placement between the bladder neck and seminal vesicles.[26] An open or robotic approach may be used, both of which procedurally mimic that of the open or robotic radical prostatectomy. In an open approach, the extravesical dissection is first performed, separating the endopelvic fascia, after which a plane is created posteriorly around the bladder neck, anterior to the seminal vesicles. Robotically, an initial posterior approach allows dissection of the seminal vesicles, after which the space of Retzius is developed. Separating the endopelvic fascia then joins our anterior and posterior dissections, creating an aperture for sling placement. Bulbar urethral slings and AUS offer a significantly less invasive option for men with ISD and will be described elsewhere in this article.

Graft choices include autografts (rectus fascia/tensor fascia lata), allografts, xenografts, and synthetic mesh. Although all are viable options, autografts are readily available, cost effective, and have significantly lower rates of perforation or urethral erosion than synthetic mesh.[27] Additionally, continued reliance on CIC increases the risk of urethral perforation in patients with nLUTD, so biological materials are preferable in patients at higher risk for urethral injury.

Outcomes and Complications

Although few series describe outcomes for PVS or bladder neck sling in adults with nLUTD, those available seem to be promising. McGuire and colleagues described intermediate outcomes in 33 adult women with ISD secondary to SB or SCI undergoing PVS, noting 25 of 33 (76%) as completely dry, 5 of 33 (15%) as markedly improved, and 30 of 33 (91%) as satisfied with the outcome of the operation. Of the 33, 3 patients (9.1%) required reoperation for sling erosion, vesicovaginal fistula, and urethral stenosis. Similarly, of the few series describing outcomes in men undergoing bladder neck sling, outcomes seem to be satisfactory, with success rates of 69% to 83% balanced by a modest 15% need for subsequent surgery.[26,28]

ARTIFICIAL URINARY SPHINCTER
Indications

First introduced in 1972, the AUS has changed minimally in design over the past 4 decades.[29] A cuff surrounds the bladder neck or bulbar urethra; the cuff is opened and closed as fluid cycles between it and a pressure regulating balloon via a pump placed in the scrotum or labia majora. Considering its occlusive mechanism, it is indicated and well-suited for patients with ISD. The ideal candidates for AUS are patients with ISD, compliant bladders of sufficient storage capacity, and retained upper extremity function. In our experience, motivated patients with lumbosacral/sacral SB often exhibit these attributes.

Contraindications

AUS is contraindicated in patients with uncontrolled, elevated detrusor pressures, inadequate bladder capacity, and in patients lacking the independent or dependent faculties to operate their device or perform CIC if needed. Additionally, bulbar urethral cuff placement should be avoided in patients with nLUTD because many spend the majority of their day seated, applying constant perineal pressure on their device, increasing the risk of cuff erosion.

Approach and Technique

The surgical approach to AUS in nLUTD is dictated by cuff location. In women, cuffs are positioned around the bladder neck using open, laparoscopic, or robotic techniques.[30,31] The space of Retzius is developed and the endopelvic fascia is incised adjacent to the urethra bilaterally.[31] The most critical portion of the case is developing the urethrovaginal space that the cuff will traverse, because the bladder, urethra, and vagina are at risk for injury.

In men, cuffs may be placed around the bladder neck or bulbar urethra. Cuff sizes span 3.5 to 11 cm, with larger cuffs designed for bladder neck application. Urethral instrumentation across smaller cuffs placed in the bulbar urethra is associated with device erosion.[32,33] When selecting location for cuff placement, considerations regarding need for CIC (per urethra or catheterizable channel) significantly impact decision making. Because patients with nLUTD often require cystoscopy, especially in the presence of an AC, bladder neck cuffs allow for larger cuffs placed around more robust tissue, minimizing the risk of erosion in these individuals.[34]

Bladder neck AUS insertion in men requires lateral bladder neck definition with posterior bladder neck dissection for cuff placement.[35] Procedural steps in bulbar AUS are well-described; however, bladder neck placement is preferable in the typical nLUTD patient because it offers a longer device survival rate.[36] Typically, the pressure regulating balloon is placed either in the retropubic or submuscular space; both of these locations can be accessed through the external inguinal ring or via a separate incision.[37]

Although not the ideal candidate, patients with small capacity, high-pressure bladders may undergo simultaneous AC and bladder neck AUS placement with the few reporting series noting comparable outcomes with AUS-only cases.[38,39] Despite the theoretic risk of positioning a prosthetic device in a contaminated field, risk of infection does not seem to be increased.[40]

Outcomes and Complications

Few studies evaluate outcomes of AUS in nLUTD. The largest available series reviewed outcomes in 51 adult men with nLUTD resulting from SB or SCI undergoing bladder neck AUS with a mean follow-up of 83 months. They found 74% of patients were dry or had mild incontinence (nocturnal leakage or safety pad).[41]

Neurogenic patients undergoing AUS must be counseled on the relatively high rate of requiring revision surgery. Revision rates in neurogenic ISD may be higher than in nonneurogenic patients (85% vs 59% at the 6-year follow-up).[42] Several other series noted the mean life span of bladder neck AUS devices was 4.7 to 6.0 years, with fewer than 10% of devices surviving more than 8 years.[41,43,44] Infections with or without erosions are feared complications requiring urgent device removal, salvage bladder neck or urethral repair if possible, and several months of healing before addressing subsequent intervention.

BULBAR URETHRAL SLINGS
Indications

Compared with bladder neck slings, bulbar urethral slings offer a significantly less invasive alternative for men with ISD resulting from nLUTD.

Contraindications

Considering that slings are designed to augment rather than replace sphincteric function, an ISD itself is considered a relative contraindication by some.[45] Similar to PVS, bulbar urethral slings are contraindicated in patients lacking the ability to perform or arrange for CIC and should only be placed as primary therapy in patients with safe bladder compliance.

Approach and Technique

Contemporary options for male urethral slings include quadratic (Virtue, Coloplast, Humlebaek, Denmark) and transobturator slings (AdVance, AMS, Minnetonka, MN), with the latter as the only sling tested in patients with nLUTD.[46] The mechanism of transobturator retrourethral slings is poorly understood. Prevailing theories for mechanism in postprostatectomy patients involve bulbar urethral repositioning resulting in enhanced urethral coaptation without obstruction.[47] This is unlike the mechanism in patients with ISD; as such, there likely is a subtle compressive effect resulting in increased outlet resistance.[45] A standard perineal approach offers rapid insertion with minimal morbidity. This approach combined with the obviated need for autologous fascia harvest results in a significantly simpler surgery when compared with autologous fascia bladder neck slings.

Outcomes and Complications

The vast majority of series describe bulbar urethral slings in patients with postprostatectomy incontinence. Groen and colleagues[46] describe the 1-year outcomes of the AdVance trans obturator sling in 20 adult men (mean age, 23 years) with nLUTD resulting from SB or SCI, noting cure in

8 of 20 (40%) and improvement in 5 of 20 (25%), with 7 of the 20 (35%) failing. Few complications were reported, including localized hematoma in 3 of 20 (15%), challenging CIC in 3 of 20 (15%) requiring change in catheter type in 2 and temporary suprapubic cystostomy in 1 patient. Given the suboptimal results with bulbar sling and the theoretic risk of erosion, the standard of care for sling placement in men should remain autologous bladder neck sling.

BLADDER NECK CLOSURE
Indications

BNC is typically a "last resort" procedure in the end-stage bladder neck that is performed concomitantly with either suprapubic cystostomy or formal lower urinary tract reconstruction. A fixed, open bladder neck can result from the neurologic insult itself, prior bladder outlet surgery, or as a sequela of chronic indwelling urethral catheters. Candidates for BNC include those with severe incontinence who (1) may not have the dexterity or support to use an AUS, (2) are refractory to prior interventions to increase outlet resistance, or (3) have incontinence deemed too severe for either sling or AUS. Some patients who are not candidates for urinary diversion may also undergo BNC with an SPC as an alternative.

Contraindications

Patients who are unable to appropriately perform or arrange for CIC via their catheterizable channels or follow-up for routine suprapubic catheter exchanges should not undergo BNC. Additionally, patients with multiple abdominal surgeries who may not have adequate tissue for interposition, prior radiation, or previous bladder neck reconstructions are at greater risk for failure. It is also important for practitioners to understand bladder compliance before BNC, because compliance loss may occur if the detrusor leak point pressure is significantly increased after closing the outlet. Of note, before considering BNC, one must stress to the patient and their caretakers that a dislodged suprapubic catheter or compromised catheterizable channel constitutes a surgical emergency requiring prompt intervention because there is no alternative route for drainage of urine.

Approach and Technique

Although the majority of patients undergo BNC transabdominally, alternative approaches include transvaginal closure in women[48] and transperineal closure in men.[49] One must ensure good bladder neck mobilization, establishing a plane between the bladder and rectum in men or vagina in women. The so-called Khoury modification that has been adopted in many published series involves elevating a lip of the posterior bladder wall that is incorporated into the AC or cystorrhaphy.[50] Care must be taken to account for the position of the ureteral orifices as excessive posterior mobilization risks kinking the ureterovesical junction or incorporating them into the closure. In these cases, bilateral cephalad ureteroneocystostomy is indicated.[51] The urethral stump is closed in 2 layers and consideration must always be given to tissue interposition to prevent recanalization. Omentum is used, when available; alternatives include peritoneum, human pericardium (Tutoplast, Tutogen Medical, Inc, Alachua, FL), and transverse rectus abdominus.[49,52]

Outcomes and Complications

Success rates for BNC, in general, are lower than those of other surgeries for sphincteric incontinence; however, a considerable selection bias exists because patients undergoing BNC have more complex and severe incontinence. When surveying published outcomes, care must be taken when fistula is considered a complication, because a fistula, by definition, indicates failure. As such, success should only be considered when patients do not manifest leakage. Early common complications included obstructed catheters, wound and urinary tract infection, and ileus.[49] Failure rates are noteworthy; Ginger and colleagues[49] note 6 of 29 patients (21%) undergoing predominately transabdominal BNC developed fistula. Stoffel and McGuire[53] described a 20-month success rate of 92% (11 of 12) in a series of patients with nLUTD and urethral destruction undergoing either transvaginal or transabdominal BNC with lower urinary tract reconstruction; however, 8 of the 11 successes required 1 or more additional surgeries to achieve continence. Postoperative vesicourethral fistula rates range from 10% to 20%.[49,51,53,54]

SURGERY TO REDUCE BLADDER PRESSURES AND OPTIMIZE CATHETERIZATION
Augmentation Cystoplasty

Indications

When paired with strict CIC, AC increases bladder capacity, reduces detrusor storage pressure, and can preserves upper tract function in patients with nLUTD. Although introduced almost a century ago, the use of AC in nLUTD became common only after the introduction of CIC as a safe and effective method of bladder emptying in the 1970s. Yet, the use of AC has recently decreased because the introduction of intradetrusor injection of botulinum toxin has provided patients with another option for medical management[55–57] Indications for AC in patients with congenital or acquired nLUTD include (1) refractory detrusor overactivity, loss of bladder compliance, and a elevated detrusor leak point pressures or (2) reduced bladder capacity requiring prohibitively frequent CIC or an indwelling catheter.

Contraindications

There are few absolute contraindications to AC; however, appropriate patient selection is paramount. Patients with inflammatory bowel disease or abdominopelvic radiation may have compromised bowel segments, which would put patient at risk for enterovesicular or enteroentero fistula. Patients with significant prior small bowel resection may experience short bowel syndrome after AC, which occurs when there is less than 200 cm of residual bowel.[58] Considering most adults have between 300 and 800 cm of small bowel, careful querying of previous operative notes is key. Bowel resection may potentiate hepatic and renal disease in patients with baseline insufficiency. Patients with advanced renal failure are also relative contraindications for bladder augment because of the risk of metabolic derangement from the absorption of urine from the augmented segment. Finally, patients with suboptimal cognitive function and caretaker support are unlikely to adhere to their CIC schedule.

Approach and technique

Technical steps for AC date back more than a century and remain principally unchanged.[59–63] Detubularized ileum is the most frequently used, studied, and generally preferred bowel segment for AC.[57,64–66] Ileum is readily available and generally mobile, with the resection and anastomosis techniques familiar to urologists. In cases of significant prior surgery where further small bowel resection may result in short gut formation, ileocolic or sigmoid augmentation can be performed. Although not all urologists may be familiar with the mesenteric blood supply of the sigmoid nor with the principles of large bowel anastomosis, it behooves the reconstructive urologist to become comfortable with using this segment of bowel in AC because it has many advantages in patients with nLUTD. First, patients with nLUTD also have chronic constipation, resulting in a relatively redundant sigmoid colon. Resecting a sigmoid section may, therefore, improve colon transit time and reduce constipation. Second, sigmoid resection avoids the malabsorption problems of terminal ileal resection. Third and final, patients with a history of ventriculoperitoneal shunt for hydrocephalus can have incredibly inflammatory small bowel adhesions. This condition can make the sigmoid colon an attractive alternative because it is rarely involved in these adhesions and its mesentery is proximate to the bladder.

Avoiding the use of irradiated bowel has dogmatically entrenched itself into an indication to use colon; however, there is a lack of evidence supporting this practice. We often use ileum provided it seems to be free of radiation changes, including serosal inflammation or ischemic changes. Minimally invasive surgical (MIS) approaches have been well-described in the pediatric literature, with more recent application in adults with nLUTD.[67–69]

Outcomes and complications

Numerous series with intermediate and long-term follow-up report significant increases in storage capacity with concomitant reductions in detrusor pressures and incontinence in patients receiving AC.[57,65,66,70–72] Complications are well-documented and highly variable (**Table 2**).

Continent Catheterizable Channels

Indications

CIC is an effective mode of bladder drainage for many patients with congenital or acquired nLUTD. Yet CIC can be technically challenging for reasons, including quadriplegia and body habitus. Additionally, although men can perform urethral self-catheterization in their wheelchairs, women must transfer to a bed or commode. Thus, particularly in women or quadriplegic men with decent residual hand function, an abdominal wall stoma can improve independence. CCCs simplify CIC and

Table 2 Complications after augmentation cystoplasty	
Complication	**Frequency (%)**
Acid–base/electrolyte disturbance	$<5^{55,64}$
Urinary stones	$5–52^{102,106}$
Perforation	$<1–14^{106,107}$
Infections	
Asymptomatic bacteriuria	Nearly 100
Clinical urinary tract infection	$4–43^{31,105}$
Malignancy	$<1.0–5.5^{29,108}$
Gastrointestinal disturbance	$<10–55^{106,109}$
Reoperation (endoscopic or open)	$30–41^{106,110}$

are indicated in patients with difficulty catheterizing their urethra or those who desire an alternative route of bladder emptying. Additionally, when indicated or preferred, simultaneous AC can be performed via a variety of approaches. Channel selection is tailormade to each patient because multiple factors including comorbidities, anatomy, and occupational function must be considered (**Fig. 1**).

Contraindications

Contraindications are similar to those for AC (see **Table 2**), except in cases where appendix alone is used, because no bowel resection is required.

Approach and technique

Broadly, CCCs are categorized in terms of their continence mechanism (**Fig. 2**) and whether AC is indicated. Tunneled, or "flap valve" channels rely on the Mitrofanoff principle, whereby continence is enhanced as the bladder fills and further compresses the channel. This is achieved by tunneling the channel, typically appendix (Mitrofanoff appendicovesicostomy) or reconfigured ileum (Yang-Monti), through the detrusor muscle and anastomosing the distal end to the urothelium. Nipple valves maintain continence via circumferential coaptation. The ileocecal valve provides a natural nipple valve and is most commonly used. Intussuscepted ileum, described by Kock and colleagues in 1982 for use in a catheterizable heterotopic diversion, is seldom used owing to technical complexity, difficult reproducibility, and suboptimal outcomes.[73,74]

Tunneled Channel and Flap Valve: Mitrofanoff Appendicovesicostomy

The Mitrofanoff appendicovesicostomy, introduced in 1980, remains the most widely used CCC in children.[75] The appendix can be tunneled into the native bladder intravesically or extravesically or into the tenia coli of a colonic AC. The appendix is well-designed for use as a CCC given its resiliency and lumenal diameter that obviates tapering requirements. Appendicovesicostomy can be successfully performed via open (midline vs Pfannenstiel), laparoscopic, or robotic-assisted approaches.[76–78] Procedural steps for appendicovesicostomy are largely unchanged since its inception and are well-described.[79,80] In adults with larger abdominal walls, the surgeon must ensure that the appendix is long enough to reach the abdominal wall. Whereas 4 to 6 cm can be long enough in children, at least 8 and preferably 10 to 12 cm are needed in adults. One can also mobilize the ascending colon in cases with restrictive mesenteric length or transect the

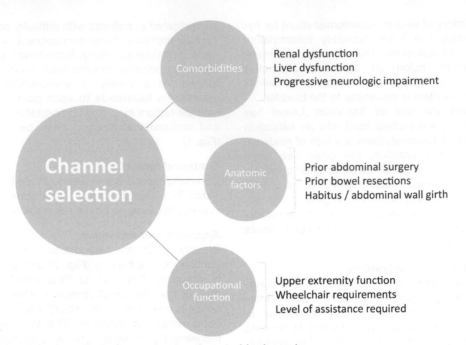

Fig. 1. Patient selection criteria for continent catheterizable channel.

appendix with a small cuff of cecum to extend the channel length and augment the stomal diameter. Unlike children, the adult umbilicus is often deep, difficult to traverse, and chronically inflamed. As such, we routinely excise the umbilical base, approximating the channel to the healthier superficial umbilical skin. Although the common practice in pediatric urology has been to bury the stoma using a Y-V flap of abdominal wall skin, we have found a rosebud stoma to be preferable because it seems to minimize stomal stenosis rates (**Fig. 3**).

Tunneled Channel and Flap Valve: Reconfigured Ileum (Yang-Monti)

The absent, retrocecal, short, or restricted appendix excludes the option of appendicovesicostomy. As such, Yang in 1993 and Monti in 1997

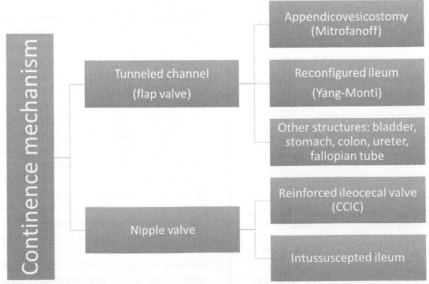

Fig. 2. Continent catheterizable channel choices, stratified by continence mechanism. CCIC, catheterizable ileal cecocystoplasty.

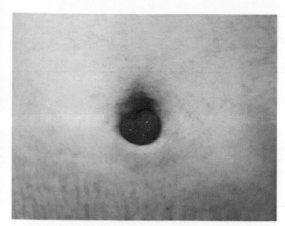

Fig. 3. Rosebud appearance of catheterizable channel after excisions of umbilical base.

described and popularized their technique of CCC creation using reconfigured ileum.[81,82] A single Yang-Monti channel involves isolating a 2-cm ileal segment that is detubularized (**Fig. 4**A) and transversely retubularized along its antimesenteric border over a catheter (**Fig. 4**B). Imbricating sutures may be placed as needed to achieve the appropriate diameter (**Fig. 4**C). Typically, a single Yang-Monti channel will result in a 6-cm channel; in adults, longer lengths are typically needed. One option involves creating a double Yang-Monti channel where a 4-cm ileal segment is isolated and divided in half, creating 2 separate channels with a sutured anastomosis.[81] Alternatively, a spiral Yang-Monti tube can be fashioned using a 3.5-cm ileal segment, which is partially divided in the center, at which point 2 separate ileal plates are created by divided each ileal segment close to the mesentery on opposing sides, resulting in a Z-shaped ileal plate that is reconfigured over a catheter, resulting in a channel length of 10 to 14 cm.[83]

Nipple Valve: Tapered Ileal Channel

Using the ileocecal valve as a continence mechanism was first described in 1950 by Gilchrist and colleagues,[84] adapted by Kock and colleagues in 1982,[74] and popularized by Rowland in 1987 by virtue of the Indiana pouch.[85] A natural extension of the Indiana pouch, reconfiguring the ileocecal segment for AC and catheterizable channel purposes was described in 1992 by Sarosdy.[86] In patients with nLUTD, the continent catheterizable ileal cecocystoplasty (CCIC) offers distinct advantages (and disadvantages) compared with appendix or small bowel when AC is indicated (**Table 3**).

Procedurally, CCIC can be performed via open or a hybrid open–MIS approach. A key step for tension-free anastomosis is appropriate mobilization of the ascending colon around the hepatic flexure. This degree of mobilization requires that a midline laparotomy be extended cephalad of the umbilicus. In our modified MIS approach, ascending colon mobilization is performed in a hand-assisted, laparoscopic fashion through a Pfannenstiel incision. A 12-mm camera port is placed through the umbilicus, which later serves as our stoma site, and a 5-mm assistant port is placed on the left side of the abdomen approximately 1 to 2 handbreadths cephalad to the camera port (**Fig. 5**). For ascending colon mobilization, our "landing zone" indicating adequate mobilization is visualization of the reflected duodenum, kidney, and inferior vena cava (**Fig. 6**). Once complete, the remainder of the procedure is performed in an open fashion. Care must be taken when placing the hand port to extend the fascial incision just beyond the width of the surgeon's hand, to prevent loss of pneumoperitoneum; the incision is extended later for the open portion of the procedure. Pfannenstiel incisions are advantageous as they carry less ventral hernia risk than midline incisions, a risk that is augmented by the often weak abdominal wall of patients with nLUTD.[87,88] Additionally, when compared with Pfannenstiel incisions, we have observed higher rates of parastomal hernia when umbilical channels are fashioned in the setting of a midline laparotomy. We reserve this Pfannenstiel approach for virgin or benign operated abdomens. In challenging abdomens, including anyone with a prior ventriculoperitoneal

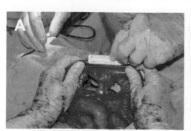
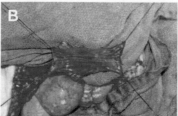
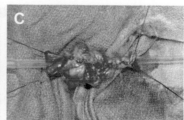

Fig. 4. Yang-Monti channel. (*A*) Isolation of small bowel. (*B*) Antimesenteric detubularization. (*C*) Transversely retubularized ileal segment.

Table 3
Outcomes and complications of continent catheterizable channels

Procedure	Continence Rates (%)	Stomal Stenosis (%)	Revision Rate (%)
Nipple valve	>95[5,80,89,90]	5–10[5,80,89–91]	5–20[5,80,89–91]
Mitrofanoff appendicovesicostomy			5–20
Reconfigured ileum			10–20
Single Yang-Monti			
Spiral Yang-Monti			
Tapered ileum	>95[92]	3–9[92,93]	5–13[79,93]
Continent catheterizable ileocecocystoplasty			

shunt, we still attempt hand-assisted laparoscopic right colon mobilization, but we do it through a lower midline incision. If we can accomplish the colon mobilization laparoscopically, then we have avoided extending the laparotomy around the umbilicus, but if we cannot accomplish it laparoscopically, it is simple to convert to a longer midline laparotomy. When a midline laparotomy is used, we prefer to place our stoma in a paramedian location, so that if a ventral hernia occurs it will not involve the stoma. Our approach to ileocecal resection, augment, and channel creation is described elsewhere in detail.[79] Briefly, approximately 10-cm segments of cecum and ileum are harvested. The cecum is detubularized and the distal ileum is tapered over a 14-F catheter with a GIA-100 (3.8 mm staple width) stapler (**Fig. 7**). Next, the native bladder is incised sagittally from the bladder neck to the trigone, in preparation for anastomosis with the cecal segment. Similar to traditional AC, a wide bladder plate is an important step in preventing hourglass deformities that may result in inefficient drainage. Once complete, the tapered ileal limb is brought through the umbilicus or in a paramedian location through the rectus muscle. We have used this approach even in some patients without an appendix who desire a CCC but do not require an AC; our rationale is that a single Monti is never long enough in an adult and that a tapered ileal channel is preferable to a double/spiral Monti. Furthermore, the fact that the tapered ileal limb exits from the dome of the AC and that there is no tunneling means that the typical final CCC length in our CCIC is only 8 cm, compared with 12 to 14 cm with a double/spiral Monti. Shorter channels are preferable because they have fewer catheterization problems.

Outcomes and complications

Table 3 highlights outcomes among patients undergoing both tunneled channels and nipple valve techniques. There are limited adult studies with

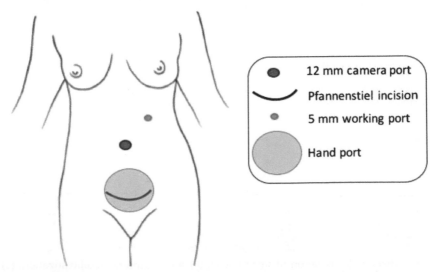

- ● 12 mm camera port
- ⌣ Pfannenstiel incision
- ● 5 mm working port
- ● Hand port

Fig. 5. Port placement for hand-assisted laparoscopic mobilization of the ascending colon.

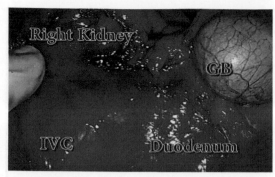

Fig. 6. "Landing zone" highlighting landmarks for mobilization of ascending colon. GB, gallbladder; IVC, inferior vena cava.

adequate follow-up, leading to heterogeneous results. Additionally, there are several, unique advantages and disadvantages when selecting CCIC for adults with nLUTD (**Table 4**).

URINARY DIVERSION
Indications

Some patients with nLUTD develop refractory symptoms that ultimately require a urinary diversion to address safety or quality of life concerns. Conditions that can necessitate this intervention include urethral erosion with a destroyed bladder outlet, chronic urinary tract infections in the setting of low bladder compliance, incontinence causing decubitus ulcers, and an inability to manage indwelling or intermittent catheterization. Chronic urethral catheterization particularly carries some morbidity, which can result in complications requiring more urgent intervention. These can include bladder perforation, pubovesical fistula, and pubic bone osteomyelitis. We have seen bladder perforation owing to chronic catheter drainage occur mostly in radiated patients.[5] These complex patients are often best served with urinary diversion, which significantly simplifies care and has been shown to enhance quality of life.[89]

Contraindications

In addition to patients "medically unfit" for major surgery, there are several, unique patient populations in whom urinary diversion may be suboptimal. Patients with significantly impaired cognitive function may repeatedly pull off their stoma appliance. Additionally, minor complications such as dehydration, electrolyte disturbances, and transient kidney injury are relatively simple to treat, provided one has access to care. Patients with geographic and/or financial barriers to receiving care are at risk for augmenting their complications from minor to major. Finally, owing to disease-limited physical activity, many patients with nLUTD are obese, with a short mesentery and thick abdominal wall, rendering diversion challenging and increasing the risk for subsequent sequelae, such as parastomal/ventral hernia, stomal stenosis, and challenging appliance management.

Approach and Technique

Major considerations during urinary diversion in this patient group include the type of diversion offered and whether to perform cystectomy. Although some may consider cystectomy an unduly morbid procedure for patients with compromised health, those who undergo diversion without cystectomy often have complications from their residual, defunctionalized bladder, many of whom require subsequent cystectomy.[90–92] Techniques for cystectomy are well-described and principally unchanged.[93,94] MIS approaches to simple cystectomy are increasingly used when feasible.[89,95] Supratrigonal cystectomy generally offers comparable outcomes while minimizing morbidity, including less blood loss and preserved potency in men.[96] Exceptions include cases when men have concomitant urethral stricture disease. In these cases, we have observed that prostatic and urethral secretions that would typically drain per urethra, build up in the obstructed urethra and residual bladder, often

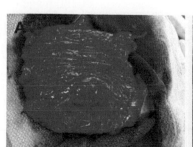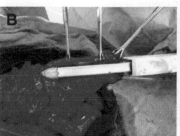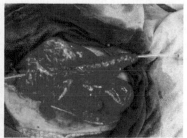

Fig. 7. (*A*) Detubularized cecum with ileocecal nipple valve. (*B*) Tapering of terminal ileum with a GIA-100 stapler. (*C*) Reinforced channel and ileocecal valve.

Table 4
Advantages and disadvantages of CCIC, compared with tunneled, flap-valve channels

Advantages	Disadvantages
A capacious cecal augment is possible with minimal bowel resection	Risk of fecal incontinence and vitamin B_{12} deficiency from ileocecal valve resection
The ileocecal pedicle supplies both the augment and channel, obviating concerns surrounding ability of the segment to reach the bladder	Colon resection/ileocolic anastomosis is less familiar to urologists
Single bowel resection	Often requires mechanical bowel preparation
Easily modifiable channel length and caliber allowing a "custom fit" for patients of varying body habitus	
Eliminates need to create a detrusor tunnel	

necessitating completion cystectomy. The decision regarding continent versus incontinent urinary diversion must be balanced by the patients' ability to catheterize and maintain their diversion. One must account for individual disease progression, because patients with progressive neurologic disease may lose their ability to maintain their diversion in the future.

Outcomes and Complications

Few available studies evaluating outcomes of cystectomy in patients with nLUTD note upper tract functional preservation in more than 90% of patients[97–99] with significant improvements in urinary quality of life after urinary diversion.[89,97,98] Similar to radical cystectomy for malignant disease, there is significant morbidity associated with simple cystectomy, with early and intermediate complication rates ranging from 30% to 70%.[93,94,97,100]

CONSIDERATIONS IN THE CONGENITAL PATIENT

Patients with congenital nLUTD present multiple challenges that complicate preoperative, intraoperative, and postoperative management. Many have multiple prior surgeries, resulting in arduous intraabdominal adhesions, often complicated by the presence of a ventriculoperitoneal shunt. These patients have particularly challenging abdomens; one can expect to spend several hours performing lysis of adhesions. When combined with unclear surgical history owing to poor recall and remote records, surgeons must be prepared for intraoperative "puzzle solving" to orient themselves properly. With respect to continent diversion, patients with SB often have short mesenteries that limit intestinal mobility for urinary diversion and thick abdominal walls making stoma maturation more difficult. Finally, most patients have concomitant neurogenic bowel dysfunction,

leading to postoperative delayed return of bowel function.

Adult patients with congenital or acquired nLUTD have heterogeneous care and support, which often complicates care; bladder reconstructions are only as effective as the maintenance they are provided.[101,102] Children often have parents that assume responsibility for their care that does not always extend into adulthood. Additionally, poor executive functioning and attention disorders in patients with SB contributes to lax adherence to bladder maintenance.[103] Older patients with acquired nLUTD may not have the volume of care that allows for CIC, irrigations, and routine physician follow-up. Still, the surgeon should never assume social support is poor and should consider the potential for continent diversion in all appropriate patient. MIS approaches are increasingly used in adults with nLUTD; this trend should continue as contemporary training programs offer a rich experience in laparoscopic and robotic techniques. Nonetheless, considerable expertise in robotics is compulsory because a steep learning curve is present with significantly longer operative times.[31,104] Sound reconstructive principles must be maintained and care must be taken to not equate "feasibility" with "reproducibility."

REFERENCES

1. Wyndaele JJ. The management of neurogenic lower urinary tract dysfunction after spinal cord injury. Nat Rev Urol 2016;13(12):705–14.
2. Loftus CJ, Wood HM. Congenital causes of neurogenic bladder and the transition to adult care. Transl Androl Urol 2016;5(1):39–50.
3. Szymanski KM, Cain MP, Hardacker TJ, et al. How successful is the transition to adult urology care in spina bifida? A single center 7-year experience. J Pediatr Urol 2017;13(1):40.e1–6.
4. Vírseda-Chamorro M, Salinas-Casado J, Rubio-Hidalgo E, et al. Risk factors of urethral diverticula

in male patients with spinal cord injury. Spinal Cord 2015;53(11):803–6.

5. Stern JA, Clemens JQ. Osteomyelitis of the pubis: a complication of a chronic indwelling catheter. Urology 2003;61(2):462.

6. Politano VA, Small MP, Harper JM, et al. Periurethral Teflon injection for urinary incontinence. J Urol 1974;111(2):180–3.

7. Stöhrer M, Blok B, Castro-Diaz D, et al. EAU guidelines on neurogenic lower urinary tract dysfunction. Eur Urol 2009;56(1):81–8.

8. Alova I, Margaryan M, Bernuy M, et al. Long-term effects of endoscopic injection of dextranomer/hyaluronic acid based implants for treatment of urinary incontinence in children with neurogenic bladder. J Urol 2012;188(5):1905–9.

9. De Vocht TF, Chrzan R, Dik P, et al. Long-term results of bulking agent injection for persistent incontinence in cases of neurogenic bladder dysfunction. J Urol 2010;183(2):719–23.

10. Sundaram CP, Reinberg Y, Aliabadi HA. Failure to obtain durable results with collagen implantation in children with urinary incontinence. J Urol 1997;157(6):2306–7.

11. Silveri M, Capitanucci ML, Mosiello G, et al. Endoscopic treatment for urinary incontinence in children with a congenital neuropathic bladder. Br J Urol 1998;82(5):694–7.

12. Dyer L, Franco I, Firlit CF, et al. Endoscopic injection of bulking agents in children with incontinence: dextranomer/hyaluronic acid copolymer versus polytetrafluoroethylene. J Urol 2007;178(4 Pt 2):1628–31.

13. Lewis RI, Lockhart JL, Politano VA. Periurethral polytetrafluoroethylene injections in incontinent female subjects with neurogenic bladder disease. J Urol 1984;131(3):459–62.

14. Bennett JK, Green BG, Foote JE, et al. Collagen injections for intrinsic sphincter deficiency in the neuropathic urethra. Paraplegia 1995;33(12):697–700.

15. Zimmern PE, Gormley EA, Stoddard AM, et al. Management of recurrent stress urinary incontinence after Burch and sling procedures. Neurourol Urodyn 2016;35(3):344–8.

16. Lee HN, Lee YS, Han JY, et al. Transurethral injection of bulking agent for treatment of failed mid-urethral sling procedures. Int Urogynecol J 2010;21(12):1479–83.

17. Sweat SD, Lightner DJ. Complications of sterile abscess formation and pulmonary embolism following periurethral bulking agents. J Urol 1999;161(1):93–6.

18. Gopinath D, Smith AR, Reid FM. Periurethral abscess following polyacrylamide hydrogel (Bulkamid) for stress urinary incontinence. Int Urogynecol J 2012;23(11):1645–8.

19. Pannek J, Brands FH, Senge T. Particle migration after transurethral injection of carbon coated beads for stress urinary incontinence. J Urol 2001;166(4):1350–3.

20. Ghoniem GM, Khater U. Urethral prolapse after Durasphere injection. Int Urogynecol J Pelvic Floor Dysfunct 2006;17(3):297–8.

21. Berger MB, Morgan DM. Delayed presentation of pseudoabscess secondary to injection of pyrolytic carbon-coated beads bulking agent. Female Pelvic Med Reconstr Surg 2012;18(5):303–5.

22. Madjar S, Sharma AK, Waltzer WC, et al. Periurethral mass formations following bulking agent injection for the treatment of urinary incontinence. J Urol 2006;175(4):1408–10.

23. Grimsby GM, Menon V, Schlomer BJ, et al. Long-term outcomes of bladder neck reconstruction without augmentation cystoplasty in children. J Urol 2016;195(1):155–61.

24. Athanasopoulos A, Gyftopoulos K, McGuire EJ. Treating stress urinary incontinence in female patients with neuropathic bladder: the value of the autologous fascia rectus sling. Int Urol Nephrol 2012;44(5):1363–7.

25. Mcguire EJ, Lytton B. Pubovaginal sling procedure for stress incontinence. J Urol 1978;119(1):82–4.

26. Herschorn S, Radomski SB. Fascial slings and bladder neck tapering in the treatment of male neurogenic incontinence. J Urol 1992;147(4):1073–5.

27. Blaivas JG, Sandhu J. Urethral reconstruction after erosion of slings in women. Curr Opin Urol 2004;14(6):335–8.

28. Daneshmand S, Ginsberg DA, Bennet JK, et al. Puboprostatic sling repair for treatment of urethral incompetence in adult neurogenic incontinence. J Urol 2003;169(1):199–202.

29. Scott FB, Bradley WE, Timm GW. Treatment of urinary incontinence by an implantable prosthetic urinary sphincter. J Urol 1974;112(1):75–80.

30. Phé V, Léon P, Granger B, et al. Stress urinary incontinence in female neurological patients: long-term functional outcomes after artificial urinary sphincter (AMS 800TM) implantation. Neurourol Urodyn 2017;36(3):764–9.

31. Biardeau X, Rizk J, Marcelli F, et al. Robot-assisted laparoscopic approach for artificial urinary sphincter implantation in 11 women with urinary stress incontinence: surgical technique and initial experience. Eur Urol 2015;67(5):937–42.

32. Seideman CA, Zhao LC, Hudak SJ, et al. Is prolonged catheterization a risk factor for artificial urinary sphincter cuff erosion? Urology 2013;82(4):943–6.

33. Anusionwu II, Wright EJ. Indications for revision of artificial urinary sphincter and modifiable risk factors for device-related morbidity. Neurourol Urodyn 2013;32(1):63–5.

34. Myers JB, Mayer EN, Lenherr S, Neurogenic Bladder Research Group (NBRG.org). Management options for sphincteric deficiency in adults with neurogenic bladder. Transl Androl Urol 2016; 5(1):145–57.

35. Yates DR, Phé V, Rouprêt M, et al. Robot-assisted laparoscopic artificial urinary sphincter insertion in men with neurogenic stress urinary incontinence. BJU Int 2013;111(7):1175–9.

36. Suarez OA, McCammon KA. The artificial urinary sphincter in the management of incontinence. Urology 2016;92:14–9.

37. James MH, McCammon KA. Artificial urinary sphincter for post-prostatectomy incontinence: a review. Int J Urol 2014;21(6):536–43.

38. Viers BR, Elliott DS, Kramer SA. Simultaneous augmentation cystoplasty and cuff only artificial urinary sphincter in children and young adults with neurogenic urinary incontinence. J Urol 2014; 191(4):1104–8.

39. Castera R, Podestá ML, Ruarte A, et al. 10-year experience with artificial urinary sphincter in children and adolescents. J Urol 2001;165(6 Pt 2): 2373–6.

40. Mor Y, Leibovitch I, Golomb J. Lower urinary tract reconstruction by augmentation cystoplasty and insertion of artificial urinary sphincter cuff only: long term follow-up. Prog Urol 2004;14(3):310–4 [in French].

41. Chartier-Kastler E, Genevois S, Gamé X, et al. Treatment of neurogenic male urinary incontinence related to intrinsic sphincter insufficiency with an artificial urinary sphincter: a French retrospective multicentre study. BJU Int 2011;107(3):426–32.

42. Murphy S, Rea D, O'Mahony J, et al. A comparison of the functional durability of the AMS 800 artificial urinary sphincter between cases with and without an underlying neurogenic aetiology. Ir J Med Sci 2003;172(3):136–8.

43. Simeoni J, Guys JM, Mollard P, et al. Artificial urinary sphincter implantation for neurogenic bladder: a multi-institutional study in 107 children. Br J Urol 1996;78(2):287–93.

44. Spiess PE, Capolicchio JP, Kiruluta G, et al. Is an artificial sphincter the best choice for incontinent boys with spina bifida? Review of our long term experience with the AS-800 artificial sphincter. Can J Urol 2002;9(2):1486–91.

45. Montague DK. Males slings: compressive versus repositioning. Eur Urol 2009;56(6):934–5 [discussion: 935–6].

46. Groen LA, Spinoit AF, Hoebeke P, et al. The AdVance male sling as a minimally invasive treatment for intrinsic sphincter deficiency in patients with neurogenic bladder sphincter dysfunction: a pilot study. Neurourol Urodyn 2012;31(8): 1284–7.

47. Rapp DE. The male suburethral sling: remaining questions. Can J Urol 2014;21(4):7350.

48. Rovner ES, Goudelocke CM, Gilchrist A, et al. Transvaginal bladder neck closure with posterior urethral flap for devastated urethra. Urology 2011; 78(1):208–12.

49. Ginger VA, Miller JL, Yang CC. Bladder neck closure and suprapubic tube placement in a debilitated patient population. Neurourol Urodyn 2010; 29(3):382–6.

50. Khoury AE, Agarwal SK, Bägli D, et al. Concomitant modified bladder neck closure and Mitrofanoff urinary diversion. J Urol 1999;162(5):1746–8.

51. Shpall AI, Ginsberg DA. Bladder neck closure with lower urinary tract reconstruction: technique and long-term followup. J Urol 2004;172(6 Pt 1): 2296–9.

52. Kavanagh A, Afshar K, Scott H, et al. Bladder neck closure in conjunction with enterocystoplasty and Mitrofanoff diversion for complex incontinence: closing the door for good. J Urol 2012; 188(4 Suppl):1561–5.

53. Stoffel JT, McGuire EJ. Outcome of urethral closure in patients with neurologic impairment and complete urethral destruction. Neurourol Urodyn 2006; 25(1):19–22.

54. Landau EH, Gofrit ON, Pode D, et al. Bladder neck closure in children: a decade of followup. J Urol 2009;182(4 Suppl):1797–801.

55. Lapides J, Diokno AC, Silber SJ, et al. Clean, intermittent self-catheterization in the treatment of urinary tract disease. J Urol 1972;107(3):458–61.

56. Mitchell ME, Kulb TB, Backes DJ. Intestinocystoplasty in combination with clean intermittent catheterization in the management of vesical dysfunction. J Urol 1986;136(1 Pt 2):288–91.

57. Biers SM, Venn SN, Greenwell TJ. The past, present and future of augmentation cystoplasty. BJU Int 2012;109(9):1280–93.

58. Buchman AL, Scolapio J, Fryer J. AGA technical review on short bowel syndrome and intestinal transplantation. Gastroenterology 2003;124(4):1111–34.

59. Goodwin WE, Winter CC, Barker WF. Cup-patch technique of ileocystoplasty for bladder enlargement or partial substitution. Surg Gynecol Obstet 1959;108(2):240–4.

60. Cibert J. Bladder enlargement through ileocystoplasty. J Urol 1953;70(4):600–4.

61. Jacobs A. Ileocystoplasty for the relief of bladder contracture. Br J Urol 1957;29(3):307–11.

62. Kay R, Straffon R. Augmentation cystoplasty. Urol Clin North Am 1986;13(2):295–305.

63. Smith JJ, Swierzewski SJ. Augmentation cystoplasty. Urol Clin North Am 1997;24(4):745–54.

64. Mundy AR, Stephenson TP. "Clam" ileocystoplasty for the treatment of refractory urge incontinence. Br J Urol 1985;57(6):641–6.

65. Gurung PM, Attar KH, Abdul-Rahman A, et al. Long-term outcomes of augmentation ileocystoplasty in patients with spinal cord injury: a minimum of 10 years of follow-up. BJU Int 2012; 109(8):1236–42.

66. Kilic N, Celayir S, Elicevik M, et al. Bladder augmentation: urodynamic findings and clinical outcome in different augmentation techniques. Eur J Pediatr Surg 2008;9(1):29–32.

67. Flum AS, Zhao LC, Kielb SJ, et al. Completely intracorporeal robotic-assisted laparoscopic augmentation enterocystoplasty with continent catheterizable channel. Urology 2014;84(6):1314–8.

68. Cohen AJ, Pariser JJ, Anderson BB, et al. The robotic appendicovesicostomy and bladder augmentation: the next frontier in robotics, are we there? Urol Clin North Am 2015;42(1):121–30.

69. Wiestma AC, Estrada CR, Cho PS, et al. Robotic-assisted laparoscopic bladder augmentation in the pediatric patient. J Pediatr Urol 2016;12(5): 313.e1–2.

70. Çetinel B, Kocjancic E, Demirdağ Ç. Augmentation cystoplasty in neurogenic bladder. Investig Clin Urol 2016;57(5):316–23.

71. Sajadi KP, Goldman HB. Bladder augmentation and urinary diversion for neurogenic LUTS: current indications. Curr Urol Rep 2012;13(5):389–93.

72. Scales CD, Wiener JS. Evaluating outcomes of enterocystoplasty in patients with spina bifida: a review of the literature. J Urol 2008;180(6):2323–9.

73. deKernion JB, DenBesten L, Kaufman JJ, et al. The Kock pouch as a urinary reservoir. Pitfalls and perspectives. Am J Surg 1985;150(1):83–9.

74. Kock NG, Nilson AE, Nilsson LO, et al. Urinary diversion via a continent ileal reservoir: clinical results in 12 patients. J Urol 1982;128(3):469–75.

75. Mitrofanoff P. Trans-appendicular continent cystostomy in the management of the neurogenic bladder. Chir Pediatr 1980;21(4):297–305.

76. Rey D, Helou E, Oderda M, et al. Laparoscopic and robot-assisted continent urinary diversions (Mitrofanoff and Yang-Monti conduits) in a consecutive series of 15 adult patients: the Saint Augustin technique. BJU Int 2013;112(7):953–8.

77. Murthy P, Cohn JA, Selig RB, et al. Robot-assisted laparoscopic augmentation ileocystoplasty and Mitrofanoff appendicovesicostomy in children: updated interim results. Eur Urol 2015;68(6):1069–75.

78. Gundeti MS, Petravick ME, Pariser JJ, et al. A multi-institutional study of perioperative and functional outcomes for pediatric robotic-assisted laparoscopic Mitrofanoff appendicovesicostomy. J Pediatr Urol 2016;12(6):386.e1–5.

79. Levy ME, Elliott SP. Reconstructive techniques for creation of catheterizable channels: tunneled and nipple valve channels. Transl Androl Urol 2016; 5(1):136–44.

80. Harris CF, Cooper CS, Hutcheson JC, et al. Appendicovesicostomy: the Mitrofanoff procedure-a 15 year perspective. J Urol 2000;163(6):1922–6.

81. Monti PR, Lara RC, Dutra MA, et al. New techniques for construction of efferent conduits based on the Mitrofanoff principle. Urology 1997;49(1): 112–5.

82. Yang WH. Yang needle tunneling technique in creating antireflux and continent mechanisms. J Urol 1993;150(3):830–4.

83. Casale AJ. A long continence ileovesicostomy using a single piece of bowel. J Urol 1999;162(5): 1743–5.

84. Gilchrist RK, Merricks JW, Hamlin HH, et al. Construction of a substitute bladder and urethra. Surg Gynecol Obstet 1950;90(6):752–60.

85. Rowland RG, Mitchell ME, Bihrle R, et al. Indiana continent urinary reservoir. J Urol 1987;137(6): 1136–9.

86. Sarosdy MF. Continent urinary diversion using cutaneous ileocecocystoplasty. Urology 1992; 40(2):102–6.

87. Le Huu Nho R, Mege D, Ouaïssi M, et al. Incidence and prevention of ventral incisional hernia. J Visc Surg 2012;149(5 Suppl):e3–14.

88. Lee L, Mappin-Kasirer B, Sender Liberman A, et al. High incidence of symptomatic incisional hernia after midline extraction in laparoscopic colon resection. Surg Endosc 2012;26(11):3180–5.

89. Guillotreau J, Castel-Lacanal E, Roumiguié M, et al. Prospective study of the impact on quality of life of cystectomy with ileal conduit urinary diversion for neurogenic bladder dysfunction. Neurourol Urodyn 2011;30(8):1503–6.

90. Fazili T, Bhat TR, Masood S, et al. Fate of the leftover bladder after supravesical urinary diversion for benign disease. J Urol 2006;176(2):620–1.

91. von Rundstedt FC, Lazica D, Brandt AS, et al. Long-term follow-up of the defunctionalized bladder after urinary diversion. Urologe A 2010; 49(1):69–74 [in German].

92. Brown ET, Cohn JA, Kaufman MR, et al. Cystectomy for neurogenic bladder. Curr Bladder Dysfunct Rep 2016;11(4):341–5.

93. Cheng JN, Lawrentschuk N, Gyomber D, et al. Cystectomy in patients with spinal cord injury: indications and long-term outcomes. J Urol 2010; 184(1):92–8.

94. Cohn JA, Large MC, Richards KA, et al. Cystectomy and urinary diversion as management of treatment-refractory benign disease: the impact of preoperative urological conditions on perioperative outcomes. Int J Urol 2014;21(4):382–6.

95. Lloyd G. V10-13 a novel technique of robotic-assisted simple cystectomy during robotic-assisted urinary diversion for benign indications. J Urol 2015;193(4):e848–9.

96. Chong JT, Dolat MT, Klausner AP, et al. The role of cystectomy for non-malignant bladder conditions: a review. Can J Urol 2014;21(5):7433–41.

97. Legrand G, Rouprêt M, Comperat E, et al. Functional outcomes after management of end-stage neurological bladder dysfunction with ileal conduit in a multiple sclerosis population: a monocentric experience. Urology 2011;78(4):937–41.

98. Stein R, Fisch M, Ermert A. Urinary diversion and orthotopic bladder substitution in children and young adults with neurogenic bladder. J Urol 2000;163(2):568–73.

99. Gobeaux N, Yates DR, Denys P, et al. Supratrigonal cystectomy with Hautmann pouch as treatment for neurogenic bladder in spinal cord injury patients: long-term functional results. Neurourol Urodyn 2012;31(5):672–6.

100. DeLong J, Tighiouart H, Stoffel J. Urinary diversion/reconstruction for cases of catheter intolerant secondary progressive multiple sclerosis with refractory urinary symptoms. J Urol 2011;185(6):2201–6.

101. Husmann DA. Long-term complications following bladder augmentations in patients with spina bifida: bladder calculi, perforation of the augmented bladder and upper tract deterioration. Transl Androl Urol 2016;5(1):3–11.

102. De la Torre GG, Martin A, Cervantes E, et al. Attention lapses in children with spina bifida and hydrocephalus and children with attention-deficit/hyperactivity disorder. J Clin Exp Neuropsychol 2017;39(6):563–73.

103. Kelly NC, Ammerman RT, Rausch JR, et al. Executive functioning and psychological adjustment in children and youth with spina bifida. Child Neuropsychol 2012;18(5):417–31.

104. Cohen AJ, Brodie K, Murthy P, et al. Comparative outcomes and perioperative complications of robotic vs open cystoplasty and complex reconstructions. Urology 2016;97:172–8.

105. Blaivas JG, Weiss JP, Desai P, et al. Long-term followup of augmentation enterocystoplasty and continent diversion in patients with benign disease. J Urol 2005;173(5):1631–4.

106. Welk B, Herschorn S, Law C, et al. Population based assessment of enterocystoplasty complications in adults. J Urol 2012;188(2):464–9.

107. Defoor W, Minevich E, Reddy P, et al. Bladder calculi after augmentation cystoplasty: risk factors and prevention strategies. J Urol 2004;172(5 Pt 1):1964–6.

108. Higuchi TT, Granberg CF, Fox JA, et al. Augmentation cystoplasty and risk of neoplasia: fact, fiction and controversy. J Urol 2010;184(6):2492–6.

109. Somani BK, Kumar V, Wong S, et al. Bowel dysfunction after transposition of intestinal segments into the urinary tract: 8-year prospective cohort study. J Urol 2007;177(5):1793–8.

110. Schlomer BJ, Copp HL. Cumulative incidence of outcomes and urologic procedures after augmentation cystoplasty. J Pediatr Urol 2014;10(6):1043–50.

New Frontiers of Basic Science Research in Neurogenic Lower Urinary Tract Dysfunction

Minoru Miyazato, MD, PhD[a,b], Katsumi Kadekawa, MD, PhD[b],
Takeya Kitta, MD, PhD[b], Naoki Wada, MD, PhD[b], Nobutaka Shimizu, MD, PhD[b],
William C. de Groat, PhD[c], Lori A. Birder, PhD[d], Anthony J. Kanai, PhD[d],
Seiichi Saito, MD, PhD[a], Naoki Yoshimura, MD, PhD[b,c],*

KEYWORDS

- Lower urinary tract • Afferents • Animal model • Central nervous system

KEY POINTS

- Due to the complexity of the neural mechanisms regulating the lower urinary tract, micturition is sensitive to a wide variety of injuries and diseases, resulting in neurogenic lower urinary tract dysfunction.
- In animal models of cerebral infarction (CI) produced by occlusion of middle cerebral artery, the balance between excitatory glutamatergic neurons and inhibitory glycinergic or GABAergic in the brain might be disrupted, leading to neurogenic lower urinary tract dysfunction.
- In animal models of parkinson disease (PD) produced by disruption of nigrostriatal dopaminergic pathways, bladder overactivity is primarily induced by disruption of D1-like dopamine receptor-mediated inhibition of the micturition reflex.
- In animal models of multiple sclerosis (MS) induced by experimental encephalomyelitis, neurogenic lower urinary tract dysfunction associated with detrusor overactivity is developed as seen in patients with MS.
- In animal models of spinal cord injury (SCI), hyperexcitability of C-fiber bladder afferents is a major pathophysiological basis of neurogenic lower urinary tract dysfunction, and various neural plasticities in peripheral and central nervous systems are identified.

Disclosure: N. Yoshimura has acted as a consultant for Astellas Pharma and Kyorin Pharmaceutical and has received research grants from Astellas Pharma and GlaxoSmithKline. The authors have no other relevant affiliations or financial involvement with any organization or entity with a financial interest in or financial conflict with the subject matter or materials discussed in the article apart from those disclosed.
The authors' research has been supported in part by grants from the National Institutes of Health (Grant Number P01DK093424 and R01DK088836), the Department of Defense (W81XWH-11-1-0763), and the Paralyzed Veterans of America (2793).
[a] Department of Urology, Graduate School of Medicine, University of the Ryukyus, Okinawa 903-0215, Japan;
[b] Department of Urology, University of Pittsburgh School of Medicine, 3471 Fifth Avenue, Pittsburgh, PA 15213, USA; [c] Department of Pharmacology & Chemical Biology, University of Pittsburgh School of Medicine, 200 Lothrop Street, Pittsburgh, PA 15216, USA; [d] Department of Medicine, University of Pittsburgh School of Medicine, 3550 Terrace Street, Pittsburgh, PA 15216, USA
* Corresponding author. Department of Urology, University of Pittsburgh School of Medicine, Suite 700, Kaufmann Medical Building, 3471 Fifth Avenue, Pittsburgh, PA 15213.
E-mail address: nyos@pitt.edu

urologic.theclinics.com

INTRODUCTION

The functions of the lower urinary tract to store and periodically eliminate urine depend on neural reflexes located in the brain, spinal cord, and peripheral ganglia.[1] Coordination between the bladder and urethra maintain storage phase and work reciprocally. Thus, urine storage and elimination depend greatly on the central nervous system. This dependence on the central nervous system distinguishes the lower urinary tract from many other visceral structures, such as the gastrointestinal tract and cardiovascular system that maintain a certain level of function because of the local pace-making mechanism inside the organ, even after elimination of extrinsic neural input. In addition, voiding is under voluntary control and depends on learned behavior that develops during maturation of the central nervous system, whereas many other visceral organs are regulated involuntary.[2,3]

Due to the complexity of the neural control of lower urinary tract, micturition is sensitive to numerous injuries, medical diseases, and drugs that affect the nervous system. Neurologic mechanisms are an important consideration in the diagnosis and treatment of voiding disorders. Thus, this article focuses on neurophysiologic mechanisms in the control of lower urinary tract function and their alterations that contribute to the pathologic conditions involved in the central nervous system, such as cerebral infarction (CI), Parkinson disease (PD), multiple sclerosis (MS), spinal cord injury (SCI), and spina bifida.

NEUROPHYSIOLOGY OF THE LOWER URINARY TRACT
Bladder and Urethra

The lower urinary tract is composed of the bladder and the urethra, the 2 functional units for storage (the bladder body, or reservoir) and elimination (the bladder neck and urethra, or outlet) of urine. The bladder and urethra function reciprocally. As the bladder fills during the urine storage phase, the detrusor remains quiescent, with a little change in intravesical pressure, adapting to the increasing volume by increasing the length of its muscle cells. Furthermore, neural pathways that stimulate the bladder for micturition are quiescent during this phase, and inhibitory pathways are active.[4,5]

In normal rats, external urethral sphincter (EUS)–electromyogram (EMG) recordings, which are widely used for evaluating the urethral function, exhibit tonic activity before onset of voiding and bursting activity during voiding (**Fig. 1**). This EUS bursting during voiding is characterized by clusters of high-frequency spikes separated by low tonic activity, and produces rhythmic contractions and a relaxation of EUS that present a pumping action of EUS.[6–12] The EUS bursting activity and pressure oscillations in cystometrograms are abolished by bungarotoxin, a neuromuscular

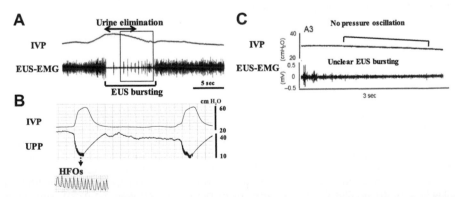

Fig. 1. Representative recordings of simultaneous measurement of intravesical pressure (IVP) and EUS-EMG activity or urethral perfusion pressure (UPP) in a rat (*A* and *B*) or a mouse (*C*). The EUS-EMG exhibits tonic activity before the onset of voiding and bursting activity during voiding (*A*). The bursting produces rhythmic contractions and relaxation of the EUS and is thought to generate a urethral pumping action during voiding, which is seen as high-frequency oscillations (HFOs) on UPP (*B*). In contrast, most mice exhibited reduced EUS activity without bursting and no obvious pressure oscillation on the cystometrogram during voiding. ([*A, C*] *Adapted from* Kadekawa K, Yoshimura N, Majima T, et al. Characterization of bladder and external urethral activity in mice with or without SCI–a comparison study with rats. Am J Physiol Regul Integr Comp Physiol 2016;310:R752–8; and [*B*] *From* Miyazato M, Sasatomi K, Hiragata S, et al. Suppression of detrusor-sphincter dysynergia by GABA-receptor activation in the lumbosacral spinal cord in spinal cord-injured rats. Am J Physiol Regul Integr Comp Physiol 2008;295:R336–42.)

blocker or pudendal nerve transection in rats,[10,13,14] suggesting that the EUS pumping activity plays an important role in efficient bladder emptying. This bursting activity is thought to generate high-frequency oscillations (HFOs) measured by urethral perfusion pressure, which are mainly shown in some species, such as rat and dog.[2] However, in normal mice, only a minority exhibits bursting-like EUS activity, and it has little impact on voiding efficiency,[11] indicating that there are species differences regarding the neural control of bladder and sphincter function during voiding. However, the precise mechanisms of voluntary and reflex controls of bladder and urethra in humans still need to be clarified, although in brain imaging studies using functional MRI, various brain regions are identified to be involved in the storage and voiding phases of micturition.[15]

The lower urinary tract is peripherally innervated by parasympathetic, sympathetic, and somatic peripheral nerves that are components of intricate efferent and afferent circuitry derived from the brain and the spinal cord. The neural circuits act as an integrated complex of reflexes that regulates micturition, allowing the lower urinary tract to be in either a storage or elimination mode.

Efferent Pathways

The smooth muscles of the bladder (the detrusor) are innervated primarily by parasympathetic nerves, whereas those of the bladder neck and urethra (the internal sphincter) are innervated by sympathetic nerves. The striated muscles of the EUS receive their primary innervation from somatic nerves (**Figs. 2** and **3**).

Parasympathetic nerves

The efferent parasympathetic pathway provides the major excitatory innervation of the detrusor.[5] Preganglionic axons emerge, as does the pelvic nerve, from the sacral parasympathetic nucleus in the intermediolateral column of sacral spinal segments S2 to S4 in humans and synapse in the pelvic ganglia, as well as in small ganglia on the bladder wall, releasing acetylcholine (ACh). Excitation of postsynaptic neurons by ACh is mediated by nicotinic receptors. Postganglionic axons continue for a short distance in the pelvic nerve and terminate in the detrusor layer where they release ACh to induce contractions of the smooth muscle fibers of the detrusor. This stimulatory effect of ACh at the postganglionic axon

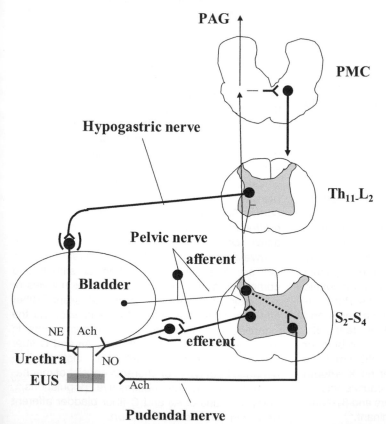

Fig. 2. Efferent pathways: Major preganglionic and postganglionic neural pathways from the spinal cord to the lower urinary tract. The sympathetic hypogastric nerve, emerging from the inferior mesenteric ganglion, stimulates urethral smooth muscle. The parasympathetic pelvic nerve, emerging from the pelvic ganglion, stimulates bladder detrusor muscle and inhibits urethral smooth muscle. The somatic pudendal nerve stimulates striated muscle of the EUS. Afferent pathways: Ascending afferent inputs from the spinal cord passes through neurons in the periaqueductal gray (PAG) to upper brain regions and the pontine micturition (PMC). ACh, acetylcholine; NE, norepinephrine; NO, nitric oxide; S_2-S_4, sacral segments of the spinal cord; T_{11}-L_2, thoracolumbar segments of the spinal cord.

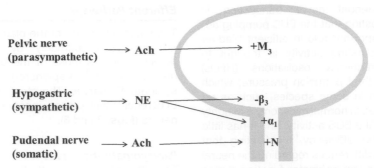

Fig. 3. Innervation of the lower urinary tract: The parasympathetic pelvic nerve stimulates the bladder detrusor muscle, mediated by muscarinic receptors (M_3) being activated by ACh. The sympathetic hypogastric nerve stimulates urethral smooth muscle and inhibits bladder detrusor, mediated by α_1-adrenergic and β_3-adrenergic receptors, respectively. The somatic pudendal nerve stimulates striated muscle of the EUS, mediated by ACh activating nicotinic (N) receptors. ACh, acetylcholine; NE, norepinephrine. Plus and minus signs indicate neural stimulation and inhibition, respectively.

terminal is mediated by muscarinic receptors in detrusor cells. Two muscarinic subtypes, M2 and M3, are known to be present in the bladder; although M2 is most abundant in detrusor cells, the M3 subtype is the major receptor mediating stimulation of detrusor contractions.[5,16,17] Parasympathetic postganglionic nerves also release nonadrenergic, noncholinergic transmitters (adenosine triphosphate [ATP]), which act on $P2X_1$ purinoceptors.[18]

In addition to the parasympathetic stimulation of bladder smooth muscle, some postsynaptic parasympathetic neurons exert a relaxation effect on urethral smooth muscle, most likely via transmission of nitric oxide (NO).[5,17,19,20] Thus, as the bladder contracts during the elimination phase, the internal urethral sphincter relaxes to facilitate the bladder emptying.

Sympathetic nerves

Sympathetic nerves stimulate smooth muscle contraction in the urethra and bladder neck and cause relaxation of the detrusor. Preganglionic sympathetic neurons are located in the intermediolateral column of thoracolumbar cord segments T11 to L2 in humans.[5,17] Most of the preganglionic fibers synapse with postganglionic neurons in the inferior mesenteric ganglia. The preganglionic neurotransmitter is ACh, which acts via nicotinic receptors in the postganglionic neurons. Postganglionic axons travel in the hypogastric nerve and release norepinephrine (NE) at their terminals. The major terminals are in the urethra and bladder neck, as well as in the bladder body. NE stimulates contraction of urethral and bladder neck smooth muscle via α_1-adrenoceptors and causes relaxation of detrusor via β_2-adrenoceptors and β_3-adrenoceptors, the latter being predominant.[21]

Somatic nerves

Somatic nerves provide excitatory innervation to the striated muscles of the EUS and pelvic floor. The efferent motoneurons are located in Onuf nucleus, along the lateral border of the ventral horn in sacral spinal cord segments S2 to S4 in humans.[5,22] The motoneuron axons are carried in the pudendal nerve and release ACh at their terminals. The ACh acts on nicotinic receptors in the striated muscle, inducing muscle contraction to maintain closure of the EUS.[5,22,23]

Afferent Pathways

The pelvic, hypogastric, and pudendal nerves carry sensory information in afferent fibers from the lower urinary tract to the lumbosacral spinal cord.[22,24,25] The most important afferents for initiating micturition are those passing in the pelvic nerve to sacral spinal cord. These afferents are small myelinated Aδ and unmyelinated C fibers, which convey information from receptor in the bladder wall to second-order neurons in the spinal cord.[26] Aδ bladder afferents in the cat respond in a graded manner to passive distension, as well as to active contraction of the bladder. In contrast, unmyelinated C-fiber bladder afferents in the cat are insensitive to mechanical stimuli and commonly do not respond to even high levels of intravesical pressure.[27,28] In the cat, silent C-fiber afferents have specialized function, such as the signaling of inflammatory or noxious events in the lower urinary tract. In the rat, Aδ and C-fiber bladder afferents cannot be distinguished because both types of afferents consist of mechanosensitive and chemosensitive populations.[27] The properties of Aδ and C-fiber bladder afferent nerves in humans are unknown.

Bladder Urothelium

The urothelium, which has been traditionally viewed as a passive barrier, also has specialized sensory and signaling properties that allow it to respond to chemical and mechanical stimuli and to engage in chemical communication with neighboring nerves or myofibroblasts in the underlying lamina, which comprises the bladder mucosa with the urothelial layer.[18,29,30] These urothelial properties include (1) expression of receptors for ACh, NE, tachykinins, and agonists for transient receptor potential (TRP) channels, such as TRPV1, TRPV4, and TRPV8; (2) close physical association with afferent nerves; and (3) ability to release chemical mediators, such as ATP, ACh, nerve growth factor (NGF), and NO, which also can influence reflex bladder contractions.[18,29] The somata of the pelvic and pudendal afferent nerves are located in dorsal root ganglia at sacral segments S2 to S4; the somata of the hypogastric nerve are located in dorsal root ganglia at thoracolumbar segments T11–L2.

Neural Circuits Controlling Micturition

Coordination between the bladder and urinary sphincter is mediated by a complex neural control system that is located in the brain, spinal cord, and peripheral ganglia (**Fig. 4**). Storage function is primarily maintained by the spinal-cord reflex, which enhances the activity of the sympathetic and somatic nerves innervating the EUS. This function is also facilitated by the pontine storage center, which lies ventrolateral to the pontine micturition center (PMC), the hypothalamus, the cerebellum, the basal ganglia, and the frontal cortex. In those without neurologic deficits, the micturition reflex depends on the spinobulbospinal reflex, which involves the periaqueductal gray (PAG) in the midbrain and in the PMC.[31] The PAG is thought to mediate switching from storage to voiding, and the PMC, which is located in or adjacent to the locus coeruleus, has spinal descending fibers containing glutamate as a major excitatory neurotransmitter, which project to the sacral cord intermediate column. Fibers that contain γ-aminobutyric acid (GABA) and glycine as inhibitory neurotransmitters also project from the PMC to the Onuf nucleus. These fibers are able to suppress urethral sphincter activity during voiding. In addition, the mechanism of switching from storage to voiding in the PAG is thought to be regulated by higher brain structures, such as the hypothalamus and prefrontal cortex. Overall, owing to the complexities of the neural mechanisms regulating the LUT, a wide variety of neurologic diseases, such as CI, PD, MS, SCI, and spina bifida, affect micturition and are able to induce lower urinary tract (LUT) dysfunction (see **Fig. 4**).

DISEASE-INDUCED CHANGES IN MICTURITION-ANIMAL MODELS
Terminology

This section summarizes the findings of basic science research in neurogenic lower urinary tract dysfunction using animal models of human diseases, such as CI, PD, MS, spinal cord injury, and spina bifida. At present, the terminology of lower urinary tract dysfunction in basic animal research is not yet standardized. Also, it is not known which urodynamic findings in animals directly correspond to human conditions of neurogenic lower urinary tract dysfunction. Therefore, this article avoids the use of the term overactive bladder, which is a symptom-based disease definition, when describing the urodynamic findings of animal models. Also, based on the international continence society standardization, detrusor overactivity (DO) in humans is defined as the unexpected bladder muscle (the detrusor) contraction during bladder filling. Thus, the term DO is used only when animals exhibit nonvoiding bladder contractions during the storage phase in cystometric analyses. In other cases in which frequent voiding with reduced voided volume in voiding behavior studies or reduced intercontraction intervals with decreased bladder capacity during cystometry are observed, the condition is called bladder overactivity to avoid the confusion with DO. In addition, the term detrusor sphincter dyssynergia (DSD) is used when the tonic activity of EUS-EMG is increased or the urethral pressure becomes positive values above $0 \, cmH_2O$ in urethral perfusion pressure measurements during voiding bladder contractions.

Cerebral Infarction

Cerebrovascular accident is a serious neurologic event and it can cause temporary or permanent neurogenic lower urinary tract dysfunction to patients.[32] In CI survivors, there is also a high prevalence of urinary incontinence varying from 12% to 79%, depending on time after CI.[33,34] In CI, the neurologic dysfunction is caused by a focal brain damage due to ischemia and/or hemorrhage. When the brain damage is located in a small area in the right frontal region of cerebrum, which is involved in the control of micturition, it may predominantly result in bladder overactivity and urgency urinary incontinence.[1,35,36]

A rat model of CI produced by occlusion of the middle cerebral artery with a flamed 4-0 monofilament nylon inserted into the internal carotid artery has been shown to exhibit bladder overactivity as

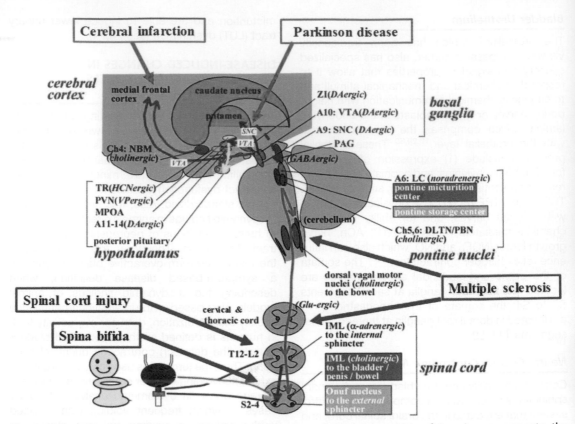

Fig. 4. Neural circuitry relevant to micturition. The lower urinary tract consists of 2 major components: the bladder, and the urethra. The bladder is mainly innervated by the parasympathetic pelvic nerve. The urethra is innervated by the sympathetic hypogastric nerve and somatic pudendal nerve, respectively. Urinary storage depends on the reflex arc of the sacral spinal cord. The storage reflex is thought to be tonically facilitated by the brain, particularly the pontine storage center. The storage function is thought to be further facilitated by the hypothalamus, cerebellum, basal ganglia, and frontal cortex. Central cholinergic fibers from the nucleus basalis Meynert (NBM; also called the Ch4 cell group) seem to facilitate urinary storage. Micturition depends on the reflex arc of the brainstem and spinal cord, which involves the midbrain PAG and the PMC (located in or adjacent to the locus coeruleus [LC]). The voiding function is thought to be initiated by the hypothalamus and prefrontal cortex, which overlap the storage-facilitating area. CI induces the neural damage in the cerebrum. PD is primarily induced by degeneration of dopaminergic (DAgic) neurons in the substantia nigra pars compacta (SNC). MS is induced by focal demyelization of the central nervous system at various levels. SCI is induced by complete or incomplete neural damages of the spinal cord at different levels. Spina bifida is caused by a failure of the caudal neural tube to fuse normally in early development, thus often inducing the damage of the lumbosacral spinal cord and resulting in myelomeningocele, in which the spinal cord and neural elements are exposed. A, adrenergic or noradrenergic; DLTN, dorsolateral tegmental nucleus; GABA, γ-aminobutyric acid; HCN, hypocretinergic; IML, intermediolateral cell column; L, lumbar; MPOA, medial preoptic area; PBN, parabrachial nucleus; PVN, paraventricular nucleus; S, sacral; SNC, substantia nigra pars compacta; T, thoracic; TR, tuberous region; VTA, ventral tegmental area; ZI, zona incerta.

evidenced by reduced bladder capacity during awake cystometry.[37] In another rat model of bladder overactivity without brain damage, midbrain ischemia is induced by anastomosis between the right external jugular vein and the right common carotid artery with partial obstruction of the left common carotid artery.[38] The mechanism underlying lower urinary tract dysfunction after CI remains unclear. However, using animal models of CI, it has been reported that N-methyl-

D-aspartate (NMDA) glutamatergic excitatory mechanisms play an important role in bladder overactivity induced by CI. Pretreatment with MK-801, an NMDA receptor agonist, can prevent bladder overactivity in CI rats.[39] Rats with CI also exhibit the upregulation of D_2-like dopamine receptor-mediated excitatory mechanisms and alteration in dopaminergic-glutamatergic interaction in the brain.[40–42] Disruption of GABAergic[43] and glycinergic[44] inhibitory mechanisms in the brain is also involved to enhance the micturition reflex. Thus, the balance between excitatory glutamatergic neurons and inhibitory glycinergic or GABAergic might be impaired after CI, which results in bladder overactivity.

In addition to bladder dysfunction, CI reportedly induces urethral dysfunction. In a recent study in CI rats, leak point pressure was 29% lower compared with normal rats,[45] and duloxetine, an NE and serotonin reuptake inhibitor, failed to enhance the sneeze-induced urethral continence reflex,[45] suggesting that CI impairs the urethral continence mechanism to induce stress urinary incontinence. Robinson and Bloom[46] postulated that ischemic lesions may interrupt the biogenic amine-containing axons ascending from the brainstem to the cerebral cortex, leading to decreased availability of biogenic amines in limbic structures of the frontal and temporal lobes, as well as in the basal ganglia. The monoamine theory postulates that depression is associated with low levels of monoamines, particularly NE, serotonin, and dopamine.[47] In addition, monoaminergic descending pathways projecting through the dorsolateral spinal column are instrumental in the regulation of pain.[48] Thus, ascending and descending pathways through the raphe nuclei and the locus coeruleus, which are the major sources of spinal serotonergic and noradrenergic pathways, respectively,[49] in the brain stem may be disrupted by the stroke lesion, which may result in impaired urethral continence function.

Parkinson Disease

PD is a degenerative disorder of central nervous system characterized by muscle rigidity, tremor, and a slow physical movement. These symptoms result from decreased stimulation of the motor cortex by the basal ganglia, usually caused by the insufficient formation and action of dopamine, which is produced in the pathways from the substantia nigra to the striatum in the midbrain. Patients with PD also often have lower urinary tract symptoms, such as nocturia, increased urinary frequency, and urinary incontinence, which overlap with those of overactive bladder symptoms. The reported incidence of such symptoms ranges from 27% to 63.9% across different studies.[50] The most common finding in the urodynamic study is DO, shown by uninhibited contractions during bladder filling, which result from impaired activity of the central nervous system, especially in the nigrostriatal dopaminergic pathways.[51,52] A previous functional brain imaging study has shown some overlaps (PAG, thalamus, putamen, and insula), as well as differences (pons or anterior cingulate gyrus only in healthy volunteers) in brain activation sites during filling between healthy volunteers and subjects with PD who had DO.[53]

The underlying mechanisms inducing bladder dysfunction in PD have been investigated in animal studies. **Fig. 5** shows a hypothetical diagram drawn from animal models of bladder dysfunction in PD. In monkeys, disruption of nigrostriatal dopaminergic pathways induced by the neurotoxin 1-methyl-4-phenyl-1,2,3,6-tetrahydropyridine (MPTP) produces PD-like motor symptoms accompanied by bladder overactivity shown by frequent urination with reduced voided volume.[54–56] A rat model of PD induced by a unilateral 6-hydroxydopamine injection into the substantia nigra exhibits a similar type of bladder overactivity.[57,58] In these animal models, bladder overactivity was suppressed by enhancement of D_1-like receptors with SKF 38393 or pergolide,[55–57] suggesting that bladder overactivity in PD is primarily induced by disruption of D_1-like dopamine receptor-mediated inhibition of the micturition reflex.

Levodopa for treatment of PD patients often worsens DO due to activation of dopamine D_2-receptors.[59] In addition, in a rat model of PD, bladder overactivity was suppressed by an adenosine A_{2A} receptor antagonist, ZM 241385, suggesting that enhanced activity of the adenosine A_{2A} system in the brain contribute to bladder overactivity associated with PD.[60] The adenosine A_{2A} receptor-expressing neural pathways are very likely located downstream of D_1 receptor expressing pathways in the control of micturition because inhibition of bladder activity by D_1 receptor activation can induce the partial suppression of adenosine A_{2A} receptor-mediated excitatory mechanisms in the rat model of PD.[60] Kitta and colleagues[61] also reported that intravenous ZM 241385 dose-dependently increased the amplitude of evoked potentials in the anterior cingulate cortex in a rat PD model but not in sham operated rats, suggesting that anterior cingulate cortex neurons have an inhibitory role in bladder control and an executive function, including decision-making in the micturition reflex. Clinical studies of adenosine A_{2A} receptor antagonists also provided promising results of motor dysfunction in PD subjects.[62,63] Istradefylline, an adenosine A_{2A} receptor antagonist, has been already approved and launched for patients with PD, which also may be a promising candidate for treatment of lower urinary tract dysfunction in patients with PD.[64] To support this assumption, a recent open-labeled clinical study reported that treatment with istradefylline, a selective adenosine A2A receptor antagonist, for 12 weeks significantly improved lower urinary tract symptoms in 13 male PD patients[64]

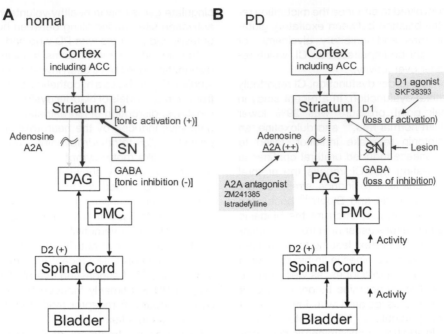

Fig. 5. A hypothetical diagram demonstrates working model of bladder dysfunction in PD. Micturition reflex is controlled by spinobulbospinal pathways through PAG in midbrain and PMC in brainstem. This neural circuit is under control of higher centers, including anterior cingulate cortex (ACC) and other cortex regions. (*A*) Under normal conditions tonic inhibition from ACC suppress micturition reflex. Tonic firing (+) of dopaminergic neurons in SN activates dopamine D_1 receptors expressed on GABAergic inhibitory neurons in the striatum to induce tonic GABAergic inhibition (−) of the micturition reflex at the level of PAG. At the same time, D_1 receptor stimulation suppresses the activity of adenosinergic neurons, which exert an excitatory effect on micturition via adenosine A_{2A} receptors (+). (*B*) In PD, dopaminergic neurons in the substantia nigra pars compacta (SN) are lost (lesion), leading to the loss of dopamine D_1 receptors activation (D_1 [loss of activation]), which results in reduced activation inhibitory GABAergic neurons in the striatum (GABA [loss of inhibition]). At the same time, reduced D_1 receptor stimulation enhances the adenosinergic mechanism to stimulate adenosine A_{2A} receptors (adenosine A_{2A} [++]), leading to facilitation of the spinobulbospinal pathway controlling the micturition reflex pathway. Administration of dopamine D_1 receptor agonist (SKF 38393) can restore the GABAergic nerve activity and suppress A_{2A} receptor-mediated activation to reduce bladder overactivity in PD. Also, administration of adenosine A_{2A} antagonists (ZM241385 or istradefylline) can suppress A_{2A} receptor-mediated activation of the micturition reflex to reduce bladder overactivity in PD. Dopamine D_2 receptors (D_2 [+]) expressed in the spinal cord enhances the micturition reflex. (*Modified from* Kitta T, Chancellor MB, de Groat WC, et al. Role of the anterior cingulate cortex in the control of micturition reflex in a rat model of Parkinson's disease. J Urol 2016;195:1613–20.)

although a larger-sized, placebo-controlled randomized study is needed to confirm the results.

In addition, a previous study[65] shows that the injection of human amniotic-fluid-derived stem cells and bone-marrow-derived mesenchymal stem cells into the medial forebrain bundle improves bladder dysfunction in rat models of PD and stem-cell injection did improve cystometric parameters 14 days after implantation. This effect is not sustained and the number of stem cells gradually decreases with time. After injection, human stem cells were found to express superoxide dismutase-2, and modulated the expression of interleukin-6 and glial cell–derived neurotrophic factor by host cells. Thus, the injected stem cells

seem to act on the juxtacrine or paracrine system, although the precise mechanism is yet to be determined.

Multiple Sclerosis

MS is a chronic disease with focal demyelization of the central nervous system at various levels, causing a wide spectrum of neurologic manifestation. The onset of MS ranges from 20 to 40 years, with more than 80% patients suffering from lower urinary tract symptoms.[66] The storage symptoms, such as frequency, urgency, and urge incontinence, are more common but voiding symptoms, such as weak stream, straining, and large residual urine, are also commonly seen in MS patients.[67–69] The exact causes of the development of MS are still unknown; however, experimental autoimmune encephalomyelitis is among the most commonly used and characterized animal model of MS using mice or rats.[70–72] Coronavirus-induced encephalomyelitis in mice was also reported to develop neurogenic lower urinary tract dysfunction that is compatible with DO, often seen in patients with MS.[73,74] Thus, these findings are in line with the current view that bladder dysfunction in MS is associated with spinal cord demyelination and, subsequently, disruption of pathways between the lumbosacral spinal cord and the PMC.

In addition to the neurogenic dysfunction in the central nervous system, there is also evidence showing the damage in peripheral nerves and urothelial function of the bladder. For example, Lamarre and colleagues[74] demonstrated a deficit in the nerve-evoked cholinergic component of bladder contraction. Negoro and colleagues[75] also reported that pannexin1, a member of the gap junction protein expressed in the bladder urothelium, provides a positive feedback loop for inflammatory responses in bladder dysfunction in an MS mouse model with experimental autoimmune encephalomyelitis.

Spinal Cord Injury

SCI initially induces areflexic bladder and urinary retention, followed by the emergence of automatic micturition and, eventually, DO mediated by spinal reflex mechanisms. This reflex mimics a neonatal exteroceptive micturition reflex that is activated by the mother licking the perineal region for the expelling of urine.[76,77] Maximal voiding pressure is increased, voiding efficiency is reduced, and bladder undergoes marked hypertrophy.[6,8,78] Bladder-sphincter coordination is impaired, leading to DSD.[79–83] Thus, the organization of the micturition reflex shows marked changes after SCI (**Fig. 6**). Any injury to the spinal cord, such as blunt, degenerative, developmental, vascular, infectious, traumatic, and idiopathic injury, can cause voiding dysfunction. In cats with chronic thoracic spinal cord transection, micturition is induced by C-fiber afferent pathways. It has been demonstrated that in chronic spinalized cats, desensitization of TRPV1-expressing C-fiber afferent pathways by subcutaneously administered capsaicin, a C-fiber neurotoxin that binds to TRPV1 receptors, completely blocked DO shown by nonvoiding bladder contractions during the storage phase, whereas capsaicin had no inhibitory effects on reflex bladder contractions in spinal intact cats.[80,84] Thus, it is plausible that C-fiber bladder

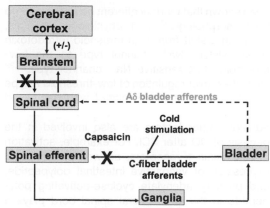

Fig. 6. A hypothetical diagram demonstrates micturition reflex pathways after SCI. SCI rostral to the lumbosacral spinal cord level eliminates voluntary and supraspinal control of voiding. Over a period of several weeks following SCI, a spinal reflex mechanism emerges, which is triggered by unmyelinated C-fiber bladder afferents. Aδ-fiber bladder afferent inputs are ineffective. Stimulation of C-fiber afferents by instillation of ice water into the bladder (cold stimulation) activates voiding responses. Pretreatment with capsaicin that desensitizes TRPV1-expressing C-fiber afferent pathways reduces detrusor overactivity in chronic SCI rats but does not block the micturition reflex in normal rats.

afferents that usually do not respond to bladder distension[27,28] become mechanosensitive and initiate automatic micturition after SCI.

In a rat model of SCI induced by complete transection of the thoracic spinal cord, increased excitability of C-fiber bladder afferents after SCI also induces DO, as evidenced by nonvoiding bladder contractions before micturition, because desensitizing C-fiber afferents by systemic capsaicin administration completely suppressed these nonvoiding bladder contractions without affecting the voiding reflex.[6,85] Desensitization of C-fiber afferent pathways by capsaicin pretreatment also reduces DSD in chronic SCI rats.[86] Furthermore, it has also been shown in the cat that C-fiber bladder afferents are responsible for cold-induced bladder reflexes via TRPM8 receptors.[29,87] Chronic SCI in humans also causes the emergence of an unusual bladder reflex that is elicited by infusion of cold water into the bladder, which is blocked by intravesical capsaicin treatment.[88–90] Thus, it is likely that cold-sensitive and capsaicin-sensitive C-fiber bladder afferents contribute to the emergence of DO and DSD after SCI.

The mechanisms inducing hyperexcitability of C-fiber afferent pathways after SCI has also been investigated in SCI animal models. In rats, it has been shown that bladder afferent neurons undergo both morphologic[91] and physiologic changes, including a shift from high-threshold tetrodotoxin (TTX)-resistant Na^+ channel type to the low-threshold, TTX-sensitive Na^+ channel type,[83,92] as well as downregulation of low-threshold A-type K^+ channels that is associated with decreased expression of Kv1.4 α-subunit following SCI.[93] In addition, other factors are also involved in the genesis of DO after SCI. For example, activation of neurokinin-1 receptors, as well as increased expression of vasoactive intestinal polypeptide, and pituitary adenylate cyclase-activating polypeptide in the lumbosacral spinal cord plays a role in the emergence of DO after SCI.[86,94] TRP receptors in the suburothelial nerve fibers, such as TRPV1 or TRPA1, are also involved in C-fiber bladder hyperexcitability that contributes to neurogenic DO in SCI.[95,96]

It has also been speculated that SCI-induced DO is mediated by the action of neurotrophic factors, such as NGF or brain-derived neurotrophic factor (BDNF). Animal studies demonstrated that chronic administration of NGF into the spinal cord or into the bladder wall induced DO and increased excitability of bladder afferent neurons.[97–99] Immunoneutralization of NGF in the spinal cord reduced NGF levels in the L6 to S1 dorsal root ganglia, which contain bladder afferent neurons, and also suppressed DO and DSD.[86,100] Thus, a combination of peripheral and central NGF action is likely to be involved in the emergence of DO or DSD. In addition, although the role of BDNF has not been well-defined, a previous study by Frias and colleagues[101] demonstrated that BDNF may be an important regulator of neurogenic DO appearance and maintenance because the early-phase administration of BDNF inhibited neurogenic DO, whereas, at later stages, BDNF sequestration reduced neurogenic DO in a rat model of SCI.

Furthermore, SCI can induce peripheral changes in urothelial and detrusor muscle function in the bladder to stimulate bladder afferents and induce bladder overactivity. For example, the urothelial release of ATP that can activate bladder afferents through $P2X_{2/3}$ ATP receptors is shown to be increased in a rat model of SCI.[102,103] Also, previous studies have reported that urothelially activated intrinsic detrusor contractions that are sensitive to L-type Ca^{2+} channels blockers, such as nifedipine, are enhanced in the SCI rat bladder[104] and that the SCI-induced intrinsic detrusor activity is linked to the increased firing of single unit bladder afferent fibers in SCI mice.[105]

In the central nervous system, glutamate is a major excitatory amino acid, whereas glycine and GABA are major inhibitory neurotransmitters and act to inhibit the micturition reflex at supraspinal and/or spinal sites.[106] Intravenous application of an α-amino-3-hydroxy-5-methyl-4-isoxazole-propionic acid (AMPA) glutamatergic receptor antagonist is reported to eliminate DSD.[107] Glycine and GABA have additive or synergistic inhibitory effects on bladder activity.[108] Hypofunction of glycinergic or GABAergic mechanisms in the lumbosacral spinal cord induces lower urinary tract dysfunction, such as DO or DSD, after SCI in rats.[12,109,110] Intrathecal, intravenous, or dietary glycine inhibits both bladder and urethral activity in normal and SCI rats.[109,111] Therefore, glycine might be useful agent for the treatment of DO. Also, intrathecal muscimol and baclofen (GABA$_A$ and GABA$_B$ agonists, respectively) in SCI rats inhibit nonvoiding bladder contractions by suppressing C-fiber bladder afferents,[110] and they improve DSD as well.[12] Baclofen is approved for treatment of DO in SCI patients,[112] but this agent has not been widely used because the therapeutic window of this drug is modest with the limited dose range due to side effects. Gene delivery of glutamic acid decarboxylase (GAD), the GABA synthesis enzyme, by using nonreplicating herpes simplex virus vectors inhibits DO or DSD without affecting voiding contraction in SCI rats.[113,114] Therefore, GAD gene therapy can restore urine storage function without affecting voiding function; therefore, it would be more beneficial than drug therapy for the treatment of urinary problems in SCI patients. In addition, a recent study using rats with partial SCI induced by bilateral dorsal lesions of the thoracic spinal cord has demonstrated that the treatment with a $P2X_7$ ATP receptor antagonist at the injured spinal cord region reduced DO induced after SCI and that $P2X_7$ receptors were expressed in CD11b-positive microglia cells.[115] Because the ATP release from the spinal cord during bladder distension is reportedly increased in SCI rats compared with spinal intact rats,[116] it is conceivable that the ATP-mediated excitatory mechanism in the spinal cord via $P2X_7$ receptors expressed in microglia cells is enhanced to induce neurogenic DO after SCI. Overall, various levels of changes in both central and peripheral nervous systems, as well as in the lower urinary tract seem to contribute to neurogenic lower urinary tract dysfunction such as DO after SCI.

Although DO during urine storage is similarly observed in both rats and mice after SCI,[105,117] the behavior of EUS during voiding is quite different in these 2 species.[11] In SCI rats, EUS bursting occurs during voiding bladder contractions, which coincides with small-amplitude intravesical pressure oscillations during cystometry. However, SCI mice do not exhibit clear EUS bursting or intravesical pressure oscillation but rather exhibit intermittent voiding with slow large-amplitude reductions in intravesical pressure, which occur during periods of reduced EUS activity.[11] α-Bungarotoxin improved voiding by reducing urethral outlet resistance in SCI rats[14]; however, in normal rats, the toxin reduced voiding, probably by suppressing high-frequency phasic sphincter activity necessary for efficient urine elimination in normal animals. Thus, the reflex EUS pumping activity recovers and enables achieving efficient voiding, even after SCI in rats, whereas it is not the case in SCI mice.[11] These results suggest that the difference in voiding efficiency after SCI in these 2 species might be due to the difference in urethral activity during the voiding phase, which should be taken into account in the basic research of SCI-induced neurogenic lower urinary tract dysfunction such as DSD. In addition, bilateral transection of hypogastric nerve, which provides the major sympathetic input to the urinary bladder and proximal urethra, improved voiding dysfunction in SCI rats[118] although the role of hypogastric nerves in SCI mice has not been investigated.

Spina Bifida

The birth prevalence of spina bifida is at approximately 30 per 100,000 in the United States. Spina bifida is caused by a failure of the caudal neural tube to fuse normally in early development, thus often inducing the damage of the lumbosacral spinal cord. Myelomeningocele, in which the spinal cord and neural elements are exposed, is the most common and clinically severe of the open spina bifida defects. Thus, it causes variable impact on the somatic, parasympathetic, and sympathetic innervation of the lower urinary tract to affect the ability to store and empty urine.[119]

Although the basic research on neurogenic lower urinary tract dysfunction induced by spinal bifida is limited, fetal rats with retinoic acid-induced myelomeningocele[120] have been used as an animal model of spina bifida to investigate bladder dysfunction. It has been reported that fetuses with myelomeningocele from pregnant Sprague-Dawley rats that were gavage fed with retinoic acid showed a reduction in KCl or bethanechol-induced muscle strip contractility and decreased nerve density in the bladder, whereas bladder smooth muscle of fetal myelomeningocele rats was morphologically normal.[121,122] A recent study has also shown that the number of interstitial cells of Cajal in the bladder is decreased in fetal myelomeningocele rats.[123] Thus, this animal model of spinal bifida and myelomeningocele seems to be useful to study the denervation process in the bladder and the possible damage of coordinating activity of bladder smooth muscles, although it is not likely to be suitable for the postnatal investigation of spina bifida-induced lower urinary tract dysfunction.

SUMMARY

The lower urinary tract has 2 main functions, storage and elimination of urine. These highly, coordinated functions are regulated by a complex neural control system located in the brain and spinal cord (ie, central nervous system). Due to the complexity of these systems, micturition is sensitive to various diseases, such as CI, PD, MS, SCI, and spinal bifida. Studies in animals for these diseases are helpful to investigate the mechanism involved in the genesis and the plasticity in reflex pathways to the lower urinary tract after lesions, although care should be taken in extrapolating observations made in animals when applying them to human disease conditions.

REFERENCES

1. Fowler CJ, Griffiths D, de Groat WC. The neural control of micturition. Nat Rev Neurosci 2008;9: 453–66.
2. de Groat WC, Griffiths D, Yoshimura N. Neural control of the lower urinary tract. Compr Physiol 2015; 5:327–96.
3. de Groat WC, Yoshimura N. Anatomy and physiology of the lower urinary tract. Handbook Clin Neurol 2015;130:61–108.
4. Park JM, Bloom DA, McGuire EJ. The guarding reflex revisited. Br J Urol 1997;80:940–5.
5. Yoshimura N, de Groat WC. Neural control of the lower urinary tract. Int J Urol 1997;4:111–25.
6. Cheng CL, de Groat WC. The role of capsaicin-sensitive afferent fibers in the lower urinary tract dysfunction induced by chronic spinal cord injury in rats. Exp Neurol 2004;187:445–54.
7. Chen SC, Fan WJ, Lai CH. Jason Chen JJ, Peng CW. Effect of a 5-HT(1A) receptor agonist (8-OH-DPAT) on the external urethral sphincter activity in the rat. J Formos Med Assoc 2012;111:67–76.
8. Kruse MN, Belton AL, de Groat WC. Changes in bladder and external urethral sphincter function after spinal cord injury in the rat. Am J Physiol 1993; 264:R1157–63.
9. Liu G, Lin YH, Yamada Y, et al. External urethral sphincter activity in diabetic rats. Neurourol Urodyn 2008;27:429–34.
10. Maggi CA, Giuliani S, Santicioli P, et al. Analysis of factors involved in determining urinary bladder

voiding cycle in urethan-anesthetized rats. Am J Physiol 1986;251:R250–7.

11. Kadekawa K, Yoshimura N, Majima T, et al. Characterization of bladder and external urethral activity in mice with or without spinal cord injury–a comparison study with rats. Am J Physiol Regul Integr Comp Physiol 2016;310:R752–8.

12. Miyazato M, Sasatomi K, Hiragata S, et al. Suppression of detrusor-sphincter dysynergia by GABA-receptor activation in the lumbosacral spinal cord in spinal cord-injured rats. Am J Physiol Regul Integr Comp Physiol 2008;295:R336–42.

13. Peng CW, Chen JJ, Cheng CL, et al. Role of pudendal afferents in voiding efficiency in the rat. Am J Physiol Regul Integr Comp Physiol 2008;294:R660–72.

14. Yoshiyama M, deGroat WC, Fraser MO. Influences of external urethral sphincter relaxation induced by alpha-bungarotoxin, a neuromuscular junction blocking agent, on voiding dysfunction in the rat with spinal cord injury. Urology 2000;55:956–60.

15. Griffiths D. Functional imaging of structures involved in neural control of the lower urinary tract. Handbook Clin Neurol 2015;130:121–33.

16. Chapple CR, Yamanishi T, Chess-Williams R. Muscarinic receptor subtypes and management of the overactive bladder. Urology 2002;60:82–8 [discussion: 88–9].

17. de Groat WC, Yoshimura N. Pharmacology of the lower urinary tract. Annu Rev Pharmacol Toxicol 2001;41:691–721.

18. Birder L, de Groat W, Mills I, et al. Neural control of the lower urinary tract: peripheral and spinal mechanisms. Neurourol Urodyn 2010;29:128–39.

19. Bennett BC, Kruse MN, Roppolo JR, et al. Neural control of urethral outlet activity in vivo: role of nitric oxide. J Urol 1995;153:2004–9.

20. Yono M, Yamamoto Y, Yoshida M, et al. Effects of doxazosin on blood flow and mRNA expression of nitric oxide synthase in the spontaneously hypertensive rat genitourinary tract. Life Sci 2007;81:218–22.

21. Nomiya M, Yamaguchi O. A quantitative analysis of mRNA expression of alpha 1 and beta-adrenoceptor subtypes and their functional roles in human normal and obstructed bladders. J Urol 2003;170:649–53.

22. Thor KB, Morgan C, Nadelhaft I, et al. Organization of afferent and efferent pathways in the pudendal nerve of the female cat. J Comp Neurol 1989;288:263–79.

23. Blaivas JG. The neurophysiology of micturition: a clinical study of 550 patients. J Urol 1982;127:958–63.

24. Morgan C, deGroat WC, Nadelhaft I. The spinal distribution of sympathetic preganglionic and visceral primary afferent neurons that send axons into the hypogastric nerves of the cat. J Comp Neurol 1986;243:23–40.

25. Andersson KE, Wein AJ. Pharmacology of the lower urinary tract: basis for current and future treatments of urinary incontinence. Pharmacol Rev 2004;56:581–631.

26. Mallory B, Steers WD, De Groat WC. Electrophysiological study of micturition reflexes in rats. Am J Physiol 1989;257:R410–21.

27. de Groat WC, Yoshimura N. Afferent nerve regulation of bladder function in health and disease. Handb Exp Pharmacol 2009;194:91–138.

28. Habler HJ, Janig W, Koltzenburg M. Activation of unmyelinated afferent fibres by mechanical stimuli and inflammation of the urinary bladder in the cat. J Physiol 1990;425:545–62.

29. Birder LA. Urothelial signaling. Auton Neurosci 2010;153:33–40.

30. Andersson KE, McCloskey KD. Lamina propria: the functional center of the bladder? Neurourol Urodyn 2014;33:9–16.

31. Kakizaki H, Kita M, Wada N. Models for sensory neurons of dorsal root ganglia and stress urinary incontinence. Neurourol Urodyn 2011;30:653–7.

32. Sakakibara R. Lower urinary tract dysfunction in patients with brain lesions. Handbook Clin Neurol 2015;130:269–87.

33. Brittain KR, Peet SM, Castleden CM. Stroke and incontinence. Stroke 1998;29:524–8.

34. Kolominsky-Rabas PL, Hilz MJ, Neundoerfer B, et al. Impact of urinary incontinence after stroke: results from a prospective population-based stroke register. Neurourol Urodyn 2003;22:322–7.

35. Griffiths D. Clinical studies of cerebral and urinary tract function in elderly people with urinary incontinence. Behav Brain Res 1998;92:151–5.

36. Griffiths DJ. Cerebral control of bladder function. Curr Urol Rep 2004;5:348–52.

37. Yokoyama O, Komatsu K, Ishiura Y, et al. Change in bladder contractility associated with bladder overactivity in rats with cerebral infarction. J Urol 1998;159:577–80.

38. Yotsuyanagi S, Narimoto K, Namiki M. Mild brain ischemia produces bladder hyperactivity without brain damage in rats. Urol Int 2006;77:57–63.

39. Yokoyama O, Yoshiyama M, Namiki M, et al. Glutamatergic and dopaminergic contributions to rat bladder hyperactivity after cerebral artery occlusion. Am J Physiol 1999;276:R935–42.

40. Yokoyama O, Yoshiyama M, Namiki M, et al. Interaction between D2 dopaminergic and glutamatergic excitatory influences on lower urinary tract function in normal and cerebral-infarcted rats. Exp Neurol 2001;169:148–55.

41. Yokoyama O, Yoshiyama M, Namiki M, et al. Role of the forebrain in bladder overactivity following cerebral infarction in the rat. Exp Neurol 2000;163:469–76.

42. Yokoyama O, Yoshiyama M, Namiki M, et al. Changes in dopaminergic and glutamatergic

excitatory mechanisms of micturition reflex after middle cerebral artery occlusion in conscious rats. Exp Neurol 2002;173:129–35.

43. Kanie S, Yokoyama O, Komatsu K, et al. GABAergic contribution to rat bladder hyperactivity after middle cerebral artery occlusion. Am J Physiol Regul Integr Comp Physiol 2000;279:R1230–8.

44. Sugaya K, Nishijima S, Miyazato M, et al. Central nervous control of micturition and urine storage. J Smooth Muscle Res 2005;41:117–32.

45. Miyazato M, Kitta T, Kaiho Y, et al. Effects of duloxetine on urethral continence reflex and bladder activity in rats with cerebral infarction. J Urol 2015;194:842–7.

46. Robinson RG, Bloom FE. Pharmacological treatment following experimental cerebral infarction: implications for understanding psychological symptoms of human stroke. Biol Psychiatry 1977;12:669–80.

47. Krishnan V, Nestler EJ. The molecular neurobiology of depression. Nature 2008;455:894–902.

48. Loubinoux I, Kronenberg G, Endres M, et al. Poststroke depression: mechanisms, translation and therapy. J Cell Mol Med 2012;16:1961–9.

49. Holstege JC, Kuypers HG. Brainstem projections to spinal motoneurons: an update. Neuroscience 1987;23:809–21.

50. Ogawa T, Sakakibara R, Kuno S, et al. Prevalence and treatment of LUTS in patients with PD or multiple system atrophy. Nat Rev Urol 2017;14(2):79–89.

51. Araki I, Kitahara M, Oida T, et al. Voiding dysfunction and Parkinson's disease: urodynamic abnormalities and urinary symptoms. J Urol 2000;164:1640–3.

52. Araki I, Kuno S. Assessment of voiding dysfunction in Parkinson's disease by the international prostate symptom score. J Neurol Neurosurg Psychiatry 2000;68:429–33.

53. Kitta T, Kakizaki H, Furuno T, et al. Brain activation during detrusor overactivity in patients with Parkinson's disease: a positron emission tomography study. J Urol 2006;175:994–8.

54. Albanese A, Jenner P, Marsden CD, et al. Bladder hyperreflexia induced in marmosets by 1-methyl-4-phenyl-1,2,3,6-tetrahydropyridine. Neurosci Lett 1988;87:46–50.

55. Yoshimura N, Erdman SL, Snider MW, et al. Effects of spinal cord injury on neurofilament immunoreactivity and capsaicin sensitivity in rat dorsal root ganglion neurons innervating the urinary bladder. Neuroscience 1998;83:633–43.

56. Yoshimura N, Mizuta E, Kuno S, et al. The dopamine D1 receptor agonist SKF 38393 suppresses detrusor hyperreflexia in the monkey with parkinsonism induced by 1-methyl-4-phenyl-1,2,3,6-tetrahydropyridine (MPTP). Neuropharmacology 1993;32:315–21.

57. Yoshimura N, Seki S, Erickson KA, et al. Histological and electrical properties of rat dorsal root ganglion neurons innervating the lower urinary tract. J Neurosci 2003;23:4355–61.

58. Kitta T, Matsumoto M, Tanaka H, et al. GABAergic mechanism mediated via D receptors in the rat periaqueductal gray participates in the micturition reflex: an in vivo microdialysis study. Eur J Neurosci 2008;27:3216–25.

59. Brusa L, Petta F, Pisani A, et al. Central acute D2 stimulation worsens bladder function in patients with mild Parkinson's disease. J Urol 2006;175:202–6 [discussion: 206–7].

60. Kitta T, Chancellor MB, de Groat WC, et al. Suppression of bladder overactivity by adenosine A2A receptor antagonist in a rat model of Parkinson disease. J Urol 2012;187:1890–7.

61. Kitta T, Chancellor MB, de Groat WC, et al. Role of the anterior cingulate cortex in the control of micturition reflex in a rat model of Parkinson's disease. J Urol 2016;195:1613–20.

62. Pinna A, Wardas J, Simola N, et al. New therapies for the treatment of Parkinson's disease: adenosine A2A receptor antagonists. Life Sci 2005;77:3259–67.

63. Pinna A, Volpini R, Cristalli G, et al. New adenosine A2A receptor antagonists: actions on Parkinson's disease models. Eur J Pharmacol 2005;512:157–64.

64. Kitta T, Yabe I, Takahashi I, et al. Clinical efficacy of istradefylline on lower urinary tract symptoms in Parkinson's disease. Int J Urol 2016;23(10):893–4.

65. Soler R, Fullhase C, Hanson A, et al. Stem cell therapy ameliorates bladder dysfunction in an animal model of Parkinson disease. J Urol 2012;187:1491–7.

66. Awad SA, Gajewski JB, Sogbein SK, et al. Relationship between neurological and urological status in patients with multiple sclerosis. J Urol 1984;132:499–502.

67. de Seze M, Ruffion A, Denys P, et al. Genulf. The neurogenic bladder in multiple sclerosis: review of the literature and proposal of management guidelines. Mult Scler 2007;13:915–28.

68. Betts CD, D'Mellow MT, Fowler CJ. Urinary symptoms and the neurological features of bladder dysfunction in multiple sclerosis. J Neurol Neurosurg Psychiatry 1993;56:245–50.

69. McCombe PA, Gordon TP, Jackson MW. Bladder dysfunction in multiple sclerosis. Expert Rev Neurother 2009;9:331–40.

70. Mannie M, Swanborg RH, Stepaniak JA. Experimental autoimmune encephalomyelitis in the rat. Curr Protoc Immunol 2009;Chapter: 15. Unit: 15.2.

71. McCarthy DP, Richards MH, Miller SD. Mouse models of multiple sclerosis: experimental autoimmune encephalomyelitis and Theiler's virus-induced demyelinating disease. Methods Mol Biol 2012;900:381–401.

72. Mizusawa H, Igawa Y, Nishizawa O, et al. A rat model for investigation of bladder dysfunction associated with demyelinating disease resembling multiple sclerosis. Neurourol Urodyn 2000; 19:689–99.

73. McMillan MT, Pan XQ, Smith AL, et al. Coronavirus-induced demyelination of neural pathways triggers neurogenic bladder overactivity in a mouse model of multiple sclerosis. Am J Physiol Renal Physiol 2014;307:F612–22.

74. Lamarre NS, Braverman AS, Malykhina AP, et al. Alterations in nerve-evoked bladder contractions in a coronavirus-induced mouse model of multiple sclerosis. PLoS One 2014;9:e109314.

75. Negoro H, Lutz SE, Liou LS, et al. Pannexin 1 involvement in bladder dysfunction in a multiple sclerosis model. Sci Rep 2013;3:2152.

76. de Groat WC. Plasticity of bladder reflex pathways during postnatal development. Physiol Behav 2002;77:689–92.

77. Sugaya K, De Groat WC. Micturition reflexes in the in vitro neonatal rat brain stem-spinal cord-bladder preparation. Am J Physiol 1994;266:R658–67.

78. Kruse MN, Bennett B, De Groat WC. Effect of urinary diversion on the recovery of micturition reflexes after spinal cord injury in the rat. J Urol 1994;151:1088–91.

79. de Groat WC, Yoshimura N. Mechanisms underlying the recovery of lower urinary tract function following spinal cord injury. Prog Brain Res 2006;152:59–84.

80. de Groat WC, Kawatani M, Hisamitsu T, et al. Mechanisms underlying the recovery of urinary bladder function following spinal cord injury. J Auton Nerv Syst 1990;30(Suppl):S71–7.

81. de Groat WC, Yoshimura N. Changes in afferent activity after spinal cord injury. Neurourol Urodyn 2010;29:63–76.

82. de Groat WC, Yoshimura N. Plasticity in reflex pathways to the lower urinary tract following spinal cord injury. Exp Neurol 2012;235:123–32.

83. Yoshimura N. Bladder afferent pathway and spinal cord injury: possible mechanisms inducing hyperreflexia of the urinary bladder. Prog Neurobiol 1999;57:583–606.

84. Cheng CL, Liu JC, Chang SY, et al. Effect of capsaicin on the micturition reflex in normal and chronic spinal cord-injured cats. Am J Physiol 1999;277:R786–94.

85. Cheng CL, Ma CP, de Groat WC. Effect of capsaicin on micturition and associated reflexes in chronic spinal rats. Brain Res 1995;678:40–8.

86. Seki S, Sasaki K, Igawa Y, et al. Suppression of detrusor-sphincter dyssynergia by immunoneutralization of nerve growth factor in lumbosacral spinal cord in spinal cord injured rats. J Urol 2004;171:478–82.

87. Fall M, Lindstrom S, Mazieres L. A bladder-to-bladder cooling reflex in the cat. J Physiol 1990; 427:281–300.

88. Geirsson G, Fall M, Lindstrom S. The ice-water test–a simple and valuable supplement to routine cystometry. Br J Urol 1993;71:681–5.

89. Geirsson G, Lindstrom S, Fall M, et al. Positive bladder cooling test in neurologically normal young children. J Urol 1994;151:446–8.

90. Geirsson G, Fall M, Sullivan L. Clinical and urodynamic effects of intravesical capsaicin treatment in patients with chronic traumatic spinal detrusor hyperreflexia. J Urol 1995;154:1825–9.

91. Kruse MN, Bray LA, de Groat WC. Influence of spinal cord injury on the morphology of bladder afferent and efferent neurons. J Auton nervous Syst 1995;54:215–24.

92. Yoshimura N, de Groat WC. Plasticity of Na+ channels in afferent neurones innervating rat urinary bladder following spinal cord injury. J Physiol 1997;503(Pt 2):269–76.

93. Takahashi R, Yoshizawa T, Yunoki T, et al. Hyperexcitability of bladder afferent neurons associated with reduction of Kv1.4 alpha-subunit in rats with spinal cord injury. J Urol 2013;190:2296–304.

94. Zvarova K, Dunleavy JD, Vizzard MA. Changes in pituitary adenylate cyclase activating polypeptide expression in urinary bladder pathways after spinal cord injury. Exp Neurol 2005;192:46–59.

95. Santos-Silva A, Charrua A, Cruz CD, et al. Rat detrusor overactivity induced by chronic spinalization can be abolished by a transient receptor potential vanilloid 1 (TRPV1) antagonist. Auton Neurosci 2012;166:35–8.

96. Andrade EL, Meotti FC, Calixto JB. TRPA1 antagonists as potential analgesic drugs. Pharmacol Ther 2012;133:189–204.

97. Lamb K, Gebhart GF, Bielefeldt K. Increased nerve growth factor expression triggers bladder overactivity. J Pain 2004;5:150–6.

98. Yoshimura N, Bennett NE, Hayashi Y, et al. Bladder overactivity and hyperexcitability of bladder afferent neurons after intrathecal delivery of nerve growth factor in rats. J Neurosci 2006; 26:10847–55.

99. Zvara P, Vizzard MA. Exogenous overexpression of nerve growth factor in the urinary bladder produces bladder overactivity and altered micturition circuitry in the lumbosacral spinal cord. BMC Physiol 2007;7:9.

100. Seki S, Sasaki K, Fraser MO, et al. Immunoneutralization of nerve growth factor in lumbosacral spinal cord reduces bladder hyperreflexia in spinal cord injured rats. J Urol 2002;168:2269–74.

101. Frias B, Santos J, Morgado M, et al. The role of brain-derived neurotrophic factor (BDNF) in the development of neurogenic detrusor overactivity (NDO). J Neurosci 2015;35:2146–60.

102. Smith CP, Gangitano DA, Munoz A, et al. Botulinum toxin type A normalizes alterations in urothelial ATP

and NO release induced by chronic spinal cord injury. Neurochem Int 2008;52:1068–75.

103. Munoz A, Somogyi GT, Boone TB, et al. Modulation of bladder afferent signals in normal and spinal cord-injured rats by purinergic P2X3 and P2X2/3 receptors. BJU Int 2012;110:E409–14.

104. Ikeda Y, Kanai A. Urotheliogenic modulation of intrinsic activity in spinal cord-transected rat bladders: role of mucosal muscarinic receptors. Am J Physiol Ren Physiol 2008;295:F454–61.

105. McCarthy CJ, Zabbarova IV, Brumovsky PR, et al. Spontaneous contractions evoke afferent nerve firing in mouse bladders with detrusor overactivity. J Urol 2009;181:1459–66.

106. Shapiro S. Neurotransmission by neurons that use serotonin, noradrenaline, glutamate, glycine, and gamma-aminobutyric acid in the normal and injured spinal cord. Neurosurgery 1997;40:168–76 [discussion: 177].

107. Yoshiyama M, Nezu FM, Yokoyama O, et al. Influence of glutamate receptor antagonists on micturition in rats with spinal cord injury. Exp Neurol 1999; 159:250–7.

108. Miyazato M, Sugaya K, Nishijima S, et al. Rectal distention inhibits bladder activity via glycinergic and GABAergic mechanisms in rats. J Urol 2004; 171:1353–6.

109. Miyazato M, Sugaya K, Nishijima S, et al. Inhibitory effect of intrathecal glycine on the micturition reflex in normal and spinal cord injury rats. Exp Neurol 2003;183:232–40.

110. Miyazato M, Sasatomi K, Hiragata S, et al. GABA receptor activation in the lumbosacral spinal cord decreases detrusor overactivity in spinal cord injured rats. J Urol 2008;179:1178–83.

111. Miyazato M, Sugaya K, Nishijima S, et al. Dietary glycine inhibits bladder activity in normal rats and rats with spinal cord injury. J Urol 2005;173:314–7.

112. Steers WD, Meythaler JM, Haworth C, et al. Effects of acute bolus and chronic continuous intrathecal baclofen on genitourinary dysfunction due to spinal cord pathology. J Urol 1992;148:1849–55.

113. Miyazato M, Sugaya K, Goins WF, et al. Herpes simplex virus vector-mediated gene delivery of glutamic acid decarboxylase reduces detrusor overactivity in spinal cord-injured rats. Gene Ther 2009;16:660–8.

114. Miyazato M, Sugaya K, Saito S, et al. Suppression of detrusor-sphincter dyssynergia by herpes simplex virus vector mediated gene delivery of glutamic acid decarboxylase in spinal cord injured rats. J Urol 2010;184:1204–10.

115. Munoz A, Yazdi IK, Tang X, et al. Localized inhibition of P2X7R at the spinal cord injury site improves neurogenic bladder dysfunction by decreasing urothelial P2X3R expression in rats. Life Sci 2016; 171:60–7.

116. Salas NA, Somogyi GT, Gangitano DA, et al. Receptor activated bladder and spinal ATP release in neurally intact and chronic spinal cord injured rats. Neurochem Int 2007;50:345–50.

117. Wada N, Shimizu T, Takai S, et al. Post-injury bladder management strategy influences lower urinary tract dysfunction in the mouse model of spinal cord injury. Neurourol Urodyn 2016. [Epub ahead of print].

118. Yoshiyama M, de Groat WC. Effect of bilateral hypogastric nerve transection on voiding dysfunction in rats with spinal cord injury. Exp Neurol 2002;175: 191–7.

119. Snow-Lisy DC, Yerkes EB, Cheng EY. Update on Urological Management of Spina Bifida from Prenatal Diagnosis to Adulthood. J Urol 2015;194: 288–96.

120. Danzer E, Schwarz U, Wehrli S, et al. Retinoic acid induced myelomeningocele in fetal rats: characterization by histopathological analysis and magnetic resonance imaging. Exp Neurol 2005;194:467–75.

121. Danzer E, Kiddoo DA, Redden RA, et al. Structural and functional characterization of bladder smooth muscle in fetal rats with retinoic acid-induced myelomeningocele. Am J Physiol Ren Physiol 2007; 292:F197–206.

122. Shen J, Zhou G, Chen H, et al. Morphology of nervous lesion in the spinal cord and bladder of fetal rats with myelomeningocele at different gestational age. J Pediatr Surg 2013;48:2446–52.

123. Tekin A, Karakus OZ, Hakguder G, et al. Distribution of interstitial cells of Cajal in the bladders of fetal rats with retinoic acid induced myelomeningocele. Turk J Urol 2016;42:285–9.

Mending Gaps in Knowledge
Collaborations in Neurogenic Bladder Research

Jeremy B. Myers, MD[a],*, Darshan P. Patel, MD[a],
Sean P. Elliott, MD, MS[b], John T. Stoffel, MD[c],
Blayne Welk, MD, MSc[d], Amitabh Jha, MD, MPH[e],
Sara M. Lenherr, MD, MS[a], Neurogenic Bladder Research Group

KEYWORDS

- Neurogenic bladder • Spinal cord injury • Complication • Incontinence
- Patient-reported outcomes

KEY POINTS

- Patient-reported outcomes need to be incorporated into the study design of neurogenic bladder trials.
- Prospective studies around neurogenic bladder management need to be guided by clinical outcomes and patient preferences.
- Multi-institutional collaborative groups are essential in neurogenic bladder research due to the rarity of many causes of neurogenic bladder, and due to potential institutional and individual surgeon biases that arise from single-center studies.
- A large prospective observational study of bladder-related quality of life after spinal cord injury has been initiated by the Neurogenic Bladder Research Group.

BACKGROUND

Neurogenic bladder (NGB) is a nonspecific term that encompasses many different patterns of bladder dysfunction. The term implies an underlying neurologic condition leading to bladder dysfunction, but these underlying disease states span hugely disparate conditions from elderly diabetic patients with peripheral neuropathy to childhood spinal cord problems, such as myelomeningocele. In addition, bladder dysfunction from NGB also has a huge range of clinical manifestations from benign urinary retention to high bladder storage pressures leading to complications such as renal failure, urosepsis, and death.

Disclosures: Drs S. Elliott, S. Lenherr, J.B. Myers and J. Stoffel receive salary support and B. Welk and Amitabh Jha are paid consultants from the Patient-Centered Outcomes Research Institute (CER14092138). Drs S. Elliott, S. Lenherr, J.B. Myers, and J. Stoffel receive salary support from the Department of Defense grant SCI170051. These grants are focused on spinal cord injury patients and use patient-reported outcomes.
^a Genitourinary Injury and Reconstructive Urology, Department of Surgery, University of Utah, Salt Lake City, UT, USA; ^b Department of Urology, University of Minnesota, Minneapolis, MN, USA; ^c Department of Urology, University of Michigan Health System, Ann Arbor, MI, USA; ^d Department of Surgery, Schulich School of Medicine, Western University, London, Ontario, Canada; ^e Department of Physical Medicine and Rehabilitation, Salt Lake City Veterans Medical Center, University of Utah, Salt Lake City, UT, USA
* Corresponding author. Genitourinary Injury and Reconstructive Urology, 30 North 1900 East, Room # 3B420, Salt Lake City, UT 84132.
E-mail address: Jeremy.myers@hsc.utah.edu

Urol Clin N Am 44 (2017) 507–515
http://dx.doi.org/10.1016/j.ucl.2017.04.015
0094-0143/17/© 2017 Elsevier Inc. All rights reserved.

Given the heterogeneity of disease processes causing NGB and its clinical presentations it is difficult to define best management recommendations and treatment guidelines. Two important components of research in NGB are first to define patient preferences for management via patient-reported outcome measures (PROMs) and then use this information to target these preferences with high-quality prospective studies of innovative strategies oriented to improving the clinical outcomes and quality of life (QoL) associated with the treatments. For instance, if patients within a given NGB population generally prefer indwelling catheters, efforts to try to keep them doing intermittent catheterization are futile and research should instead be focused on making indwelling catheters safer and minimizing complications, such as serious urinary tract infections (UTIs) and renal dysfunction.

Because the causes of NGB are so varied, many subpopulations of patients are rarely encountered by clinicians outside of specialty centers. For instance, although spinal cord injury (SCI) is among the leading causes of NGB, it is estimated that SCI affects fewer than 1 out of 1000 people in the United States.[1] Other causes, such as myelomeningocele, cerebral palsy, and bladder exstrophy have an even lower prevalence compared to SCI. Over the last several decades, a major step forward in the study of SCI has been establishment of several large national and international databases. Perhaps the best known of these databases is the Model System for SCI care in the United States.[2,3] The Model System of SCI treatment centers contribute to a large database, which collects longitudinal information about the incidence, prevalence, cause, bladder and bowel management, and complications associated with SCI. However, PROMs within this database are limited to general health-related QoL and are not specific to urinary incontinence or bladder-related QoL. The rarity of patients with NGB and lack of specific data about bladder-related QoL emphasizes the importance of study through collaborative multi-institutional groups.

Collaborations in Reconstructive Urology

The Neurogenic Bladder Research Group (NBRG; NBRG.org), was formed in 2015. A founding principle was to address gaps in knowledge in the treatment of NGB and provide a platform for high-quality patient-centered prospective studies. The group is currently composed of 8 high-volume centers in North America with urologists that specialize in reconstructive urology or neurourology. The impetus for the formation of NBRG was to address limitations in the study of NGB to date. First, it addressed the lack of prospective well-designed studies in NGB. In the literature, retrospective, single-center studies predominate. These studies often report patient outcomes over huge spans of time, include surgical techniques that may not be reproducible by others, and focus on surgeon-defined outcomes. These studies may be prone to bias and under-reporting of adverse effects on QoL. Second, it addressed the need to establish a framework to evaluate patient-reported outcomes, which requires sampling of a large diverse population because of the heterogeneity of NGB patient populations.

The Trauma and Urologic Reconstruction Network of Surgeons (TURNS) is an analogous group that focuses on outcomes research in trauma, urethral strictures, and male incontinence. This group was established in 2009 and served as the conceptual framework for establishment of NBRG. Universities of Utah and Minnesota are active members of TURNS, and experience gained and the lessons learned with this group were critical in the formation of NBRG. There are important design considerations in a collaborative group. First, an administrative structure for sharing clinical data in a safe way across multiple health care systems must be established. TURNS accomplished this with a centralized database, which now functions on the Research Electronic Data Capture (REDCap) platform and is housed at a participating institution. Shared databases on these types of platforms can allow patient identifiers to be removed from view other than the institution entering the data. They also allow scheduled questionnaires to be sent electronically through email to patients for longitudinal follow-up. Questionnaires can be custom-generated or standardized questionnaires can be designated from a large library housed in REDCap. Multi-institutional databases have been increasingly recognized, in many fields, as critical tools for pushing clinical outcomes research forward.[4,5] Second, full buy-in from all collaborators with commitment of time, resources, energy, and ideas is necessary. In forming collaborative research groups, many active surgeons or clinicians express interest in contributing; however, it is helpful to have clear thresholds defining active participation in the group. These requirements can include active ongoing entry of data, participation in planning and completion of studies, article preparation, and administrative tasks (ie, Web site design, budgetary considerations, and promotion of the group). Third, there must be adequate support from a participating institution. Data entry is time-consuming, as well as tracking patient compliance with follow-up, and the authors' experience with TURNS indicates these tasks will rarely be completed by busy clinicians, regardless of their commitment to the objectives of the group.

Similar to NGB, urethral stricture disease had very few high-quality multi-institutional studies. In addition, there is only 1 disease-specific PROM for urethral strictures, and this was developed by using questions from other bladder-related PROMs rather than patient focus groups.[6,7] The TURNS group understood that defining patient perceptions about their outcomes was the first step needed for prospective research studies. To accomplish this goal, first, a standardized follow-up protocol for patients after urethroplasty was established, as well as anatomic and functional definitions for successful treatment of urethral strictures.[8,9] Then, the associations between surgical and patient-perceived outcomes were investigated for satisfaction with surgery,[10] sexual function,[11] bladder symptoms,[12] and urologic pain.[13] Recognizing the limitations of the current PROMs, the group has now undertaken development of a new disease-specific PROM based on interviews with patient focus groups, which will be used in the future to follow outcomes. Once these basic associations were established, TURNS began prospective randomized studies incorporating PROMs into study outcome measures.[14,15]

In forming NBRG, the strategy was to first develop an administrative backbone based on a large observational study involving PROMs. Although prospective cohort and randomized controlled trials are ideal in determining best-care practices, the first need was to establish a working collaborative network. In addition, as previously discussed, there are not enough data on patient-reported outcomes and QoL in NGB. Establishing familiarity with this type of study design, as well as gaining a substantive knowledge base about these preferences will guide further investigation into patient-centered topics. This article presents the study design for the first large collaborative study on bladder management methods and QoL after SCI.

Study background: bladder-related quality of life after spinal cord injury

Patients with SCI report bladder management difficulties as the second leading impact on QoL,[16] with only pain having a greater impact. In addition to adverse effects on QoL, up to 40% of SCI patients have serious UTIs[17] and urinary tract complications are the leading reason for hospitalization.[18] Volitional voiding after SCI is rare and almost all patients need some method-assisted bladder drainage. These drainage methods often include condom catheters, commonly combined with sphincterotomy, chronic indwelling catheters (Foley catheter or suprapubic tube), intermittent catheterization, urinary reconstruction to facilitate intermittent catheterization, and conduit urinary diversion to bypass the NGB completely. Because NGB is a chronic condition without a cure, a patient's day-to-day QoL and preferences with different treatments are critical in choosing management strategies.

The current literature on patient-reported outcomes for the treatment of NGB is limited and often patients' management preferences are contrary to clinicians' recommendations. For instance, urologists have a strong preference for intermittent catheterization due to the low complication rate compared with chronic indwelling catheters[19–21] and a perception that this method promotes the greatest independence. Despite this strong bias among clinicians for continued management with intermittent catheterization, most patients with SCI who start with intermittent catheterization transition to a permanent indwelling catheter during the long-term course of their injury.[22] The reason these patients transition to indwelling catheters over time is not known, although it is likely that QoL issues associated with intermittent catheterization play a role (eg, urinary leakage, autonomic dysreflexia, poor bladder capacity, labor-intensive catheterization schedule, and increased UTI rate perceived to be due to intermittent catheterization). Patient-reported QoL provides the framework to finding the root of these issues and addressing modifiable factors so that clinician and patient preferences have greater harmony.

Patient-Reported Outcome Measures

Measuring patient perceptions, preferences, and outcomes is done with PROMs, which are generally validated questionnaires. Validation of questionnaires is a complex science involving the generation of questions with face validity, usually with focus groups composed of patients and sometimes clinicians. Psychometric testing is then used to test the statistical validity of these questions, their ability to test for the desired measurements within a given population of patients, reproducibility, and whether differences can be detected for patients with a range of disease states that the instrument is measuring.[23] The ideal questionnaire differentiates between patients that do very well with a given disease and those who are significantly affected by their disease.

Current Study Design

The Patient-Centered Outcomes Research Institute (PCORI; pcori.org) was funded by the United States Congress in 2010 with a mandate to improve comparative effectiveness research through patient-centered studies. A key and novel component of PCORI's mandate is engagement of patients in the research process, rather than simply funding studies using patient-centered outcomes or having a patient-centered focus. Patients are engaged throughout the research project, including during project conceptualization, grant writing, grant review, the research process, and in dissemination of results. Patients are referred to as stakeholders in this process and are often joined by other stakeholders, such as clinicians, advocacy groups, caregivers, insurers, and hospitals. For all the reasons mentioned previously, the study of NGB is ideally suited to such an inclusive design process.

The PCORI research protocol is a multicenter prospective observational trial designed to analyze SCI patients' bladder-related QoL with different bladder management strategies. The study also follows patients longitudinally, to determine how complications and changes in bladder management affect QoL. As preparatory work for this protocol, a review of current PROMs for NGB was performed to identify the available PROM and QoL instruments.[24] Patient stakeholders with SCI were identified from the investigators' clinical practices. A patient advisory meeting was convened with these patient stakeholders at which a facilitator-led semistructured qualitative group discussion was held about NGB management and QoL. Themes identified in this discussion included (1) the importance of bladder and bowel management in overall QoL, (2) the lack of high-quality information about bladder management choices and the barrier this presented to decision-making, (3) and the importance of discussion of choices about bladder management with peers with similar injuries and disabilities. These themes were used to guide the structure of the study and plan the dissemination of its results. Study design based on this input included

- Engagement of patients via social media, the Internet, and advocacy groups to engage as many diverse participants as possible
- Design of a Web-based information resource to disseminate high-quality information about bladder management, study results, and allow people with SCI the ability to interact about their bladder management with other SCI patients

- Selection of various panels within the Spinal Cord Injury Quality of Life (SCI-QoL).

During the meeting, QoL questionnaires were reviewed by the patient stakeholders in small working-groups. Their input about the relevance and experience in answering the questions was used to select between different items from 1 of the proposed PROMs, the SCI-QoL questionnaire.

A second meeting was held at which the investigators and all relevant stakeholders, including patients, individuals associated with advocacy groups, physical medicine and rehabilitation clinicians, and research coordinators met and finalized the inclusion criteria, PROMs (**Box 1**), and research protocol (**Fig. 1**).

Box 1
Inclusion criteria and final patient-reported outcome measures

Inclusion criteria

- Eighteen years or older
- Acquired SCI excluding congenital causes or progressive causes of SCI (eg, myelomeningocele, cerebral palsy, multiple sclerosis, active malignancy)
- English-speaking
- Cognitive ability to understand the questionnaires

Final PROMs

- The Neurogenic Bladder Symptom Score (NBSS)
- Medical Outcomes Study Short Form 12-Item (SF-12)
- Numeric pain scale
- Nonvalidated questions about autonomic dysreflexia
- Neurogenic Bowel Dysfunction Score
- SCI-QoL
  - Bladder management difficulties
  - Bladder complications
  - Bowel management difficulties
  - Pain interference
  - Independence
  - Basic mobility
  - Fine-motor
  - Self-care
  - Positive affect and wellbeing
  - Satisfaction with social roles and activities

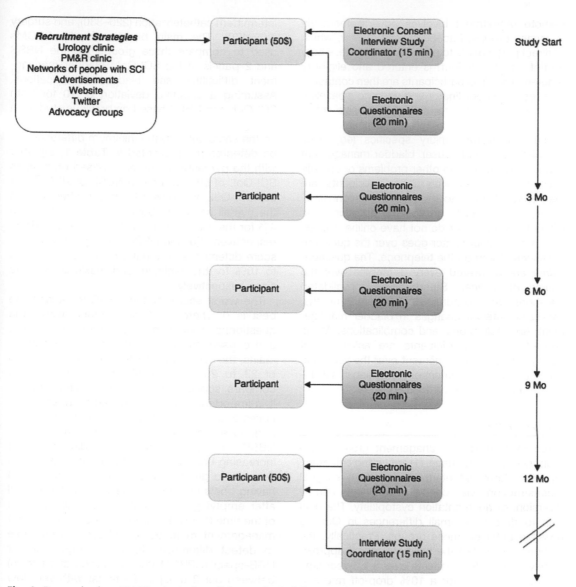

Fig. 1. Research plan. PM&R, physical medicine and rehabilitation; SCI, spinal cord injury.

Study Patient-Reported Outcome Measures

A panel of questionnaires is used to assess QoL and patient-reported outcomes. These PROMs includes 3 bladder-specific questionnaires. These are the Neurogenic Bladder Symptom Score (NBSS), bladder management difficulties, and bladder complications. The NBSS is a comprehensive questionnaire validated in NGB patients and SCI, which assess bladder management, function, complications, and psychosocial consequences from NGB. Bladder management difficulties and bladder complications come from the SCI-QoL, which is a comprehensive panel of questionnaires designed to measure all aspects of a person's experience with SCI. These 2 questionnaires are administered via computer-adaptive testing, which is a method in which the questionnaire programming selects the best questions to differentiate between QoL based on the responses of the participant. The rest of the data are meant to assess confounders and overall QoL. For example, the stakeholders were concerned that participants who had high levels of pain would have worse bladder-related QoL. This is the reason questions were included about pain interference and a numeric pain severity scale.

Research Plan

Participants are recruited via both physical rehabilitation and urology clinics, as well as remotely.

Remote recruitment involves advertisement via advocacy groups, Facebook, and Twitter, which all direct participants to the NBRG Web site, where a brief enrollment form is entered and eligibility is determined. The participants are then contacted by a research coordinator and undergo a baseline telephone interview to collect extensive information about their demographics, past medical or surgical history, injury specifics (eg, level, completeness, and cause), bladder management method over time, and other problems or complications associated with SCI. Participants are then emailed a link to the online questionnaires. If they are unable to answer the questionnaires without assistance or do not have online access, then a study coordinator goes over the questionnaires with them on the telephone. The questionnaires are answered every 3 months over the course of a year. Standardized nonvalidated questions are also administered every 3 months, assessing interval changes in bladder management, hospitalizations, and complications. At the end of a year, participants are asked about changes to their management over the year, and asked about improvement or worsening in subdomains of the NBSS on a 15-point scale.

Analysis Plan

Three main bladder management groups were proposed for comparison: (1) indwelling catheters, (2) intermittent catheterization, and (3) surgical reconstruction via conduit, continent urinary diversion, or augmentation cystoplasty. The goal was to detect as small differences in QoL as possible between these groups. Practically, the authors anticipated the ability to recruit approximately 900 to 1300 patients over a 1.5-year time frame. Accounting for a 10% drop-off rate and dividing the groups based on our clinic demographics, we came up with the following recruitment goals: indwelling catheters (370–560),

intermittent catheterization (220–330), and surgery (300–470). The main bladder-specific PROMs used to compare these groups are the NBSS and 2 panels of the SCI-QoL: bladder management difficulties and bladder complications. Assuming a standard deviation of 10 for both SCI-QoL and NBSS based on previous studies, a strong correlation between repeated measures on the same subject, the minimum differences to be detected are presented in **Table 1**, together with the percentage difference based on a mean SCI-QoL of 50 and a mean NBSS of 20.[25,26] For the SCI-QoL, we expect to detect differences in the overall score of about 4% to 5% or 3% to 4% for the minimum and maximum sample sizes, respectively. For the NBSS we expect to detect score differences of about 10% to 12% or 8.5% to 10% for the minimum and maximum sample sizes, respectively.

The worst score for the NBSS is 74 and the best is 0. There are 3 subdomains within the questionnaire: incontinence, storage and voiding, and consequences. For any of these 3 subdomains, the scores range from a maximum (worst) of 22 to 29 and a minimum (best) of 0. To compare subdomains between patients groups it is important to be able to detect these differences of about 2 points between patient groups. A good example of a 2-point difference in the NBSS subdomain storage and voiding would be increasing urinary dryness from a period of 2 to 3 hours to greater than 3 hours (1 point), and having one's bladder or reservoir still feeling full after emptying from most of the time to some of the time (1 point). In a recent study of different management methods, investigators were able to detect differences in scores from another NGB-specific PROM (the Qualiveen short form) between our 3 groups of interest with very low numbers of patients per group (indwelling catheter [39], intermittent catheterization [113], and surgery [16]).[27] The study demonstrated these

Table 1
Score difference and (% difference) at minimum and maximum sample size ranges

Questionnaire	Comparison Groups	Detected Differences n ~ 900	Detected Differences n ~ 1300
SCI-QoL Scale	Indwelling vs IC	2.34 (4.7%)	1.91 (3.8%)
	Indwelling vs surgery	2.11 (4.2%)	1.72 (3.4%)
	IC vs surgery	2.42 (4.8%)	1.98 (4.0%)
NBSS	Indwelling vs IC	2.34 (11.7%)	1.91 (9.6%)
	Indwelling vs surgery	2.11 (10.6%)	1.72 (8.6%)
	IC vs surgery	2.42 (12.1%)	1.98 (9.9%)

Assuming a minimum of approximately 900 participants, a maximum of 1300, a mean SCI-QoL of 50, and NBSS of 20.
Abbreviation: IC, intermittent catheterization.

differences on the impact of patients' QoL, despite using a single short form PROM, which is only 8 questions in length.

One of the biggest problems with the study of SCI and QoL is the number of confounders. Confounders can have a profound impact on QoL. Some of these confounders are sex, body mass index, age at injury, time since injury, completeness of SCI, paraplegia versus tetraplegia, presence of neuropathic pain, degree of spasticity, overall health, susceptibility to UTI, depression, education, social support, socioeconomic status, and independence. These are just a few. When groups start to be narrowed by some of these confounders, despite starting with a huge sample size, groups become very small. For example, a hypothetical patient is a man, paraplegic, doing intermittent catheterization, less than 10 years from injury, living at home, with less than 3 UTIs a year. He is compared with another hypothetical patient that is, tetraplegic, lives in a nursing home, is 40 years from his injury, and has a suprapubic tube. If the latter patient had a worse QoL, it would be hard to conclude that the bladder management method was to blame because of all the confounders that differ between the patients. The heterogeneity of SCI and bladder management makes it difficult to compare apples to apples and make meaningful conclusions about management recommendations for any given group. This example illustrates the need for a large study to capture as many significant subgroups as possible.

Study Update

Accrual of patients began January 2016 and will continue until July 2017. At 1-year of enrollment, approximately 1000 participants have completed the baseline interview and the first QoL questionnaires. Mean age was 45.6 plus or minus 13.9 years, with mean 31.2 plus or minus 14.2 years since SCI. Remote recruitment of participants, via the Internet and social media accounted for 55% of enrollment. SCI level was 49% paraplegia, 43% tetraplegia, and 8% unknown or other. Looking at the 3 groups of interest, the authors found 67% performing intermittent catheterization, 21% relying on an indwelling catheter, and 12% having undergone reconstructive surgery with urinary diversion or bladder augmentation.

Via remote enrollment there has been engagement of participants with SCI throughout the United States and Canada. Distribution has been heavily weighted toward states in which the 3 investigators are located, but there is wide geographic dispersal of participants (**Fig. 2**). The enrollment goal for the study is 1500 participants by July, 2017.

The goal is for the study to give an accurate picture of bladder-related QoL associated with a variety of factors related to demographics, injury level, and bladder management. The authors aim to fulfill the PCORI mandate of patient engagement by making this information freely available to people with SCI through a Web-based community forum. Ultimately, an important piece of future research is

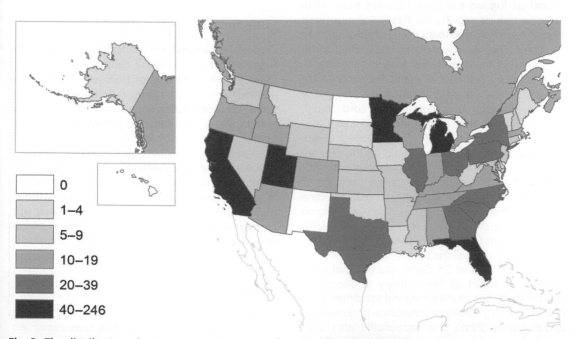

0
1–4
5–9
10–19
20–39
40–246

Fig. 2. The distribution of participants in the study of SCI bladder management.

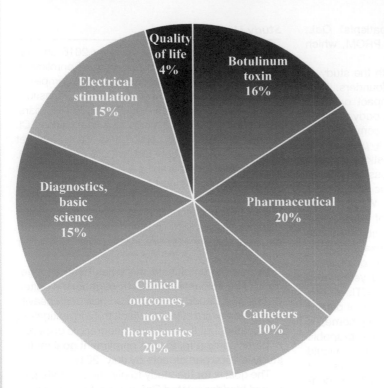

Fig. 3. Studies tabulated from the National Institutes of Health on ClinicalTrials.gov identified by the search terms: spinal cord injury and bladder, spinal cord injury and neurogenic bladder, and neurogenic bladder.

to use the information to construct shared decision-making tools for clinicians and patients with SCI guiding bladder management choices.

Other studies of neurogenic bladder

The National Institutes of Health (NIH) maintains a registry of clinical studies (clinicaltrials.gov). Almost all funded extramural studies from North America require registry via this mechanism and studies are often registered from Europe and other countries. The registry provides information about the nature of the hypothesis, trial design, investigator's origin, and primary and secondary outcomes. A search of this database using the medical subject headings spinal cord injury, neurogenic bladder, and spinal cord injury and bladder revealed a total of 69 studies (years 2010–2017) with a bladder focus as the primary or secondary outcome, in populations with SCI or NGB (**Fig. 3**). These studies were classified as involving pharmaceutics (20%), clinical outcome or novel therapeutics (20%), botulinum toxin (16%), diagnostic or basic science (15%), electrical stimulation (15%), catheters (10%), and QoL focus in only a small fraction of the studies (4%). There are a total of 21 (30%) studies that used PROMs as a part of their primary or secondary outcomes. These studies involved botulinum toxin injection (38%), electrical stimulation or novel therapeutics trials (29%), pharmaceutical trials (19%), and QoL-focused studies (14%). Only 8 (38%) of

the studies used PROMs that were validated or specific to NGB populations. Although, the NIH registry at clinicaltrials.gov is nowhere near a complete list on ongoing studies, the relative lack of basic patient-centered QoL studies using validated PROMs emphasizes one of the largest knowledge gaps in NGB research.

SUMMARY

One of the largest knowledge gaps in urologic research in NGB is patient-centered QoL studies. Effective future studies of NGB are likely to use multicenter collaborations due to the rarity of some disease processes causing NGB and the heterogeneity of bladder dysfunction and management of NGB. Organizations such as PCORI, or foundations focused on specific disease processes are ideal mechanisms to support these collaborations. The study presented in this article is a large and comprehensive study of bladder-related QoL in SCI patients and should shed light on factors, such as management choices, clinical parameters, complications, and psychosocial situation, which most affect QoL.

REFERENCES

1. NSCISC, Spinal Cord Injury (SCI) Facts and Figures at a Glance. 2016. Available at: https://www.nscisc.uab.edu/Public/Facts2016.pdf. Accessed March 1, 2017.

2. DeVivo MJ, Go BK, Jackson AB. Overview of the national spinal cord injury statistical center database. J Spinal Cord Med 2002;25(4):335–8.

3. Stover SL, DeVivo MJ, Go BK. History, implementation, and current status of the National Spinal Cord Injury Database. Arch Phys Med Rehabil 1999; 80(11):1365–71.

4. Green AK, Reeder-Hayes KE, Corty RW, et al. The project data sphere initiative: accelerating cancer research by sharing data. Oncologist 2015;20(5): 464.e20.

5. Won B, Carey GB, Tan YH, et al. The Chicago Thoracic Oncology Database Consortium: a multisite database initiative. Cureus 2016;8(3):e533.

6. Jackson MJ, Chaudhury I, Mangera A, et al. A prospective patient-centred evaluation of urethroplasty for anterior urethral stricture using a validated patient-reported outcome measure. Eur Urol 2013; 64(5):777–82.

7. Jackson MJ, Sciberras J, Mangera A, et al. Defining a patient-reported outcome measure for urethral stricture surgery. Eur Urol 2011;60(1):60–8.

8. Erickson BA, Elliott SP, Voelzke BB, et al. Multi-institutional 1-year bulbar urethroplasty outcomes using a standardized prospective cystoscopic follow-up protocol. Urology 2014;84(1):213–6.

9. Tam CA, Voelzke BB, Elliott SP, et al. Critical analysis of the use of uroflowmetry for urethral stricture disease surveillance. Urology 2016;91:197–202.

10. Bertrand LA, Voelzke BB, Elliott SP, et al. Measuring and predicting patient dissatisfaction after anterior urethroplasty using patient reported outcomes measures. J Urol 2016;196(2):453–61.

11. Patel DP, Elliott SP, Voelzke BB, et al. Patient-reported sexual function after staged penile urethroplasty. Urology 2015;86(2):395–400.

12. Hampson LA, Elliott SP, Erickson BA, et al. Multicenter analysis of urinary urgency and urge incontinence in patients with anterior urethral stricture disease before and after urethroplasty. J Urol 2016; 196(6):1700–5.

13. Bertrand LA, Warren GJ, Voelzke BB, et al. Lower urinary tract pain and anterior urethral stricture disease: prevalence and effects of urethral reconstruction. J Urol 2015;193(1):184–9.

14. Clinicaltrials.gov, Dorsal vs. Ventral Buccal Graft Dorsal vs. Ventral Buccal Graft. 2015. Available at: https://clinicaltrials.gov/ct2/show/NCT02551783?term= buccal&rank=1. Accessed March 1, 2017.

15. Clinicaltrials.gov, A study of transcorporal versus standard artificial urinary sphincter placement. 2015. Available at: https://clinicaltrials.gov/ct2/show/ NCT02524366. Accessed March 1, 2017.

16. Tulsky DS, Kisala PA, Victorson D, et al. Developing a contemporary patient-reported outcomes measure for spinal cord injury. Arch Phys Med Rehabil 2011; 92(10 Suppl):S44–51.

17. Welk B, Liu K, Winick-Ng J, et al. Urinary tract infections, urologic surgery, and renal dysfunction in a contemporary cohort of traumatic spinal cord injured patients. Neurourol Urodyn 2016;36:640–7.

18. Curtin CM, Suarez PA, Di Ponio LA, et al. Who are the women and men in Veterans Health Administration's current spinal cord injury population? J Rehabil Res Dev 2012;49(3):351–60.

19. Weld KJ, Dmochowski RR. Effect of bladder management on urological complications in spinal cord injured patients. J Urol 2000;163(3):768–72.

20. Bennett CJ, Suarez PA, Di Ponio LA, et al. Comparison of bladder management complication outcomes in female spinal cord injury patients. J Urol 1995;153(5):1458–60.

21. Weld KJ, Graney MJ, Dmochowski RR. Differences in bladder compliance with time and associations of bladder management with compliance in spinal cord injured patients. J Urol 2000;163(4):1228–33.

22. Cameron AP, Wallner LP, Tate DG, et al. Bladder management after spinal cord injury in the United States 1972 to 2005. J Urol 2010;184(1):213–7.

23. Clark R, Welk B. Patient reported outcome measures in neurogenic bladder. Transl Androl Urol 2016;5(1): 22–30.

24. Patel DP, Elliott SP, Stoffel JT, et al. Patient reported outcomes measures in neurogenic bladder and bowel: A systematic review of the current literature. Neurourol Urodyn 2016;35(1):8–14.

25. Welk B, Morrow S, Madarasz W, et al. The validity and reliability of the neurogenic bladder symptom score. J Urol 2014;192(2):452–7.

26. Cella D, Nowinski C, Peterman A, et al. The neurology quality-of-life measurement initiative. Arch Phys Med Rehabil 2011;92(10 Suppl):S28–36.

27. Adriaansen JJ, van Asbeck FW, Tepper M, et al. Bladder-emptying methods, neurogenic lower urinary tract dysfunction and impact on quality of life in people with long-term spinal cord injury. J Spinal Cord Med 2017;40(1):43–53.

Moving?

Make sure your subscription moves with you!

To notify us of your new address, find your **Clinics Account Number** (located on your mailing label above your name), and contact customer service at:

Email: journalscustomerservice-usa@elsevier.com

800-654-2452 (subscribers in the U.S. & Canada)
314-447-8871 (subscribers outside of the U.S. & Canada)

Fax number: 314-447-8029

Elsevier Health Sciences Division
Subscription Customer Service
3251 Riverport Lane
Maryland Heights, MO 63043

*To ensure uninterrupted delivery of your subscription, please notify us at least 4 weeks in advance of move.

Moving?

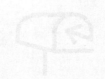

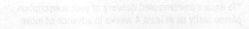